Contents

Contributors

Editors

Gwen Sherwood, PhD, RN, FAAN
Professor and Associate Dean for Academic Affairs
School of Nursing
University of North Carolina at Chapel Hill
Chapel Hill, NC

Jane Barnsteiner, PhD, RN, FAAN
Professor of Pediatric Nursing
School of Nursing
University of Pennsylvania
Philadelphia, PA

Contributors

Kathryn R. Alden, EdD, MSN, RN, IBCLC
Clinical Associate Professor
School of Nursing
University of North Carolina at Chapel Hill
Chapel Hill, NC

Elizabeth Cerbie, MSN, RN
Director of Nursing Education
Indiana University Health
Indianapolis, IN

Linda R. Cronenwett, PhD, RN, FAAN
Beerstecher-Blackwell Term Professor
School of Nursing
University of North Carolina at Chapel Hill
Chapel Hill, NC

Joanne Disch, PhD, RN, FAAN
Clinical Professor and Director
Katharine J. Densford International Center for Nursing Leadership
University of Minnesota School of Nursing
Minneapolis, MN

Mary A. Dolansky, PhD, RN
Assistant Professor
Frances Payne Bolton School of Nursing
Case Western Reserve University
Cleveland, OH

Carol F. Durham, EdD, RN, ANEF
Clinical Professor
School of Nursing
University of North Carolina at Chapel Hill
Chapel Hill, NC

Pamela M. Ironside, PhD, RN, FAAN, ANEF
Associate Professor
Director of the Center for Research in Nursing Education
Indiana University School of Nursing
Indianapolis, IN

Jean Johnson, PhD, RN, FAAN
Dean and Professor
School of Nursing
George Washington University
Washington, DC

Shirley M. Moore, PhD, RN, FAAN
Edward J. and Louise Mellen Professor of Nursing
Frances Payne Bolton School of Nursing
Case Western Reserve University
Cleveland, OH

Mary Jean Schumann, DNP, MBA, RN, CPNP
Executive Director, Nursing Alliance for Quality Care
Assistant Professor
George Washington University School of Nursing
Washington, DC

Mamta K. Singh, MD, MS
Associate Professor of Medicine
Case Western Reserve University School of Medicine
Louis Stokes Cleveland Veterans Affairs Medical Center
Cleveland, OH

Nancy Spector, PhD, RN
Director of Regulatory Innovations
National Council of State Boards of Nursing
Chicago, IL

Mary Fran Tracy, PhD, RN, CCNS, FAAN
Critical Care Clinical Nurse Specialist
University of Minnesota Medical Center, Fairview
Minneapolis, MN

Pamela Klauer Triolo, PhD, RN, FAAN
President, Principled Leadership Solutions
Houston, TX

Beth T. Ulrich, EdD, RN, FACHE, FAAN
Vice President, Hospital Services
CAE Healthcare
Houston, TX

Mary K. Walton, MSN, MBE, RN
Director, Patient and Family Centered Care
Hospital of the University of Pennsylvania
Associate Fellow
University of Pennsylvania Center for Bioethics
Philadelphia, PA

Judith J. Warren, PhD, RN, BC, FAAN, FACMI
Christine A. Hartley Centennial Professor
University of Kansas School of Nursing
Director of Nursing Informatics
University of Kansas Center for Health Informatics
Kansas City, KS

Foreword

The recent Carnegie Foundation for the Advancement of Teaching's Preparation for the Professions Program called out important changes needed in the preparation for professional work in medicine, nursing, law, engineering, and the clergy. Professor Patricia Benner led the team for nursing (Benner, Sutphen, Leonard, & Day, 2010). They began by noting that profound changes were occurring in the practice of the nursing professional that were arising from science, technology, patient activism, market-driven financing of health care, and in the settings where these forces come together and where nurses now practice. They noted a practice-to-education gap characterized by the need to match learning with the realities of the work that nursing professionals face. This book begins to address that gap by opening the knowledge and skills needed to understand and improve these new practice settings of nursing.

All professions earn societal recognition as a "profession" by the ongoing improvement of their own work (Houle, 1980). But as Benner and colleagues (2010) note, improving health care now isn't easy or simple. Health care for patients and populations today occurs in complex, interdependent systems (Batalden, Ogrinc, & Batalden, 2006). Designing and testing changes for improvement in those systems requires new knowledge and skill. This book is about developing those competencies essential for a sense of professional mastery.

"Doing quality improvement" is not necessarily the same as "improving the quality of what we do"—the profession-enabling work. This is not the work of a small department of zealots who staff offices for regulation-meeting, it is part of the work of every person who claims designation today as a health professional.

Improving the quality, safety, and value of health care invites the use of multiple knowledge disciplines (Batalden, Bate, Webb, & McLoughlin, 2011). Diverse knowledge-building traditions from biological, social, and physical sciences and the humanities come together to contribute to the development of the knowledge and science of improvement. This book is about those knowledge domains and invites attention to the scholarly and applied work of educators and researchers who develop and foster critical thinking about improving health care.

At the core of improving health for a patient is a series of interactions that can be represented by the simple logic formula:

Generalizable science + Particular patient → Measured improvement.

Each element of this logic comes together millions of times every day as clinical health professionals do their work.

We can use a similar logic representation for improving health care:

Generalizable science + Particular context → Measured performance improvement.

Each phrase or symbol of this simple logic formula is informed by knowledge that is developed and tested in customized ways. Good knowledge about "generalizable science" is developed by carefully controlling and minimizing "context" as a variable. Particular context knowledge comes from obsessing about context: the systems, processes, traditions, patterns, and so forth that characterize and give "particular" identity to contexts. Measuring performance improvement means measuring over time—not just at two points in time—and it means using balanced measures to understand the multidimensional aspects of quality, safety, and value of process and outcome of care. Even the symbols represent knowledge domains. The "+" sign signifies knowing how to construct a "good" plan that links context and science. The "→" represents the knowledge of actually executing change—making it happen. Each part and symbol of the formula invites a different way of knowing and they must all come together to make change for the improvement of health care (Batalden & Davidoff, 2007).

Benner and her colleagues (2010) also note that nurses have very diverse entries, pathways, curricula, and time frames to become a nurse. This book invites attention to that diversity by focusing on the content of what must be mastered—the competencies themselves. As health professions engage in competency-based learning, it will be important to avoid reducing all the content that is signaled by the competencies into mechanical packages that fail to invite the whole person to the learning.

What is important in health care is reducing the burden of illness for individuals and populations. What is real in health care is the people and what they are struggling to do together. The intervention for improving health care quality, safety, and value is a social change that is learned experientially (Batalden, Davidoff, Marshall, Bibby, & Pink, 2011). Improvement theories, methods, tools, and techniques are all potentially helpful—but we must never confuse them with the work of improving care, lest we make an error similar to the one of confusing a map for the territory it represents.

Creating work environments that sustain the generative, refreshing work of improving health care involves the inextricable linkage of three aims and invites the work of everyone, illustrated in Figure F.1.

Health professionals have an opportunity to help design and weave these together.

It is often noted by practicing nurses and other clinicians that their job is to protect the patient from the system of health care in which the patient and

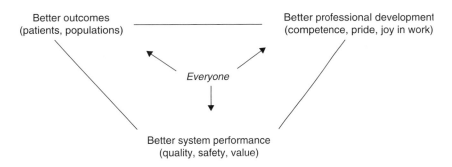

Better outcomes
(patients, populations)

Better professional development
(competence, pride, joy in work)

Everyone

Better system performance
(quality, safety, value)

Figure F.1 Creating work environments for improving health care.

clinician meet. This frames responsibility for the design of the system and its ongoing improvement as external to the working professional on the front lines of health care. I prefer a different view of professional work—one that accepts the professional responsibility for health care system quality, safety, and value. This book can help nurses and other clinicians who are not content to work in alien systems.

A nurse member of a class I was teaching many years ago said it very succinctly: "We actually have two jobs—to do our work and to improve it."

This book invites the work of improving health care—the work that helps make health care workers professionals. Enjoy it.

Paul Batalden, M.D.
Professor, The Dartmouth Institute for
Health Policy and Clinical Practice
Dartmouth Medical School
Lebanon, New Hampshire
USA

References

Batalden, P., Bate, P., Webb, D., & McLoughlin, V. (2011). Planning and leading a multidisciplinary colloquium to explore the epistemology of improvement. *BMJ Quality & Safety, 20*, i1-i4.

Batalden, P., & Davidoff, F. (2007). What is quality improvement and how can it transform healthcare? *Quality & Safety in Health Care, 16*, 2-3.

Batalden, P., Davidoff, F., Marshall, M., Bibby, J., & Pink, C. (2011). So what? Now what? Exploring, understanding and using the epistemologies that inform the improvement of health care. *BMJ Quality & Safety, 20*, i99-i105.

Batalden, P., Ogrinc, G., & Batalden, M. (2006). From one to many. *Journal of Interprofessional Care, 20*, 549-551.

Benner, P., Sutphen, M., Leonard, V., & Day L. (2010). *Educating nurses: A call for radical transformation*. San Francisco: Jossey-Bass.

Houle, C. O. (1980). *Continuing learning in the professions*. San Francisco: Jossey-Bass.

Preface

This book began almost 10 years ago as a nagging thought in the minds of a few that health care could be better. The nagging thought became a national passion with the release of a series of reports from the Institute of Medicine (IOM). Consumers and health care professionals began to realize that health care in America was far from ideal and could be better. As each report uncovered a unique part of the puzzle, it became apparent that health professionals' education must be transformed to provide all disciplines with the knowledge, skills, and attitudes (KSAs) required to improve quality and patient safety. A consensus panel from the IOM defined the core competencies for all health care professionals to be: patient-centered care, teamwork and collaboration, quality improvement, safety, evidence-based practice, and informatics.

Nursing leaders recognized that there was much work to be done within nursing. Although safety and patient-centered care have long been the cornerstones of nursing practice, the health care landscape had changed, and challenges to safe, quality care have emerged. Through a series of grants from the Robert Wood Johnson Foundation, the Quality and Safety Education for Nurses (QSEN) project was born. A steering team, a national expert panel, and an advisory board identified the KSAs for each competency and developed a train-the-trainer approach to educate hundreds of nursing faculty in the new definitions of, and KSAs associated with, the six core competencies.

These pioneers in transforming nursing education helped identify and lead early adopters through the four phases of QSEN with the belief that nurses have the *will* through a common value system if they are helped to develop the *ideas* for leading change, and are provided the tools for *execution* for the change needed. Thus, as the original two dozen pioneers leading QSEN increased to 40 early adopters and champions (QSEN facilitators; www.qsen.org) and then to hundreds of faculty who participated in the pilot schools and the AACN/QSEN Institutes, the change was underway. After six years, we see a tipping point with quality and safety firmly embedded in nursing education essential competencies in both the National League for Nurses and the American Association for Colleges of Nursing documents. We see faculty excitedly embracing the new way of thinking about quality and safety, and we see new partnerships, across professions, and between academic and service agencies, to create a bold new vision for health professions education and practice.

This book has been designed to meet the needs of faculty, practicing nurses, and nursing students at all educational levels. Each chapter tells a part of the story: Chapter 1 details the critical need for change; the numerous regulatory, policy, and consumer efforts driving change are found in chapter 2; and chapter 3 presents the first person account from Dr. Cronenwett of how QSEN began. Section 2 includes an in-depth coverage of each of the six competencies that can serve as a resource for faculty, graduate students, practicing nurses, and other leaders. Section 3 covers key content on transforming education and practice, redesigning pedagogy based on narratives, integrating the competencies in simulation, the critical nature of interprofessional teamwork to improve quality and safety, developing personal leadership to lead change, and organizational qualities that create excellence. The last chapter exposes quality and safety as a global issue, and outlines the need for sharing strategies related to education, research, and practice changes around the world. Appendices add additional resources, including the full set of prelicensure and graduate competencies, the results of a Delphi study to assist in curriculum redesign, and an extensive glossary.

Each contributor is a leader in quality and safety and offers his or her work to stimulate other work to be shared around the globe, as we rebuild health care to be a high-reliability system focused on safety and quality. It is our hope that the shared story provides motivation and *will*, that the tool kit within these pages stimulates *ideas*, and that the continuing efforts for faculty and leader development translate to *execution* as we move toward new generations of nurses fully prepared to lead and work in health care systems based on cultures of quality and safety.

Gwen Sherwood, PhD, RN, FAAN
Jane Barnsteiner, PhD, RN, FAAN
Coeditors

Acknowledgements

We dedicate this book to honor the lifelong work of nursing's thought leader in quality and safety, Linda Cronenwett, PhD, RN, FAAN. It was her insight, knowledge, and dedication that launched the Quality and Safety Education for Nurses (QSEN) project to transform nursing education by integrating the competencies that help nurses deliver safe, quality care to their patients and families. We appreciate the support of the Robert Wood Johnson Foundation and the wise counsel of Rosemary Gibson, Sue Hassmiller, and Mary Joan Ladden. We are indebted to the QSEN Faculty Expert Panel, the QSEN Advisory Board, and the hundreds of nursing faculty who have participated in the QSEN journey over these past six years, for their effort and commitment to educate tomorrow's nurses to create a safer, higher quality health care system.

Section 1

Quality and Safety:
An Overview

Chapter 1

Driving Forces for Quality and Safety: Changing Mindsets to Improve Health Care

Gwen Sherwood, PhD, RN, FAAN

In 1999, the Institute of Medicine (IOM), a not-for-profit organization sponsored by the United States National Academy of Sciences, released *To Err Is Human* (published 2000). This report revealed the gap that exists between the current status of American health care and the quality of health care that the panel believed Americans were entitled to receive. Recommendations for sweeping changes in our systems followed in the 2001 *Crossing the Quality Chasm: A New Health System for the 21st Century*. Subsequently, the 2003 IOM report, *Health Professions Education: A Bridge to Quality*, called for a radical redesign of health professions education to achieve six core competencies described as essential to improve 21st century health care: patient-centered care, teamwork and collaboration, evidence-based practice, quality improvement, safety, and informatics. The attention from the series of IOM reports over the past 10 years confirms that quality and safety are the leading contemporary issues in health care, contributing to costs and poor outcomes. Current health care reform in the United States is based on improving quality outcomes: health care mistakes cost the system between 17 and 29 billion dollars each year. Beyond the economic factors, the impact on providers is equally critical, and poor quality leads to erosion of trust with consumers.

Since the Institute of Medicine series of reports focused attention on the issues in health care quality and safety, responses have included regulatory changes, new roles and responsibilities for health care professionals, and calls for a new educational paradigm. Still, many gaps continue (Balik & Dopkiss, 2010; Cronenwett, 2012; Leape & Berwick, 2005; Wachter, 2004; Wachter, 2010). In spite of declaring education as the bridge to quality, health professions education continues to undergo transformation to include preparation in the knowledge, skills, and attitudes (KSAs) needed to improve our systems

Quality and Safety in Nursing: A Competency Approach to Improving Outcomes,
First Edition. Edited by Gwen Sherwood and Jane Barnsteiner.
© 2012 John Wiley & Sons, Inc. Published 2012 by John Wiley & Sons, Inc.

(Batalden, Leach, & Ogrinc, 2009). What are issues in redesigning our systems of care? What do health professionals need to know? What are the organizational characteristics for a culture of quality and safety? This chapter will examine the impact of the driving forces for the changes needed, application of quality and safety science to reframe organizational cultures for quality improvement and safety, and how these reframe the education needs for nurses. The framework of the new paradigm shifts from individual performance to system initiatives and redesigns to monitor outcomes of care, and situates the patient as a full partner in care.

The compelling case for quality and safety

The data revealed in the IOM reports that comprise the Quality Chasm series sent shock waves throughout the industry and grabbed the attention of consumers (Textbox 1.1). The evidence reported in this series identified the imperative for changing mindsets to include quality and safety as part of the everyday work of nurses and other health professionals. Prior to release of the first report in 1999, the issues were wrapped in silence; without a reporting system there was not an evidence base to establish the scope or depth of system issues that contributed to poor quality and safety. There was no national tracking system and little pressure to improve quality and safety outcomes from regulators, health care purchasers, or thirdparty payers. Although the United States spends more than any other country on health care, the system has significant shortcomings, particularly in efficiency, quality, access, safety, and affordability (Davis, Schoen, & Stremikis, 2010). The fragmentation and decentralization of the health care system is a barrier to quality and safety; for example, patients may see multiple providers who may not be able to share critical patient information due to a lack of technology infrastructure or have a feeling of ownership that precludes sharing and consultation. While most data are based on acute care in patient settings, errors can occur in physician offices, out-patient settings, nursing homes, patient homes, and so forth. An annotation of the reports with their recommendations is in Textbox 1.1.

The data are startling, particularly related to medication errors, one of the most common according to *Identifying and Preventing Medication Errors* (Aspen, Walcott, Bootman, & Cronenwett, 2007). Medication errors particularly impact nurses. Nurses have the primary responsibility for medication administration with patients in a complex environment. Medication errors account for over 7,000 deaths annually. On average, in-patients may experience at least one medication error per day. At least 1.5 million preventable adverse drug events occur each year. Almost 2% of admissions experience a preventable adverse drug event, which increases hospital costs by $4,700 per admission or about $2.8 million annually for a 700-bed hospital; multiplied, this would account for $2 billion nationally.

The costs associated with quality and safety are complex; accounting includes lost income, health care costs, and other expenses. The national cost

Textbox 1.1 Summary: The Institute of Medicine
(IOM) Quality Chasm Series (www.iom.edu)

- *To Err Is Human: Building a Safer Health System* (2000)
This first IOM report presented the first aggregate data on the depth
and breadth of quality and safety issues in U.S. hospitals. Analysis of
outcomes from hospitals in Colorado and Utah concluded that 44,000
people die each year as a result of medical errors, and that in New York
hospitals, the number is 98,000. Even using the lower number, more
people die annually from medical error than from motor vehicle accidents, breast cancer, or AIDS. Medical errors are the leading cause of
unexpected deaths in health care settings. Communication is the root
cause of 65% of sentinel events. The report presents a strategy for
reducing preventable medical errors with a goal of a 50% reduction
over five years.
- *Crossing the Quality Chasm: A New Health System for the 21st Century*
(2001)
The IOM issued a call for sweeping reform of the American health care
system. A set of performance expectations for 21st century health care
seeks to assure that patient care is Safe, Timely, Effective, Efficient,
Equitable, and Patient centered (STEEEP). These aims provide the
measures of quality to align incentives for payment and accountability
based on quality improvements. The report includes causes of quality
gaps and barriers to improve care. Health care organizations are analyzed as complex systems with recommendations for how system
approaches can help implement change.
- *Health Professions Education: A Bridge to Quality* (2003)
Education is declared as the bridge to quality based on five competencies
identified as essential for health professionals of the 21st century: patient-
centered care, teamwork and collaboration, evidence-based practice,
quality improvement (and safety), and informatics. Recommendations
include developing a common language to use across disciplines,
integrate learning experiences, develop evidence-based curricula and
teaching approaches, initiate faculty development to model the core
competencies, and implement plans to monitor continued proficiency in
the competencies.
- *Keeping Patients Safe: Transforming the Work Environment of Nurses*
(2004)
The 2004 IOM report links nurses and their work environment with
patient safety and quality of care. The findings of this report have
helped shape the role of nurses in patient care quality and safety
efforts. Key recommendations are creating a satisfying and rewarding
work environment for nurses, providing adequate nurse staffing,

(Continued)

Textbox 1.1 (*Continued*)

focusing on patient safety at the level of organizational governing boards, incorporating evidence-based management in the management of nursing services, building trust between nurses and organizational leaders, giving nurses a voice in patient care delivery through effective nursing leadership and participation in executive decision making, providing organizational support to promote learning for both new and experienced nurses, promoting interdisciplinary collaboration, and designing work environments and culture that promote patient safety.

- *Identifying and Preventing Medication Errors* (2006)
  Medication errors make up the largest category of error with as many as 3%–4% of patients experiencing a serious medical error while hospitalized. This report presents a national agenda for reducing medication errors and the huge costs associated with medication errors. Changes across the health care industry require collaboration from doctors, nurses, pharmacists, the Food and Drug Administration and other government agencies, hospitals and other health care organizations, and patients.

for preventable adverse events ranges between $17 billion and $29 billion; additional health care accounts for more than half these totals because tests and treatments may have to be repeated or others added, and patients may need to extend their hospital stay. In addition to these costs, there are immeasurable ones: patients may suffer or be inconvenienced, have lower satisfaction with care, and lose trust in the system. Most of what is known about the financial and other burdens are hospital related. Data are just beginning to emerge on costs associated with quality and safety across the continuum of care, including ambulatory, home health care, and skilled care.

Health care workers are also affected by the quality of care in the systems in which they work; they may experience loss of morale and lower satisfaction when they are not able to provide the best care possible. *Keeping Patients Safe: Transforming the Work Environment of Nurses* (Page, 2004) is a comprehensive analysis of the factors influencing nurses' work. Health care is value based; as professionals we pledge, first, to do no harm. Quality is an essential value. Professionals take pride in doing the right thing, but quality is more than *will*; it is a mindset of inquiry and the capacity to use appropriate tools to improve systems in which we work. Quality improvement intersects all areas of health care from economic issues to the moral basis undergirding quality for doing our best. It builds on the shared values and moral commitment common to all health professionals. Health professionals have the motivation and ability to *improve* systems if they have the necessary education and training and work in organizations where quality improvement is integrated as part of daily work.

Consumers have helped motivate changes in health care. Patients and families who experienced adverse events have called for reform in how health care systems identify, investigate, report, and share information related to errors. Patients and families who experience health care mistakes leverage their influence to prevent similar events happening to others. National organizations such as the National Patient Safety Foundation (www.npsf.org) serve both consumers as well as health professionals. Numerous nonprofit organizations created in response to adverse events focus attention on particular care delivery issues as well as broader issues, establishing patient advocacy with an increasing influence in health care. Many patients or their family members now serve on hospital boards or consumer panels, share their stories in learning situations, and bring growing pressures to have systematic participation in all areas of health care.

The health care industry is applying lessons from other industries, particularly those known as high-reliability organizations (www.ahrq.gov). A key difference is that most other industries that have had dramatic improvements in quality and safety were supported by a designated agency that sets and communicates goals, brings visibility, and systematically collects and analyzes error reports for root cause analysis; however, health care lacks a single designated agency, as responsibilities are spread among various groups. Although numerous agencies developed in the decade following the publication of *To Err Is Human* was first published, none have the purpose of collecting safety or quality data for systematic analysis with broad dissemination to assure that best practice and safety alerts are implemented across all settings. Schumann (2012) offers a summary of these federal, regulatory, professional, and consumer agencies and organizations.

With lack of information on how and what errors occur and systematic dissemination of the information we do have, health care has lagged behind other high-risk industries in establishing a safety focus. Aviation has focused on safety for more than 50 years with significant reduction in fatalities. Health care has adopted and adapted principles and approaches from aviation as well as other high-reliability organizations that have similar characteristics, such as intermittent, intense tasks that demand exacting responses. By systematically collecting data on sentinel events for review through standardized processes, these industries have been able to monitor and improve safety in their systems.

Health care delivery organizations have a significant role in safety. Systems are a set of interdependent components that interact to achieve a common goal. For example, a hospital is a system composed of service lines, nursing care units, ancillary care departments, out-patient care clinics, and so forth. The way in which these separate but united system components interact and work together is a significant factor in delivering high-quality, safe care. Organizational leadership helps align quality and safety goals with mission and vision so that it is practiced consistently throughout all areas and levels of the system (Triolo, 2012). High-reliability organizations focus on safety; it is pervasive in their culture to be mindful of where the next error may occur to increase vigilance, establish check lists, or implement other preventions (Barnsteiner, 2012).

New meanings for familiar terms: the science of quality and safety

Quality and safety are intertwined, complex concepts with multiple dimensions. Lack of a comprehensive understanding of the full scope of these terms is but one barrier for implementing quality and safety strategies. It is difficult to reshape the mental model of these broad terms held by health care workers. The historic definitions and overuse of the terms are part of the change in mindset for adopting new KSAs derived from the science of quality and safety.

Though interrelated, quality and safety comprise different concepts. Quality improvement uses data to monitor outcomes of care processes that help guide improvement methods to design and test changes in the system to continuously improve outcomes (Compas, Hopkins, & Townsley, 2008; Johnson, 2012). The goal of quality is to reach for the best practice, and the goal is determined by measuring the reality of the care delivered compared with benchmarks or the ideal. Continuous quality monitoring is the mechanism by which the health care system can be transformed through the collaboration of health care professionals, patients and their families, researchers, payers, planners, and educators. All are working toward a triangle of improvements that lead to better patient outcomes (health), better system performance (care), and better professional development (education) (Bataldan & Davidoff, 2007). All health professionals must know how to assess the scientific evidence to determine what constitutes good care, identify gaps between good care and care delivered in their setting, and implement actions to close gaps (Sherwood & Jones, 2011).

Safety science embraces an organizational framework to minimize risk of harm to patients and providers through both system effectiveness and individual performance by applying human factors as discussed more fully by Barnsteiner in another chapter (2012) and Sammer and colleagues (2010). Safety science builds on Reason's model of errors (2000). Error is the failure of a planned action to be completed as intended or the use of an incorrect plan to achieve an aim. Reason identified two kinds of failure that constitute error:

1. Error of execution in which the correct action does not proceed as intended
2. Error of planning in which the original intended action is not correct.

An adverse event is the injury that results from care delivered or from care management, not from the underlying patient condition or the reason the patient was seeking care. Preventable adverse events are those attributed to error. There are also various types of errors. Diagnostic errors delay diagnosis, prevent use of appropriate tests, or result in failure to act. Treatment errors can occur while administering treatment, include errors in administering medication, lead to avoidable delay in treatment or response to treatment, or contribute to inappropriate care. Other examples are failure to provide prophylactic treatment, inadequate monitoring or follow-up, failure to communicate, equipment malfunction, or other system failure.

With multiple components in defining errors, it is a challenge to develop a unified reporting system that can be used across settings or nationally, in the same way that the aviation industry aggregates reports of airline events. Inconsistent nomenclature of a long list of terms adds to the difficulty of consistently reporting the same events in a central system. Through implementation of a culture of safety, organizations implement processes through risk management to collect error reports for root cause analysis. Carefully detailing all steps and decisions leading to an error or near miss can formulate a system redesign of processes that lessens the chance of future occurrence. The focus is on improving the system to prevent future errors rather than blaming individuals by acknowledging the influence of complex systems and human factors that influence safety. In a just culture, the focus is to determine what went wrong rather than identifying exactly who committed the error to establish blame and punishment. Just culture establishes an environment in which errors and near misses are acknowledged, reported, and analyzed for ways to improve the system. Accountability remains a critical aspect of a culture of safety; recognizing and acknowledging one's actions is a trademark of professional behavior.

Nurses are in the forefront of examining the work environment to identify where quality and safety are issues and how it is influenced by human factors, the interrelationship between people, technology, and the environment in which they work (Page, 2004). Human factors consider the ability or inability to perform exacting tasks while attending to multiple things at once. For system improvements, organizational leadership must give attention to human factors such as managing workload fluctuations, seeking strategies to minimize interruptions in work, and attending to communication and care coordination across disciplines. Effective care coordination includes checklists and other strategies to assure safe handoffs between providers and settings. Nurses are challenged by other human factors that impact quality and safety, such as multitasking, distractions, fatigue, task fixation that limits environmental scanning, and hierarchy and authority gradients. Staffing, interpersonal relationships, and the lack of education on quality and safety are among the multiple human factors that impact quality and safety.

Assuring quality and safety involves more than individual accountability because it requires considering how system designs can prevent error as part of the continuous cycle of improvements (Hughes, 2008). Focusing on safety helps eliminate discrepancies in care that are the result of provider actions in delivering care, that is, error prevention. Quality improvement is a critical aspect of safety—it requires assessing safety issues for prevalence, comparisons across areas, and using benchmark data to help clinicians improve their own practice as well as the system. When principles and strategies from quality improvement are applied, the rate of medication errors occurring in a given setting can be measured and compared with a peer unit or industry benchmark. Root cause analysis can determine reasons for errors in medication administration to change the system to prevent or lessen the possibility of errors occurring.

National organizations for quality and safety

Many of the improvements in our health care systems are the result of regulatory mandates from groups such as the Joint Commission (www.jointcommission.org), which grants institutional accreditation and opens the possibility of different aspects of federal funding (Wachter, 2004; Wachter, 2010). The Joint Commission also established the National Patient Safety Goals, updated annually. The goals provide guidance in key areas of high vulnerability and share evidence for solutions by emphasizing a systematic process for quality improvement, patient safety, and outcomes monitoring. The Joint Commission also established regulations to eliminate disruptive behavior among health care professionals and required organizations to have a code of conduct to define acceptable and inappropriate behavior as well as a process for managing such behaviors.

The Institute for Healthcare Improvement (IHI; www.ihi.org) has been a strong advocate for quality and safety innovations, bringing collaboration among all professions. The IHI's 100,000 and 5 Million Lives campaigns are but two examples of focused collective efforts for improving outcomes. Schumann (2012) provides a comprehensive description of national groups and their goals of quality and safety.

Professional nursing organizations have responded to the imperative to improve quality and safety in health care systems. The American Nurses Association, following a long history of promoting quality assurance, and the International Council of Nurses (2002) developed a new framework on quality improvement distributed nationally and globally (Doran, 2010). The Magnet recognition program recognizes organizational quality in nursing care delivery (Triolo, 2012) with standards based on continuous quality improvement. The standards reinforce conditions in the organization and practice environment that support and facilitate nursing excellence. Recognition is linked to improvement in nurse recruitment, retention, quality outcomes, and patient satisfaction scores. The American Nurses Association also established the National Database of Nursing Quality Indicators in 1998, which maintains data on sustained improvement in a designated nursing-sensitive indicator such as staffing, hospital-acquired pressure ulcers, falls and prevention of injury from falls, staff satisfaction, and pediatric and psychiatric mental health data (Montalvo & Dunton, 2007; Schumann, 2012).

Federal programs in Medicare and Medicaid have helped define nurses' roles and revised the payment structure for health care. Medicare and Medicaid subsequently developed programs to reduce hospital-acquired conditions, or those conditions that were not present at the time of a patient's hospital admission (Bodrock & Mion, 2008; Centers for Medicare and Medicaid Services, 2008). Hospitals are no longer reimbursed for 10 preventable hospital-acquired conditions, many of which were part of nursing care interventions (Hines & Yu, 2009). Other third-party payers and large employers have "pay for performance" plans in which health systems receive additional economic incentives when specific quality targets are met, many of which are nurse driven.

A progress report: where are we now more than a decade later?

The IOM (2001) issued four recommendations to change the system:

- Create a national focus through leadership, research, tool kits, and protocols to enhance knowledge about safety.
- Identify and learn from errors by establishing a vigorous error reporting system to assure a safer health care system.
- Increase standards and expectations for safety improvements through oversight groups, professional organizations, and health care purchasers.
- Improve the safety system within health care organizations to assure care improves.

There are progress reports 5 years and 10 years since the release of *To Err Is Human* (IOM, 2000) that examine progress based on these goals. Longo, Hewett, Ge, and Schubert (2005) used a 91-item survey to assess changes over time between two survey points in 2002 ($N = 126$) and 2004 ($N = 128$) in hospitals in Missouri and Utah that had collaborated on a patient safety project funded by the Agency for Healthcare Research and Quality (AHRQ). Assessment included seven variables: computerized physician order entry systems and test results, and assessments of safety procedures; specific safety policies; use of data in patient safety programs; drug handling procedures; manner of handling adverse events reporting; prevention policies; and root cause analysis. At the five-year mark, the report concludes that hospitals are not satisfactorily meeting the IOM recommendations, progress is slow, and technology applications that could improve safety lag.

Another study by Wachter (2004) measured five areas of patient safety five years after the the first IOM report and also found progress insufficient. Stronger regulation stimulated early improvements, but that impact has slowed. While there was some progress by 2004 in information technology applications and workforce organization and training, there was little demonstrable impact from error reporting systems and only small improvement in accountability, leading Wachter to declare that at the five-year mark from this galvanizing report, "we are at the end of the beginning," indicating there remains much work ahead.

In 2010 Wachter added another analysis to assess 10-year progress following publication of *To Err Is Human* (2000). Using a report card grading system from A (highest) to D (lowest), he assessed 10 key patient safety domains based on 1999–2004 and 2004–2009. Overall, Wachter graded the progress in safety as a B-, a modest improvement from a C+ based on data in the 2004 report. Leadership engagement from provider organizations and reporting systems were gauged as having made the most progress. There is a stronger business case for hospitals to concentrate on their safety efforts due to stronger accreditation standards and error reporting requirements. Interventions across national and international organizations receive the highest grade, including major campaigns from groups such as IHI, AHRQ, the Joint Commission, the National Quality Forum, and the World Health Organization. Few hospitals have moved to fully implement information technology applications. More systems are implementing a safety culture that balances no blame with accountability. Research is advancing in spite of inadequate funding. Progress in workforce and training is limited as few organizations have robust teamwork or culture change, but some impact has been felt from reducing residents' duty hours and easing of the nursing shortage. Patient engagement and involvement remains small, with more progress related to disclosure policies and procedures, also addressed by Balik and Dopkiss (2010). Payment system intervention is uncertain, as pay for performance is only beginning. Wachter concludes that our limited ability to measure safety outcomes is a major barrier to progress.

Progress is reported in several areas of nursing practice. Many nursing organizations have identified and developed programs to improve quality and safety. For example, the American Association of Critical-Care Nurses (2010) developed multiple approaches including a program on healthy work environments focused on teamwork and collaboration. Competencies were developed for prelicensure and graduate nurses by the Quality and Safety Education for Nurses (QSEN) project (Cronenwett, 2012). The Nursing Alliance for Quality Care (Schumann, 2012) was formed to bring one organized nursing voice to ensure that (a) patients receive the right care at the right time by the right professional; (b) nurses actively advocate and are accountable for consumer-centered, high-quality health care; and (c) policymakers recognize the contributions of nurses in advancing consumer-centered, high-quality health care.

Strategies to change mindsets: nurses' roles in improving quality and safety

While quality and safety improvements are goals for practitioners in all levels and areas of health care, nurses have particular roles. The IOM website has the following quote from the 2010 report *The Future of Nursing: Leading Change, Advancing Health*:

> Overcoming challenges in nursing is essential to overcoming the challenges in the health care system as a whole. Nurses are the largest segment of the health care workforce, and their skills and availability can directly affect quality, safety, and efficiency. Most nurses work in hospitals or other acute settings, where they are patients' primary, professional caregivers and the individuals most likely to intercept medical errors. However, because hospital systems and acute care settings are often complex and chaotic, many nurses spend unnecessary time hunting for supplies, filling out paperwork, and coordinating staff time and patient care, reducing the time they are able to spend with patients and delivering care.

Considering the scope of the recommendations and the limited progress, what is the nursing response to the IOM Quality Chasm series? Wachter's (2010) review of progress to achieve the IOM recommendations cites moderate progress in addressing workforce and training issues, reporting systems, and research. What does it mean for nursing? Three primary goals can guide nurses in leading change. First, all nurses must develop a mindset of questioning to constantly improve their work and increase their capacity to recognize and acknowledge quality and safety issues in their own work and in the systems in which they work. Second, educational programs must be transformed to address quality and safety competencies to help learners with changes in KSAs. Third, advancing scholarship to determine best practices in education, practice, and systems applications will establish an evidence base to implement effective approaches to transform health care.

Change mindset

Increasing nurses' awareness of quality and safety developed within new science applications will help nurses recognize quality and safety concerns in their practice and in their settings. Many remain largely unaware of the scope of the problems and have not been taught how to identify, report, and systematically analyze a near-miss or sentinel event or lead a quality improvement team (Chenot & Daniel, 2010). A mindset of inquiry, of asking questions can lead to improvements in the systems. Day and Smith (2007) demonstrate inquiry-based clinical learning by focusing on patient-centered care to ask, "What is the most important thing to do right now for this patient?" Reflection is another learning approach that helps with change; reflection asks questions; questions are the first step in change (Horton-Deutsch & Sherwood, 2008). Asking questions opens the way to innovative approaches, application of evidence-based practice standards, and various methods of quality improvement. Learning the concepts of new safety science refocuses how errors are reported. Rather than using incident reports to establish blame on an individual provider, organizations committed to quality and safety create a culture in which nurses and other professionals are empowered to disclose near misses and mistakes through a reporting system, and to identify areas in which outcomes do not match benchmarks.

It is a challenge, however, to build the awareness that empowers nurses to make the first step and acknowledge a near miss or mistake. Nurses then need to know what to report, and how, as well as how to follow the steps in the organization's safety plan. In a just culture, there is a shift from establishing blame and punishing someone for a mistake to a systematic analysis for the purpose of learning and change. All providers who had any part in the event come together, led by trained professionals, to establish the chain of actions, decisions, and circumstances that may have contributed to an error so there is the opportunity to learn and develop system changes to prevent future occurrences. Patients and their families should be informed and included in the process to achieve transparency in the system, to have full disclosure of the event. Quality improvement teams can collect information to monitor occurrences of the problem in other parts of the system, compare data, and initiate strategies to eliminate variances. Asking questions can lead to conducting an annual safety culture survey to identify areas for workplace improvement and priorities for improving quality, or it can lead to using scorecards to collect data on services to identify areas for improvement. In academic settings, educators establish a culture of safety and quality for their own educational processes such as a reporting system of learner near misses and errors to assess processes and increase safety awareness.

Transform education to integrate competencies

The second focus area is transforming nursing education to integrate the competencies based on the KSAs developed from the Quality and Safety Education for Nurses (QSEN) project. The project goal for the QSEN project in the United States (www.qsen.org) is to (a) change the mindset of nurses to a practice based on inquiry in which questions are raised about the whys of nursing care, (b) develop and use evidence-based standards and interventions, and (c) investigate outcomes and critical incidents from a system perspective (Cronenwett, 2012; Cronenwett et al., 2007; Cronenwett et al., 2009; Sherwood, 2012). These competency statements can guide educators in developing educational programs that help learners achieve the KSAs necessary to work in redesigned health care settings built around quality and safety. The IOM (Greiner & Knebel, 2003) identified five competencies as essential for all health professionals if we are to improve health care with quality and safety combined; subsequent definitions list quality improvement and safety separately based on the knowledge base for each. The six competencies are not isolated concepts but are interrelated and apply across all health disciplines. The goal of the competencies is to enable health professionals to deliver patient-centered care, work as part of interdisciplinary teams, practice evidence-based health care, implement quality improvement measures and strategies, and use information technology (Cronenwett et al., 2007; Cronenwett et al., 2009; Finkelman & Kenner, 2009; Greiner & Knebel, 2003). Brief descriptions of the competencies are in Textbox 1.2, complete definitions and the KSAs are in Appendixes A and B, and each competency is discussed in separate chapters in Section 2 of this book.

Education transformation cannot happen in isolation. The IOM recommendations demand interprofessional learning experiences for both academic and clinical learning situations. Nursing education most often occurs in silos–independent departments–with few shared learning opportunities between the many health disciplines with which nurses are expected to work. Knowing what each discipline contributes is crucial to high performance and flexible team leadership that works through authority gradients so all team members have equal opportunity to share information in establishing patient care goals (Disch, 2012a). These educational changes must happen in all settings to prepare nurses in practice as well as those in academic programs.

Textbox 1.2   Descriptions of six competencies
to improve quality and safety*

- Patient-centered care
  In patient-centered care, care decisions are based on knowledge of patient values, beliefs, and preferences so that patients and their families are treated with respect and honor, included as partners in care, and treated as safety allies (Walton & Barnsteiner, 2012). Their familiarity with their treatment plan makes them an important part of the team by helping alert clinicians when care is not according to their usual routine, and thus helps prevent errors.
- Teamwork and collaboration
  How well health care professionals work together accounts for as much as 70% of health care errors (Institute of Medicine, 2000), yet nurses and physicians have few educational experiences together. Coordinating complex care requires cross-disciplinary communication, knowing scope of responsibility, and organizational support for speaking up when safety is compromised (Disch, 2012b). Nurses need skills in problem solving, conflict resolution, and negotiation to be able to coordinate care across interprofessional teams (Moore, Dolansky, & Singh, 2012). A health professional who develops emotional intelligence can apply his or her personal strengths to foster effective team functioning. Flexible leadership, standardized communication, mutual support, and constant environmental scans contribute to effective team leadership (Disch, 2012a).
- Evidence-based practice
  Patient care should be based on evidence-based practice standards, not tradition or trial and error (Tracey & Barnsteiner, 2012). Nurses who practice from a spirit of inquiry with reflection on the care delivered will apply informatics skills to seek current evidence to determine best practices and clarify care decisions. Patient-centered care considers patient preferences, values, and beliefs within an evidence-based approach. Nurses use evidence-based standards and quality improvement tools to measure how care in their own setting compares with benchmark data to determine areas to improve.
- Quality improvement
  The spirit of inquiry promotes a practice attitude of continuously improving care every day with every patient. Quality improvement is an approach to practice that measures variance in ideal and actual care and implements strategies to close the gap (Johnson, 2012). Nurses use quality improvement tools, informatics to seek evidence and measure care outcomes, and benchmark data to assess current practice. The ethical responsibility of quality improvement includes commitment to provide the best known care as well as the ethical conduct of the process itself.

(Continued)

Textbox 1.2   (*Continued*)

- Safety
  Safety is the effort to minimize the risk of harm to patients and providers through both system effectiveness and individual performance (Barnsteiner, 2012). Competency in safety is based on constantly asking how actions affect patient risk, where the next error is likely to occur, and what actions can prevent near misses. Safety science redirects the examination of errors from the person approach in which the individual is blamed for forgetfulness, lack of attention, or moral weakness, to one that examines the system in which the error occurred. A systems approach examines the conditions in the environment that may have contributed to the error and designs defenses to prevent errors or mitigate effects.
- Informatics
  Informatics is a thread through all the competencies to help manage care through documentation in electronic health records, decision support tools, and safety alerts (Warren, 2012). Providers apply skills in informatics to retrieve information, search for the latest evidence, manage quality improvement data and strategies, and share information across the interprofessional team. Nurses also use informatics knowledge, skills, and attitudes to help guide development of informatics applications, purchases, and ways to use it on the unit.

*Appendixes A and B have definitions with knowledge, skill, and attitude objectives.

Educators have help available in making the transition. To assist educator development, the American Association of Colleges of Nursing has offered a series of QSEN faculty development workshops, and the QSEN project team leads an annual national forum to share outcomes and strategies. The QSEN website offers teaching strategies, annotated bibliographies, demonstration projects, videos, learning modules, and a facilitator panel to assist with educator development. Educators and organizations responsible for accreditation, licensing and certification of health professionals have embedded the competencies into nursing education standards to help lead transformation of how we prepare students and nurses to be proficient in these competencies essential to quality and safety (Sherwood, 2012).

Advancing scholarship

A third area of focus is advancing the scholarship in all areas of quality and safety. Research is imperative to develop the scientific evidence of quality and safety issues to know how and to what extent patients are harmed and ways to mitigate. We need evidence-based educational strategies to determine best practices for teaching and implementing quality and safety concepts in practice. Traditional education methods relying on lecture have not demonstrated the capacity to achieve the KSAs needed to redesign health care across multiple settings (Sherwood, 2012; Ironsides & Cerbie, 2012). To integrate the competencies, educators need evidence-based curricula and teaching strategies to derive innovative educational interventions, whether as part of their formal education or as staff in clinical settings (www.qsen.org). Examples of work include the following:

- Hobgood et al. (2010) compared four pedagogical approaches including high and low fidelity to measure changes in knowledge and attitude of nursing and medical students from an educational intervention for interdisciplinary teamwork.
- Welsh, Flanagan, and Ebright (2010) compared two methods of end-of-shift handoffs to examine communication and potential for adverse events.
- Varkey, Reller, Smith, Ponto, and Osborn (2006) used the QI Knowledge Application Tool to measure effectiveness of a 4-week quality improvement learning experience with interprofessional learners.
- A QSEN-led 15-school Pilot Learning Collaborative demonstrated integration of the competencies in which the schools worked with a clinical partner (Cronenwett, Sherwood, & Gelmon, 2009; www.QSEN.org).

These few examples illustrate opportunities to develop evidence-based approaches to achieving the IOM recommendations. We have an unparalleled opportunity for nursing leadership and scholarship to help improve our health systems. We need to determine the effectiveness of what we are teaching about quality and safety, measure the long-term behavior change, and assess the skills needed in the workplace that will drive curricular changes. Benner, Sutphin, Leonard, and Day (2010) call for nurses to claim this opportunity for radical redesign of nursing education that can match the radical changes needed in health care delivery. Scholarly investigation can determine effective pedagogies, outcomes of care interventions, strategies for reporting and investigating errors, system malfunctions that lead to work-arounds, and communication that promotes interprofessional teamwork.

Summary

Ten years later, the United States still has no lead organization for quality and safety in spite of the recommendation for a comprehensive strategy, and other changes are being implemented slowly. Various organizations, including professional and consumer groups, have developed regulations, educational programs, and initiatives for leading change. There is progress in establishing a culture conducive for pursuing health care quality and reporting; clinicians are replacing the fear of a punitive response and cover-up with a focus on accountability and reporting events so that through analysis the organization can implement improvements and prevention strategies. Nurses have new roles and responsibilities in continuous quality improvement that encourages a culture of inquiry and asking questions, and investigates outcomes and critical incidents from a system perspective. The QSEN project continues to lead integration of quality and safety competencies in all levels of nursing education. Progress in evidence-based education approaches and pedagogies will help determine ways to prepare clinicians with new mindsets and lasting behavior change based on the six quality and safety competencies.

References

American Association of Critical-Care Nurses. (2010). *Clinical practice resources: Healthy work environment.* Retrieved July 10, 2011, from http://www.aacn.org/

Aspen, P., Walcott, J., Bootman, L., & Cronenwett, L. (Eds.) and the Committee on Identifying and Preventing Medication Errors. (2007). *Identifying and Preventing Medication Errors.* Washington, DC: National Academies Press.

Balik, B., & Dopkiss, F. (2010). 10 years after To Err Is Human: Are we listening to patients and families yet? *Focus on Patient Safety, Newsletter of the National Patient Safety Foundation, 13*(1), 1–3. Retrieved June 29, 2010, from http://www.npsf.org/paf/npsfp/fo/pdf/Focus_vol_13_1_2010.pdf

Barnsteiner, J. (2012). Safety. In G. Sherwood & J. Barnsteiner (Eds.), *Quality and safety in nursing: A competency approach to improving outcomes.* Hoboken, NJ: Wiley-Blackwell.

Batalden, P. B., & Davidoff, F. (2007). What is "quality improvement" and how can it transform healthcare? *Quality & Safety in Health Care, 16*(1), 2–3.

Batalden, P. B., Leach, D., & Ogrinc, G. (2009). Knowing is not enough: Executives and educators must act to address challenges and reshape healthcare. *Healthcare Executive, 24*(2), 68–70.

Benner, P., Sutphen, M., Leonard, V., & Day, L. (2010). *Educating nurses: A call for radical transformation.* San Francisco, CA: Jossey-Bass.

Bodrock, J. A., & Mion, L.C. (2008). Pay for performance in hospitals: Implications for nurses and nursing care. *Quality Management in Health Care, 17*(2), 102–111.

Centers for Medicare and Medicaid Services. (2008). *Roadmap for Implementing Value Driven Healthcare in the Traditional Medicare Fee-for-Service* Program. Retrieved July 14, 2010, from https://www.cms.gov/QualityInitiativesGenInfo/downloads/VBPRoadmap_OEA_1-16_508.pdf

Chenot, T., & Daniel, L. (2010). Frameworks for patient safety in the nursing curriculum. *Journal of Nursing Education, 49*(10), 559–568. DOI:10.3928/01484834-20100730-02.

Compas, C., Hopkins. K., & Townsley, E. (2008). Best practices in implementing and sustaining quality of care: A review of the quality of improvement literature. *Research in Gerontological Nursing, 1*(3), 209–215.

Cronenwett, L. (2012). A National Initiative: Quality and Safety Education for Nurses (QSEN). In G. Sherwood & J. Barnsteiner (Eds.), *Quality and safety in nursing: A competency approach to improving outcomes.* Hoboken, NJ: Wiley-Blackwell.

Cronenwett, L., Sherwood, G., Barnsteiner, J., Disch, J., Johnson, J., Mitchell, P., et al. (2007). Quality and safety education for nurses. *Nursing Outlook, 55*(3), 122–131.

Cronenwett, L., Sherwood, G., & Gelmon, S. (2009). Improving quality and safety education: The QSEN learning collaborative. *Nursing Outlook, 57*(6), 304–312.

Cronenwett, L., Sherwood, G., Pohl, J, Barnsteiner, J., Moore, S., Sullivan, D. T., et al. (2009). Quality and safety education for advanced practice nursing practice. *Nursing Outlook*, *57*(6), 338–348.

Davis, K., Schoen, C., & Stremikis, K. (2010). *Mirror, mirror on the wall: How the performance of the U.S. health care system compares internationally, 2010 Update*. Retrieved July 14, 2010, from http://www.commonwealthfund.org/~/media/Files/Publications/Fund%20Report/2010/Jun/1400_Davis_Mirror_Mirror_on_the_wall_2010.pdf

Day, L., & Smith, E. L. (2007). Integrating quality and safety content into clinical teaching in the acute care setting. *Nursing Outlook*, *55*(3), 138–143.

Disch, J. (2012a). Leadership to create change. In G. Sherwood & J. Barnsteiner (Eds.), *Quality and safety in nursing: A competency approach to improving outcomes*. Hoboken, NJ: Wiley-Blackwell.

Disch, J. (2012b). Teamwork and collaboration. In G. Sherwood & J. Barnsteiner (Eds.), *Quality and safety in nursing: A competency approach to improving outcomes*. Hoboken, NJ: Wiley-Blackwell.

Doran, D.M. (2010). *Nursing outcomes: The state of the science* (2nd ed.). Sudbury, MA: Jones & Bartlett Learning.

Finkelman, A., & Kenner, C. (2009). *Teaching IOM*. Silver Spring MD: American Nurses Association.

Greiner, A. C., & Knebel, E., Institute of Medicine Committee on the Health Professions Education Summit. (2003). *Health Professions Education: A Bridge to Quality*. Washington, DC: National Academies Press.

Hines, P. A., & Yu, K. M. (2009). The changing reimbursement landscape: Nurses' role in quality and operational excellence. *Nursing Economic*, *27*(1), 345–352.

Hobgood, C., Sherwood, G., Frush, K., Hollar, D., Maynard, L., Foster, B., et al., on behalf of the Interprofessional Patient Safety Education Collaborative. (2010). Teamwork training with nursing and medical students: Does the method matter? Results of an interinstitutional interdidsciplinary collaboration. *Quality and Safety in Health Care*, *19*, 1–6.

Horton-Deutsch, S., & Sherwood, G. (2008). Reflection: An educational strategy to develop emotionally competent nurse leaders. *Journal of Nursing Management*, *16*(8), 946–954.

Hughes, R. G. (2008). Tools and strategies for quality improvement and patient safety. In Hughes, R. G. (Ed.), *Patient safety and quality: An evidence-based handbook for nurses*, Vol. 3, pp. 3-1-3-40. Rockville, MD: Agency for Healthcare Research and Quality. Also retrieved from http://www.ahrq.gov/qual/nurseshdbk

Institute of Medicine. (2000). *To err is human: Building a safer health system*. Washington, DC: National Academies Press.

Institute of Medicine. (2001). *Crossing the quality chasm: A new health system for the 21st century*. Washington, DC: National Academies Press.

Institute of Medicine. (2010). *The future of nursing: Leading change, advancing health*. Institute of Medicine and the Robert Wood Johnson Foundation. Washington, DC: National Academies Press. Retrieved from http://www.iom.edu/Reports/2010/A-Summary-of-the-October-2009-Forum-on-the-Future-of-Nursing-Acute-Care.aspx

International Council of Nurses. (2002). *Position statement on patient safety*. Retrieved July 14, 2010, from http://www.icn.ch/images/stories/documents/publications/position_statements/D05_Patient_Safety.pdf

Ironsides, P., & Cerbie, E. (2012). Narrative teaching strategies to foster quality and safety. In G. Sherwood & J. Barnsteiner (Eds.), *Quality and safety in nursing: A competency approach to improving outcomes*. Hoboken, NJ: Wiley-Blackwell.

Johnson, J. (2012). Quality improvement. In G. Sherwood & J. Barnsteiner (Eds.), *Quality and safety in nursing: A competency approach to improving outcomes*. Hoboken, NJ: Wiley-Blackwell.

Leape, L. L., & Berwick, D. M. (2005). Five years after *To Err Is Human*: What Have We Learned? *Journal of the American Medical Association*, *293*, 2384–2390.

Longo, D. R., Hewett, J. E., Ge, B., & Schubert, S. (2005). The long road to patient safety: A status report on patient safety systems. *Journal of the American Medical Association*, *294*(22), 2858–2865.

Montalvo, I., & Dunton, N. (2007). *Transforming nursing data into quality care: Profiles of quality improvement in U.S. healthcare facilities*. Silver Spring, MD: American Nurses Association.

Moore, S., Dolansky, M., & Singh, M. (2012). Interprofessional approaches to quality and safety education. In G. Sherwood & J. Barnsteiner (Eds.), *Quality and safety in nursing: A competency approach to improving outcomes*. Hoboken, NJ: Wiley-Blackwell.

Page, A. (2004). *Keeping patients safe: Transforming the work environment of nurses*. Committee on the Work Environment for Nurses and Patient Safety, Board on Health Care Services. Washington, DC: National Academies Press.

Reason, J. (2000). Human error: Models and management. *BMJ*, *320*(7237):768–770.

Sammer, C. E., Lykens, K., Singh, K. P., Mains, D. A., & Lackan, N. A. (2010). What is patient safety culture? A review of the literature. *Journal of Nursing Scholarship*, *42*(2), 156–165.

Schumann, M. J. (2012). Policy implications driving national quality and safety initiatives. In G. Sherwood & J. Barnsteiner (Eds.), *Quality and safety in nursing: A competency approach to improving outcomes*. Hoboken, NJ: Wiley-Blackwell.

Sherwood, G. (2012). The imperative to transform education to transform practice. In G. Sherwood & J. Barnsteiner (Eds.), *Quality and safety in nursing: A competency approach to improving outcomes*. Hoboken, NJ: Wiley-Blackwell.

Sherwood, G., & Jones, C. (2010). Quality improvement in nursing. In W. Sollecito & J. Johnson (Eds.), *CQI in healthcare*, 4th ed. (pp. 485–511). San Francisco: Jossey-Bass.

Tracey, M. F., & Barnsteiner, J. (2012). Evidence-based practice. In G. Sherwood & J. Barnsteiner (Eds.), *Quality and safety in nursing: A competency approach to improving outcomes*. Hoboken, NJ: Wiley-Blackwell.

Triolo, P. (2012). Creating cultures of excellence: Transforming organizations. In G. Sherwood & J. Barnsteiner (Eds.), *Quality and safety in nursing: A competency approach to improving outcomes*. Hoboken, NJ: Wiley-Blackwell.

Varkey, P., Reller, M. K., Smith, A., Ponto, J., & Osborn, M. (2006). An experiential interdisciplinary quality improvement education initiative. *American Journal of Medical Quality*, *21*(5), 317–322.

Wachter, R. M. (2004). The end of the beginning: Patient safety five years after "To Err Is Human." *Health Affairs*, W4-534–W4-545.

Wachter, R. M. (2010). Patient safety at ten: Unmistakable progress, troubling gaps. *Health Affairs*, *29*(1), 165–173.

Walton, M. K., & Barnsteiner, J. (2012). Patient-centered care. In G. Sherwood & J. Barnsteiner (Eds.), *Quality and safety in nursing: A competency approach to improving outcomes*. Hoboken, NJ: Wiley-Blackwell.

Warren, J. (2012). Informatics. In G. Sherwood & J. Barnsteiner (Eds.), *Quality and safety in nursing: A competency approach to improving outcomes*. Hoboken, NJ: Wiley-Blackwell.

Welsh, C. A., Flanagan, M. E., & Ebright, P. (2010). Barriers and facilitators to nursing handoffs: Recommendations for redesign. *Nursing Outlook*, *58*(3), 148–154.

Resources

Agency for Healthcare Research and Quality: www.ahrq.gov

American Association of Colleges of Nursing: www.aacn.nche.edu

American Association of Critical Care Nurses, Clinical Practice Resources: www.aacn.org/DM/MainPages/PracticeHome.aspx?lastmenu=divheader_clinical_practice

American Nurses Association. The National Center for Nursing Quality Indicators: www.nursingquality.org

American Organization of Nurse Executives: www.aone.org

Center for Studying Health System Change: www.hschange.org

Commonwealth Fund: www.commonwealthfund.org

Consumers Advancing Patient Safety: www.patientsafety.org

Empowered Patient Care Coalition: www.empoweredpatientcoalition.org

Institute for Healthcare Improvement: www.ihi.org

Institute of Medicine: www.iom.edu

Institute for Safe Medication Practices: www.ismp.org

International Council of Nurses. www.icn.ch

Joint Commission: www.jointcommission.org

Nursing Alliance for Quality Care: http://www.gwumc.edu/healthsci/departments/nursing/naqc/

National League for Nursing: www.nln.org

National Quality Forum: www.qualityforum.org

National Patient Safety Foundation: www.npsf.org

Quality and Safety Education for Nurses: www.qsen.org

Robert Wood Johnson Foundation: www.rwjf.org

Robert Wood Johnson Foundation (2008). *Transforming care at the bedside toolkit*. Retrieved July 10, 2011, from http://www.rwjf.org/pr/product.jsp?id=30051.

Chapter 2

Policy Implications Driving National Quality and Safety Initiatives

Mary Jean Schumann, DNP, MBA, RN, CPNP

While individual providers and clinicians of every discipline can elect to improve their own practice, strive to provide higher quality care, and reduce errors in their own work environments, much of the effort to reach higher levels of quality and safety must also occur through high-level policy setting. Without policies that focus prioritization of resources on quality health care as a goal, individual efforts will be subsumed by other challenges such as stressful working conditions, short staffing and limited access, and demands for cost containment. This chapter addresses the policy strategies and initiatives that have emerged since 1990, from coalition building, to standard setting, to rule making and regulation, to the development of new incentives, and even legislation. Nurses' roles in these efforts will also be described, as well as opportunities to influence policy, priorities, outcomes, and implementation today and in the decade that follows. While quality and safety are distinct, the inclusion of safety is considered in any discussion of health care quality. Since so many measures of health care quality seem rooted in the absence of negative outcomes, such as falls, development of infections, pressure ulcers, and harm as a result of medication errors, safety has become synonymous with quality improvement in many discussions.

Policy in the context of health care quality and safety

From the outset, this chapter is based on the premise that policy encompasses many strategies and certainly is not limited to or even best achieved in most instances by legislation. Simon (1966) defines policy as "a set of processes,

Quality and Safety in Nursing: A Competency Approach to Improving Outcomes, First Edition. Edited by Gwen Sherwood and Jane Barnsteiner.
© 2012 John Wiley & Sons, Inc. Published 2012 by John Wiley & Sons, Inc.

including at least (1) setting the agenda, (2) the specifying alternatives from which to choose, (3) an authoritative choice among those specified alternatives, as in a legislative vote or a presidential decision, and (4) implementing the decision." Although Kingdon (2003) ascribes multiple definitions to the term *agenda setting*, one is most applicable in the arena of health care quality. He includes as a definition of agenda setting "a coherent set of proposals, each related to the others and forming a series of enactments its proponents would prefer." There is considerable evidence in this chapter to support the value of that definition.

For purposes of this chapter's discussion, policy encompasses alternatives that include not only legislative action but also rule making, statements of positions, establishment of standards, the adoption of guidelines or principles of best practice, and national consensus strategies. While policy is not confined to federal or national actions, the policy initiatives and opportunities discussed here will be largely at that level, given the scope and nature of the quality issues.

Another important concept espoused by Kingdon (2003), useful to understanding not only policy formation but also nursing's role in shaping it, is that multiple process streams exist. Kingdon describes these as streams of problems, policies, and politics. Indeed, accurate formulation of problems is often a crucial first step to figuring out how to move toward solutions that derive from useful policy. Unless the problem is correctly identified, one can chase many alternative solutions without getting to any that might lead to resolution of the real problem. Kingdon concludes that the greatest policy changes grow out of that coupling of problems, policy proposals, and politics. If we think more broadly about the recent passage of health care reform legislation, policy emerged where there was a convergence of health care delivery challenges, support of stakeholder groups and alliances around policy proposals to improve care, and the political will to enact legislation, modify funding streams, and adjust priorities.

The landscape of formal stakeholders in the ongoing quality dialogue

Many collective efforts have been initiated over the last 20 years to drive quality and safety improvement through policy channels. This chapter will describe formalized efforts that grew out of a need to address health delivery challenges, using organizational structures or alliances whose missions were substantially focused on quality. The list is necessarily broad and incorporates federal agencies as well as others. Certainly this list is not exhaustive; the intent has been to include those efforts in which nursing has or needs to have a voice in the formal agenda, solutions, and policy formulations.

While this chapter will begin with a discussion of the result of two decades of effort—the passage and early efforts to implement the Affordable Care Act and the many provisions within it that support health care quality and safety–the subsequent discussion centers around understanding what other policy efforts were required to achieve convergence and successful legislation.

Affordable Care Act (ACA) emerged where efforts converged

In March 2010, the U.S. Congress passed and the president signed into law the Affordable Care Act. While the provisions are many and remain controversial, from the perspective of driving improvements in quality, several key provisions of the law are underway that provide significant opportunity to reshape the future delivery of care. Nurses were critical to designing and supporting passage of these provisions and now have significant opportunity to influence and suggest innovations in care delivery that are consistent with these provisions and with implementation of various aspects of the law focused on the improvement of quality. The following are some of the key provisions specific to quality.

Improving health care quality and efficiency

The law established a new Center for Medicare and Medicaid Innovation that has begun pilot demonstrations to test new ways of delivering care to patients. In addition, this new center is looking for existing and promising innovative programs that can be replicated or scaled up to improve the quality of health care delivered and also reduce the rate of growth in health care costs for Medicare, Medicaid, and the Children's Health Insurance Program. Included in this provision, the Department of Health and Human Services (HHS) was required to submit a National Strategy for Quality Improvement in Health Care that would include these programs in addition to those of third party payers. This National Strategy is a strategic plan for improving the delivery of health care services, achieving better patient outcomes, and improving the health of the U.S. population. The ACA called for the establishment of an Interagency Working Group on Health Care Quality, composed of senior officials representing 23 federal agencies with major responsibility for health care quality and quality improvement. The working group's function is to provide a platform for collaboration, cooperation, and consultation among relevant agencies regarding quality initiatives as a means to ensure alignment and coordination across federal efforts and with the private sector.

Linking payment to quality outcomes

ACA establishes a Hospital Value-Based Purchasing program for traditional Medicare participants. This program offers financial incentives to hospitals to improve the quality of care. In keeping with the intent of transparency and accountability, hospital performance will be required to be publicly reported, beginning with measures relating to heart attacks, heart failure, pneumonia, surgical care, health care–associated infections, and patients' perception of care. Early in 2011, stakeholders and quality alliances, including nursing, submitted public comments regarding the proposed rules that would implement this provision. The work of developing and endorsing performance measures that meet the intent of this provision are the result of work in which various entities, alliances, and individual stakeholder organizations engage.

Encouraging integrated health systems

ACA provides incentives for physicians and other providers to join together to form Accountable Care Organizations (ACOs), which will allow physicians and other providers to better coordinate patient care and improve health care quality, help prevent disease and illness, and reduce unnecessary hospital admissions. If an ACO provides high-quality care while reducing costs to the health care system, rules allow the ACO to keep some of the money saved. Key stakeholder groups, including nursing, have been engaged in public comments in response to controversial ACO rules proposed by the Centers for Medicare and Medicaid Services (CMS). While ACOs clearly would benefit from the services of RNs, APRNs, and other clinicians, certain exclusions in the rules could have negative impact in recognizing their contributions or sharing cost savings.

Paying providers based on value, not volume

A new provision will tie provider payments to the quality of care they provide. Providers are expected to see their payments modified so that those who provide higher value care will receive higher payments than those who provide lower quality care. This provision is scheduled to occur in 2015, leaving open the opportunity to yet influence the shape of this program and urge inclusion of nurse providers.

Partnership for patients

Partnership for Patients is a new national partnership initiated in April 2011 by HHS that will help save 60,000 lives by preventing injuries and complications in patient care over the next three years. HHS states that the Partnership for Patients also has the potential to save up to $35 billion in health care costs, including up to $10 billion for Medicare. Over the next ten years, the Partnership for Patients could reduce costs to Medicare by $50 billion and save billions more in Medicaid. More than 3,500 hospitals, physician and nurse groups, consumer groups, and employers have already pledged their commitment to the new initiative. CMS is implementing this program under its Center for Medicare and Medicaid Innovations.

Funding for this public-private partnership will be invested in reforms that help achieve two shared goals:

- **Keeping hospital patients from getting injured or sicker:** By the end of 2013, preventable hospital-acquired conditions would decrease by 40% compared to 2010. Achieving this goal would mean approximately 1.8 million fewer injuries to patients, with more than 60,000 lives saved over the next three years.
- **Helping patients heal without complication:** By the end of 2013, preventable complications during a transition from one care setting to another would be decreased so that all hospital readmissions would be reduced by 20 compared with those of 2010. Achieving this goal would mean that more than 1.6 million patients will recover from illness without suffering a preventable complication requiring rehospitalization within 30 days of discharge.

The partnership will target all forms of harm to patients but will start by asking hospitals to focus on nine types of medical errors and complications where the potential for dramatic reductions in harm rates has been demonstrated by pioneering hospitals and systems across the country. Examples include preventing adverse drug reactions, pressure ulcers, childbirth complications, and surgical site infections. The CMS Innovation Center will help hospitals adapt effective, evidence-based care improvements to target preventable patient injuries on a local level, developing innovative approaches to spreading and sharing strategies among public and private partners in all states. Members of the partnership will identify specific steps they will take to reduce preventable injuries and complications in patient care.

National quality strategy is the future

In compliance with ACA, the National Quality Strategy was released via a report to Congress in March 2011. Consistent with the initiatives of the National Quality Forum and the National Priorities Partners Goals and Priorities, the National Quality Strategy will pursue three broad aims—similar to those referenced by the Institute for Health Care Improvement as the Triple Aims—to guide and assess local, state, and national efforts to improve the quality of health care. The aims include the following:

- **Better Care:** Improve the overall quality by making health care more patient centered, reliable, accessible, and safe.
- **Healthy People/Healthy Communities:** Improve the health of the U.S. population by supporting proven interventions to address behavioral, social, and environmental determinants of health in addition to delivering higher quality care.

- **Affordable Care:** Reduce the cost of quality health care for individuals, families, employers, and government.

The priorities are identified as the following:

- Making care safer
- Ensuring person-and-family-centered care
- Promoting effective communication and coordination of care
- Promoting the most effective prevention and treatment of the leading causes of mortality, starting with cardiovascular disease
- Working with communities to promote wide use of best practices to enable healthy living
- Making quality care more affordable

The National Quality Strategy is based on recognition that in the end, all health care is local, and its intent is to help assure that these local efforts remain consistent with shared national aims and priorities. The Secretary of HHS developed this initial strategy and plan through a participatory, transparent, and collaborative process that reached out to more than 300 groups, organizations, and individuals who provided comments. A full summary of all of the comments is available at www.ahrq.gov/workingforquality.

The Agency for Healthcare Research and Quality (AHRQ) is tasked with supporting and coordinating the implementation plan and further development and updating of the strategy. At the federal level, the National Quality Strategy will guide the development of HHS programs, regulations, and strategic plans for new initiatives, in addition to serving as a mechanism for evaluating the full range of federal health efforts. While the first year strategy does not include HHS-specific plans, goals, benchmarks, and standardized quality metrics, they will be developed through collaboration of the participating agencies and private sector consultations. AHRQ has engaged with the National Priority Partnership to begin this phase. The National Quality Strategy will be updated continually as the ACA implementation proceeds.

Building the momentum for quality

The inclusion of such far-reaching provisions related to quality and safety in the ACA was made possible largely because of efforts over two decades of health care industry stakeholders to identify the challenges and build multiple supportive allegiances, leading to addressing the issues through policies at every level. As by-products, professionals in the health care industry became educated about quality principles, and consumer awareness of the complexities of health care systems was raised. The following pages describe how powerful such efforts would be.

National Quality Forum (NQF): a strategic model

In 2000, following the Institute of Medicine reports on medical errors and the quality chasm, the NQF, a new private not-for-profit entity, became central to the establishment of standards and policy relative to health care quality. NQF grew out of the Presidential Advisory Commission on Consumer Protection and Quality in Health Care Industry convened in 1996. The advisory commission was one of many ways that entities concerned about the eroding quality of care began to consider how they might drive improvement. Ultimately, the commission recommended the creation of a private sector entity, which then became the NQF. The expanding role of NQF over the next decade is an instructive example of the collective efforts of many entities, whether professions, consumers, insurers or others, working to shape and implement national policy, including the National Quality Strategy.

NQF's overall purpose is to provide key leadership for a national health care quality measurement and reporting system. Its mission is focused on three themes: (1) build consensus on priorities and goals for health care quality, (2) play a major role in the endorsement of national consensus standards, and (3) use its collective membership to promote attainment of these standards in the delivery of care to consumers. From inception, the CMS, the Office of Personnel Management, and the AHRQ have been part of NQF. In addition, standard setting bodies like the Joint Commission, the National Commission for Quality Assurance, the Institute of Medicine, the National Institutes of Health, and PCPI-AMA have had key liaison roles as well. Today, there are nearly 450 NQF organizational members.

The development and expansion of NQF has included input from nurses with representation from organizational membership in NQF from its inception and at the 23-member board by nursing experts. The American Nurses Association was the first NQF nursing organization member, with others following suit over the next decade. Today, 23 entities representing nursing are NQF members, and nursing continues to hold a seat on the NQF Executive Board.

The NQF employs three strategies to collectively move quality as a national priority as well in driving performance improvement. These three strategies have been used by other coalitions and individual professions as well: (1) convening experts across the industry to define quality by developing standards and measures, (2) gathering information from measurement of performance through data reporting and analysis, and (3) identifying gaps that are provided back to providers, institutions, and others about performance to initiate performance improvement and public reporting. In addition, NQF, as do other collective efforts, places ongoing focus on dissemination of tools and educational activities that promote health care improvement in the United States.

The expansiveness of the NQF structure has provided many touch points for nursing to influence its direction. Calls for endorsement of standards or measures require formal comment and ballot-type voting. Calls for nominations to work groups based on content expertise or representation allows for formally nominating nursing leaders who can speak on behalf of quality through a nursing lens. Nursing leaders have had opportunities to serve in leadership roles within committees and work groups, to react to the work of colleagues from other disciplines, and to inform, persuade, or dissent as needed, in the shaping of policy.

Measure Applications Partnership (MAP) driving selection of measures

The National Quality Forum has been named as the consensus-based entity, as required by Section 3014 of the ACA. In the habit of convening multistakeholder groups, it is expected to provide input to the U.S. Secretary of Health and Human Services through federal government appointment, on the selection of performance measures for public reporting and performance-based payment programs. An NQF board work group met in early 2010 to consider the charge and structure for a potential new partnership to serve this purpose, called the Measure Applications Partnership (MAP). MAP has been designed as a two tiered structure that includes a standing multistakeholder Coordinating Committee to provide direction to and synchronize with the second tier of advisory work groups. The Coordinating Committee establishes the strategy for the partnership. The work groups advise on measures needed for specific uses. NQF through the Coordinating Committee recommends measures for use in public reporting, performance-based payment, and other programs to HHS. At least one nursing organization, the American Nurses Association (ANA), is a member of the Coordinating Committee, while several nursing organizations have representatives and individual nursing leaders appointed to the work groups.

National Database of Nursing Quality Indicators (NDNQI): capturing the data

Even before the release of *To Err is Human* (Institute of Medicine, 2000) and *Crossing the Quality Chasm* (Institute of Medicine, 2001), the nursing profession had begun to speak up about the eroding of the quality of care patients received. Not surprisingly, this concern surfaced early at the national nursing policy level. In 1994, the ANA House of Delegates at its annual meeting approved a house resolution that urged ANA leadership to address the problem of declining patient care quality experienced in many institutions, perceived by nurses to be due in part to reductions in staffing levels implemented following declining revenue. ANA, when addressing this problem with its interdisciplinary colleagues, was repeatedly asked to show the evidence that reduced nursing staffing led to such declines in quality care. Nurse leaders determined that not only was there a need for education about principles of quality, but that in fact, data was required that would put to rest the criticisms of those claiming that the value of nursing could not be substantiated.

In the mid-1990s, ANA began a national effort to educate nurses about the value of data and quality through regional conferences. ANA simultaneously convened nurse experts Dr. Norma Lang, Dr. Marilyn Chow, and others to identify structural, process, and outcome measures that would support the relationship between staffing levels, skill mix, and the quality of nursing care. Those initial measure definitions became the basis for the NQF-endorsed nursing sensitive measures. As a result of recommendations from this group of experts, ANA funded a contract to develop a national database with Dr. Nancy Dunton as principal investigator, that could receive and aggregate data collected via these measures. In 1998, ANA awarded grants to seven state nurses associations to encourage hospitals in those states to collect and submit data to this new database, NDNQI, a proprietary database of the ANA (Montalvo & Dunton, 2007). Since 1998, the number of acute and specialty hospitals that submit quarterly nursing-related quality data has grown to more than 1,800, more than one-third of all U.S. acute care facilities.

The impact of NDNQI on policy conversations at the institutional, state, or national level has been far reaching. Studies published at the national level utilizing the aggregated data support the impact of the quantity and skill mix on the quality of nursing care, the link between nursing satisfaction and improved satisfaction of patients with their care, and the impact of levels of nursing education with the outcomes of care. It has provided comparisons of similar institutions and unit types, both within the state and across the country, to assist chief nursing officers and nurse managers to defend the appropriate levels and skill mix of nurse staffing in their institutions, describe the impact of decreased levels on patient outcomes, and drive performance improvements at unit and institutional levels. NDNQI data reports provided back to the institutions point to opportunities for deeper examination of the processes of care and the need for evidence that supports care decisions.

Data from NDNQI has been used at the state level for public reporting, driving state initiatives, and supporting staffing legislation that defends the hospital and the nursing unit-level leaderships' rights to make decisions about safe staffing levels based on the evidence, rather than on state-mandated ratios. Major insurers provide higher ratings to those institutions that participate in NDNQI, based on their conviction that institutions that care about nursing care quality are more likely to have positive outcomes.

Institute for Healthcare Improvement (IHI) focused on system improvement

Founded in 1991, IHI has been a major driver of quality care and health care change based on the philosophy that almost any product or service, including health care, can be improved. The IHI encouraged thinking in systems with improvement a systems idea; if one can change the way things are done, one can get better results. IHI aims to improve the lives of patients, the health of communities, and the joy of the health care workforce by focusing on the Institute of Medicine's six improvement aims for the health care system: Safety, Effectiveness, Patient-Centeredness, Timeliness, Efficiency, and Equity (Institute of Medicine, 2001). IHI may be best known for its campaigns to Save 100,000 Lives, later to Save Five Million Lives, and currently the Triple Aim initiatives of better care, better health, at lower cost. IHI provides a variety of services and educational programs and tools to assist hospitals and other stakeholders to achieve these aims. IHI's structure and campaigns have enabled institutions and individual providers of care, including nurses, to share their "near misses" and successes in instructive ways. Nursing organizations have participated in IHI to contribute to discussions and to influence actions that have global and national consequences.

Informatics, electronic health records, and impact of technology on quality and policy

While also helping align the health care industry with quality expectations in other industries, dialogue about the use of technology, nursing terminologies, and consistent specifications for data capture, including physician order entry, diagnoses, interventions, and decision support, became part of the quality discussion. Harnessing complex technology for quality improvement and reporting purposes has become crucial. While NDNQI has been able to function successfully in a manual data capture environment to accommodate institutions with insufficient progress toward electronic health records, driving policy changes that impact future quality requires the ability to capture that data electronically according to widely agreed upon specifications. Unless data for measures are able to be gathered as well as submitted electronically, the ability of nurse leaders to drive progress in the policy world of quality will erode.

Data collection burdens, the accuracy of electronic data extractions, the timeliness of the data reporting and analysis, the ability to have timely comparisons to benchmarks, all impact not only the performance improvement process but also the ability to ensure that patients are receiving the care they deserve within a safety culture. The challenge of many electronic systems, as may have already been mentioned, is that while much data goes into the system, particularly in the delivery of nursing care, it can be nearly impossible to extract it for reporting and analysis. Further, decision supports based on data that identifies a patient with a stage two pressure ulcer, for instance, must also incorporate in a timely way from the patient perspective, an evidence-based appropriate plan of action to both prevent further skin breakdown and begin healing. From a public reporting perspective, is it enough to know a patient is at risk of experiencing a pressure sore while hospitalized? Engaged consumers and insurers will want to know what the data shows about not only the prevention of decubiti but also the appropriateness of treatment, the speediness of recovery, lost work days, and impact on the quality of life. Policy makers are interested in lengths of stay and other factors that drive up the cost of such hospital-acquired conditions.

Nursing informatics and the use of nursing terminologies are central to capturing key data elements in a consistent way. Adherence to consensus-based terminologies, both for the collection of data around the nursing sensitive measures, but also the processes of care, are necessary to articulate the actual contributions of nurses, their importance in keeping patients safe, and improving the quality of care, as identified in both the Institute of Medicine reports and the Quality and Safety Education for Nurses (QSEN) competencies (Cronenwett et al., 2007; Cronenwett et al., 2009).

A major contributor to this agenda is the Technology Informatics Guiding Education Reform (TIGER Initiative), launched as a result of a 2006 conference convened to create a vision for the future of nursing, bridging the quality chasm with information technology, enabling nurses to use informatics in practice and education to provide safer, high-quality patient care (Warren, 2012). Laying the groundwork for an interdisciplinary collaborative, TIGER is implementing phase 3 to integrate TIGER recommendations for a virtual learning network on health information technology, for the nursing community as well as the larger interdisciplinary health care community. While at first this may seem to be about education and practice, the implications for policy are clear. As national initiatives improve electronic interoperability and the development and implementation of health records, the collection of meaningful data that can be used to influence improvements in care has the potential to revolutionize nurses' care delivery. At the same time, issues of privacy and confidentiality of data confront every nurse practicing or teaching in such environments, necessitating policies that address these issues and electronic patient data for research and quality improvement.

National Priorities Partnership and implementation of the National Quality Strategy

The National Priorities Partnership is another national collaborative effort, initially including 28 national health care organizations, convened in 2008 as an initiative of the National Quality Forum. Its role is to join stakeholders from both public and private sectors to influence policy encompassing every aspect of the health care system. Stakeholder groups currently include consumer groups, employers, government, health plans, health care organizations, health care professions, scientists, accrediting and certifying bodies, and quality alliances. Since 2008, the number of organizations has expanded to more than 40 stakeholder groups. Nursing was represented only by ANA in the initial stakeholder group, but the newly formed Nursing Alliance for Quality Care was added as the group expanded. The partnership took the early step of identifying a set of national priorities and goals to coalesce efforts toward achieving performance improvement by stakeholders on high-leverage areas

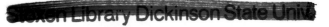

with the potential to make the most substantial contributions in the near term to the health care delivery systems of the nation and ultimately to consumers. In 2011 the National Priorities Partnership expanded its focus. Significantly, the full list of priorities and goals, consistent with the QSEN competencies identified earlier, had substantial impact on the final recommendations of the National Quality Strategy. The list included:

- Engaging patients and families in managing their health and making decisions about their care
- Improving the health of the population
- Improving the safety and reliability of America's health care system
- Ensuring patients receive well-coordinated care within and across all health care organizations, settings, and levels of care
- Guaranteeing appropriate and compassionate care for patients with life-limiting illnesses,
- Eliminating overuse while ensuring the delivery of appropriate care
- Improving access
- Improving the health care infrastructure

As a second step, the partnership agreed to align the drivers of change and the performance measures around goals for each priority. Each goal reflects those aspects that will most likely lead to achievement of the priority, along with a road map consisting of examples of successful actions and targets for describing success. Taking an important step, the partnership agreed to commit its leadership to support the drivers (below) in order to effect change at the federal, state, and local levels:

- Performance measurement
- Public reporting
- Payment systems
- Research and knowledge dissemination
- Professional development: education and certification
- System capacity

In 2009, the ANA and NQF nursing member organizations, supported by NQF and the Robert Wood Johnson Foundation, hosted the Invitational Conference on Nursing and the National Priorities Partnership Goals: Next Steps. Its purpose was to examine each of the priorities, goals, and drivers to (1) identify priorities for nursing quality measurement to align nursing measures with current national quality initiatives, (2) develop specific strategies to fast-forward achievement of these priorities; and (3) envision new frameworks that would advance performance measurement to improve health and well-being. As a result of that conference, two American Academy of Nursing scholars summarized the proceedings, detailing the nursing opportunities and action plans for each of the priority areas.

Quality alliances influence policy actions through a professional lens

Various professions have followed a model similar to that of NQF while determining their own efforts to influence the measurement of quality, support quality improvements, and take action at a national policy level. From a positive perspective, these alliances create a pipeline for their profession's or specialty's representation at national stakeholder tables, for grooming nominees with the expertise to inform measure development and policy setting, and for providing national leadership for the overall quality agenda. Each faces similar challenges, including that of determining membership and governance structures and dues for long-term financial sustainability. Each needs to coordinate with other stakeholders and standard setters among its own discipline in order to lead with one voice. Externally, each alliance forms a coherent, coordinated, and consistent approach to quality and measurement that moves the health care system forward as a whole, without becoming counterproductive. Most alliances have some combination of stakeholders among their membership or board that reflects other disciplines, as well as federal agencies such as AHRQ, CMS, or NQF, so as to provide some level of transparency, consistency, and connectedness.

Nursing Alliance for Quality Care (NAQC)

Nursing through the Nursing Alliance for Quality Care (NAQC) has created its own alliance of national nursing stakeholder organizations in partnership with patient care advocacy organizations representing consumers. NAQC's membership continues to grow and to find that space where nursing can collectively make the largest contribution to the quality arena. Although formed only in early 2010 from an earlier Robert Wood Johnson Foundation–funded planning grant, NAQC is committed to advancing the highest quality, safety, and value of consumer-centered health care for patients, their families, and their communities. Governed by an independent board of directors, NAQC first sought long-range expected outcomes that include:

- Patients receiving the right care at the right time by the right professional
- Nurses actively advocating and being accountable for consumer-centered, high-quality health care
- Policymakers recognizing the contributions of nurses in advancing consumer-centered, high-quality health care.

NAQC focused on four goals to accomplish these three outcomes: (1) support consumer-centered health care quality and safety goals to achieve care that is safe, effective, patient-centered, timely, efficient, and equitable; (2) performance measurement and public reporting that strengthens the role of nursing in transparency and accountability activities; (3) advocacy, by serving as a resource to partners and stimulating policy reform that reflects evidence-based nursing practice and advances consumer-centered, high-quality health care; and (4) building nursing's capacity to serve in leadership roles that advance consumer-centered, high-quality health care.

Other similar alliances are included here to provide a perspective on the interdisciplinary reach and nursing's inclusion in those efforts to improve quality.

The Hospital Quality Alliance (HQA)

In 2002, the HQA was formed from organizations representing America's hospitals, consumer representatives, physician and nursing organizations, employers and payers, oversight organizations, and governmental agencies. It is a national public-private collaboration that is committed to making meaningful, relevant, and easily understood information about hospital performance accessible to the public and to informing and encouraging efforts to improve quality. HQA has been effective in initiating changes in national policy, perhaps most visibly in terms of quality reporting.

HQA facilitates continuous improvement in patient care through implementation of measures that portray the quality, cost, and value of hospital care; the development and use of measurement reporting in the nation's hospitals; and sharing of useful hospital performance information with the public through Hospital Compare. Hospital Compare (www.hospitalcompare.hhs.gov) contains performance information about more than 4,000 hospitals, and data are updated quarterly. Hospital Compare is a voluntary national report card of the performance among hospitals, evolved with the support and strong encouragement from HQA, while retaining the right to suppress data it deems not appropriate to share.

The Ambulatory Care Quality Alliance (AQA)

Shortly after the formation of HQA, the American Academy of Family Physicians, the American College of Physicians, America's Health Insurance Plans, and AHRQ joined together in 2004 to initiate efforts to improve performance measurement, data aggregation, and reporting in the ambulatory care setting. Since then, the mission and membership have grown to a broad-based collaborative of over 100 organizations, and include all areas of physician practice as well as a variety of other stakeholders, now known simply as AQA. To distinguish itself from the HQA, this collaborative focused initial efforts on physician or other clinician performance. AQA's most recent strategic plan focuses on being a convener to promote and facilitate alignment among the public and private sector efforts, on promoting best practice quality improvement strategies that address the gap between measurement and improvement, and on advising HHS as it implements health care reform initiatives. While ANA has sent representatives to monitor this alliance's activities, no nursing organizations are listed among its current membership.

Pharmacy Quality Alliance

The Pharmacy Quality Alliance, in place since 2006, focuses on its intersection with the health care system. Its stated mission is to improve the quality of medication use across health care settings through a collaborative process in which key stakeholders agree on a strategy for measuring and reporting performance information related to medications. This alliance, like many of its counterparts, includes representatives from CMS and NQF among its board, as well as at least one consumer representative. Once again, nursing organizations are not listed among its members, yet it has issued an invitation to NAQC to learn more about its structure and work efforts, with the potential for future collaboration.

Alliance for Pediatric Quality

Four national organizations formed the Alliance for Pediatric Quality to establish a unified voice for improving the quality of pediatric health care. These organizations are the American Academy of Pediatrics, the American Board of Pediatrics, the Child Health Corporation of America, and the National Association of Children's Hospitals and Related Institutions (NACHRI). The focus is to improve the quality of care for children by promoting effective, systematic efforts to improve children's health care and to ensure that health information technology works for children by developing standards that incorporate pediatric requirements and advocating for health information technology that enables systematic improvement. Both NACHRI and the Child Health Corporation of America include nursing in their purview, but neither organization focuses primarily on nursing. There is, however, collaboration on measures that reflect nursing in pediatric quality care, such as pediatric falls and skin breakdown. ANA and NACHRI are working together to align specifications for pediatric measures and to strengthen opportunities to measure improvements in nursing care for children.

Long-Term Quality Alliance

The Long-Term Quality Alliance was established in 2010 to respond to increasing demands for long-term services and support and for expanding the field of providers delivering that care in the United States. It is governed through a broad-based board of 30 of the nation's leading experts on long-term care and related care issues including consumers, family caregivers, health care providers, private and public purchasers, federal agencies, and others. This alliance is focused on identifying and supporting quality measures of best practices that enhance quality of life, improve care, and reduce costs. More specifically, it focuses on the goal of improving transitions in care and avoiding unnecessary hospital admissions among the more than 10 million frail and chronically ill. Nursing is well represented and has been a key player in the formation of this alliance.

Kidney Care Quality Alliance

Active since 2006, this alliance was formed by the kidney care community and the health care community at large to involve patients and their advocates, care professionals, providers, suppliers, and purchasers in developing performance measures focused on institutions and physicians. The intent is to also focus on developing data collection and aggregation strategies while promoting transparency by reporting performance measures. The broad membership includes two specialty nursing organizations that serve that patient population and nurses specializing in nephrology care.

Quality Alliance Steering Committee (QASC)

The Quality Alliance Steering Committee was formed in 2006 through a collaboration of HQA and AQA to better coordinate the promotion of quality measurement, transparency, and improvement in care. This alliance includes close relationships with CMS and AHRQ, already members of both AQA and HQA. The new steering committee is expected to expand several ongoing pilot projects focused on combining public and private information to measure and report on performance in new ways to enhance the goals of transparency and meaningful information. Nursing organizations and the NAQC are included as members of this alliance.

Institute of Pediatric Nursing

Gaining status as a private not-for-profit entity in early 2011, the Institute of Pediatric Nursing is an alliance of diverse pediatric nursing organizations and major children's hospitals, acting collaboratively to maximize pediatric nursing's contribution to child and youth health through unified leadership, knowledge, and expertise. It expects to influence (1) nursing education, (2) health care access, (3) child and youth advocacy, (4) care coordination, and (5) safe, quality evidence-based care. Governed by an independent board that reflects the various major settings of care for children and youth, this alliance serves as a catalyst and collaborative voice in addressing key issues in pediatric health care and the pediatric nursing specialty. Early efforts have focused on ensuring that Medicaid provisions are actually resulting in high-quality care by meeting the medical needs of children. The group has also helped create new partnerships to support the quality of transitions from acute to school-based care for many chronically ill children.

Alliance for Home Health Quality Innovation

The Alliance for Home Health Quality Innovation is dedicated to improving the nation's health care system by supporting research and education to demonstrate the value of home-based care. Nursing is engaged in this alliance, both through the Visiting Nurse Association of America and through the National Association of Home Care and Hospice.

Federal agencies engage with alliances

It becomes clear from studying the configuration of most of the alliances that allegiance and partnerships with federal agencies such as AHRQ and CMS are critical to any strategy driving health care system change focused on higher quality. CMS, at the behest of Congress, holds the purse strings to reimbursement for services, to rewards for higher quality care, and in making deductions due to preventable negative outcomes of care. NQF has been made the arbiter of measure endorsement and of which measures' data, gathered by institutions and providers, point to the outcomes that either get rewarded or penalized. And AHRQ plays a major role from a federal perspective in the creation and validation of standards, guidelines for best practice, and research related to quality, safety, and best practice. Any professional alliance looking to develop measures or to suggest that given measures are or are not appropriate for considerations of payment would do well to bring these entities along to the discussion, keep them informed of challenges and lessons learned, and either heed or shape the future they want to see.

Centers for Medicare and Medicaid Services (CMS)

CMS is a federal agency that administers Medicare, Medicaid, and the Children's Health Insurance Program. CMS reports to the Department of Health and Human Services. Even though Medicaid services are provided by each state, CMS provides guidance for administering services and can audit services provided to Medicare recipients. CMS has several newly created offices as a result of the Affordable Care Act, including the Center for Medicare and Medicaid Innovation, and the Center for Dual Eligibles. In recent years, CMS has created a Nursing Steering Committee that includes several CMS officials willing to address concerns that arise from external nursing organizations about Medicare and Medicaid reimbursement and service issues for Medicare or Medicaid recipients. This steering committee includes a number of nursing organizations and meets quarterly by conference call.

Agency for Healthcare Research and Quality (AHRQ)

AHRQ is the lead federal agency charged with improving the quality, safety, efficiency, and effectiveness of health care for all Americans. AHRQ is one of 12 agencies within the Department of Health and Human Services. AHRQ supports research that helps people make more informed decisions and improves the quality of health care services. AHRQ is committed to improving care safety and quality and does this through successful partnerships and the development of knowledge and tools needed for long-term improvement. AHRQ's research goals include measurable improvements in health care, with a focus on improved quality of life, improved patient safety and outcomes, and high-value care for each dollar spent.

Standard setting by nonfederal agencies

Accreditation bodies such as the Joint Commission, the National Commission on Quality Assurance, the Utilization Review Accreditation Commission, and others impact how quality is recognized in practice settings. They drive quality through formal policy mechanisms of setting, monitoring, and evaluating accreditation standards and recognition criteria. Although accreditation is voluntary and paid for by the institution seeking it, accreditation processes wield a great deal of power in shaping expectations of quality and safety. To ensure the reasonableness of standards and evaluation criteria, professional organizations and alliances participate in the development and revision of accreditation and recognition criteria and measures. ANA and others seek to ensure that nurses provide board representation, public comments, or advocacy efforts as a check and balance on the rigor of the accreditation standards and recognition criteria these entities use as the yardstick by which performance is evaluated.

The Joint Commission

The Joint Commission is a 100-year-old independent, not-for-profit organization that accredits and certifies more than 19,000 health care organizations and programs in the United States, including acute care and long-term care facilities, ambulatory care services, hospice and home care programs, behavioral health programs, managed care entities, and health care staffing services. The Joint Commission states that these activities are undertaken to continuously improve the safety and quality of care provided to the public. The Joint Commission uses Professional-Technical Advisory Committees to establish or modify existing standards and determine patient safety goals. Nursing input into these activities occurs through multiple professional nursing organizations with representation on the various advisory committees, through ongoing dialogues and via a separately established Nursing Advisory Council that meets periodically to consider nursing issues where the Joint Commission standards play a role in shaping policy. The Joint Commission has at least one board seat held by a nurse.

The National Committee for Quality Assurance (NCQA)

Founded in 1990, the NCQA is a private, not-for-profit organization dedicated to improving health care quality and elevating health care quality to the top of the national agenda. NCQA is governed by an independent board composed of multiple stakeholder groups. NCQA develops quality standards and performance measures for a broad range of health care entities that are the tools that organizations and individuals can use to identify opportunities for improvement. Annual reporting of performance against such measures provides direction for improvement. NCQA collects HEDIS data from more than 700 health plans; conducts accreditation, certification, and state plan surveys; and develops and conducts formal recognition programs including the Primary Care Medical Home Recognition Program. No nursing organizations are included in the governance of NCQA. However, nursing organizations have actively engaged with NCQA to urge acceptance of APRNs as leaders of medical homes, such that several nurse-led medical homes are now recognized by NCQA's programs.

Utilization Review Accreditation Commission (URAC)

URAC, initiated in 1990, is a not-for-profit organization promoting health care quality by accrediting health care organizations, developing measurement, and providing education. URAC's mission is to protect and empower the consumer. URAC's first mission was to improve the quality and accountability of utilization review programs. Its spectrum of services has grown to include a larger range of service functions, including the accreditation of integrated health plans. URAC is governed by a board with representatives from multiple constituencies including consumers, providers, employers, regulators, and industry experts. Nursing has a long well-established presence on URAC's Board.

"Stand for Quality in Health Care"–focused health reform efforts

A driving force for the inclusion of vital principles for quality in health reform legislation emerged from the various quality alliances. This joint effort, formed in 2008 and known as Stand for Quality in Health Care, was composed of more than 200 health care organizations, including nursing organizations. It achieved consensus around the most important features of quality as the health care reform initiatives took shape—consensus that was so strong it evoked bipartisan support. Stand for Quality established recommendations for building a foundation for high-quality affordable health care that linked performance measurement to health reform. In addition, it linked the investment in health information technology to the improvement of the quality of care and helped drive a quality agenda during the framing of the ACA. It outlined the case for supporting performance measurement, reporting, and improvement through the articulation of Core Principles Linking Performance Measurement, Improvement, and Health Reform; through identification of the Key Functions of the Performance Measurement, Reporting, and Improvement

Enterprise; and through the development of deliverables. The key functions included the following:

- Function 1. Set national priorities and provide coordination
- Function 2. Endorse and maintain national standard measures
- Function 3. Develop measures to fill gaps in priority areas
- Function 4. Effective consultative processes so stakeholders can inform policies on use of measures
- Function 5. Collect, analyze, and make performance information available and actionable
- Function 6. Supporting a sustainable infrastructure for quality improvement

Based on the final provisions of ACA, the above functions are driving the creation of the various commissions and strategies for quality.

Common strategies run through formalized initiatives

There are common strategies each collective effort employs to gain political will for change. The various alliances and other collaborative initiatives have several strategies in common, which in and of themselves contribute to a set of tactics around quality that may be applied to other policy discussions. Strategic themes among these initiatives include the following, which are critical when considering quality and safety:

- Most formal entities include consumers on their governing bodies or among the stakeholder groups they convene to ensure that the needs of the recipients of the care are heard and addressed.
- The inclusion of a broad base of stakeholders is almost universally applied, acknowledging the complexity of the challenges facing health care.
- The inclusion of multiple disciplines in most formal collaboratives reinforces that developing policy solutions is a team sport, with no discipline having the political clout to dictate or finalize solutions independently.
- Most formal collective efforts include one or more federal agencies among its board members in some capacity to ensure federal efforts and others are moving in concert.
- Professional organizations and other stakeholder groups participate in multiple efforts, maximizing their opportunities to influence policy.
- Participants on the various alliances, agencies, and accrediting bodies often participate with multiple groups. Questions remain whether this is more expeditious or not.
- Consensus building is the preferred approach to derive proposed solutions.
- Convergence on proposed solutions occurs among stakeholders and alliances, with the result that while the details might look a bit different, the same conceptual underpinnings run similarly across many collaborative efforts.

Challenges all collective efforts face in improving the quality of care

With approximately 200 national entities, including professional organizations, consumer groups, and many others engaged in the effort to improve quality, there has been substantial investment of financial and other resources, including manpower, over the last two decades. The timing of many of these efforts in the early 1990s suggests that long before the publication of *To Err is Human* and *Crossing the Quality Chasm*, leaders in the health care industry understood that the lack of quality was a significant problem. Nurses were early adopters in hospital efforts to identify opportunities for continuous quality improvement. Many engaged in dialogue with individual physicians who were being challenged by state performance review boards and utilization review committees. Then the focus was primarily on local quality improvement and policy initiatives rather than state or national efforts. Global quality leaders (Deming, 1986; Juran, 1998) stated that 85% of errors in complex organizations were due to system design rather than to inadequate individual job performance. But even their discussions were addressed in departmental, corporate, or institutional policy terms. Twenty years later in 2011, the magnitude of the current efforts to transform the health care system into one of high quality dwarfs all previous efforts. Why has this exploded to such mammoth proportions?

Looking at any acute care facility, large or small, the number of outpatient procedures and the revenue generated from them has kept pace or overtaken the revenue from acute care services. Numbers of providers in even the smallest facility have increased, including increases in specialists, whether providing virtual or face-to-face medicine. The enormity and complexity of the system needing improvement does not differ all that much, whether one considers the problems of the critical access hospital or the largest multihospital system. The technology needs of the solo practitioner bear an alarming resemblance to technological capabilities needed by larger health service plans to which many providers belong. At the same time, fewer and fewer patients see their own primary provider once they enter an acute care facility, regardless of the size of the institution. The hospitalist providing their care may have never seen them previously and will have no connection to their care once they are discharged. Home care and hospice programs may use technology to replace the face-to-face time that nurses and others have traditionally relied upon with homebound patients to determine their unspoken needs and vulnerabilities, including electronic profiles on patient caseloads and communication about patients only via electronic records.

The challenges of ensuring effective care transitions, care coordination, and engagement of patients are difficult without effective communication systems. But alas, one electronic system in a hospital department is often unable to share information with another department, let alone in a timely manner with someone outside the institution. Faxes and phone calls may seem antiquated by comparison to today's technology, but they did work. Electronic records and communications are expected to have filled the gap, but they have not. Patients suffer from the lack of effective communication with and among professional staff. The situation is magnified when ineffective communication couples with the payment system and reimbursement that rewards undesired outcomes of care, such as continued disease rather than wellness or health, or complications of hospitalization rather than speedy recovery and discharge. One begins to see how local policies and regulations have little effect. As the interconnectedness has grown, so have the problems and the solutions required to correct them.

These are the challenges faced by the various collaboratives striving to put policies, regulations, and incentives into place in every community hoping to improve the quality of care. The challenge resembles the analogy of the global epidemic, which nonetheless requires "immunity in every community" (American Nurses Association, 2011) to bring order out of the chaos.

What can every nurse do to influence policy that improves quality?

The Quality and Safety Education for Nurses (QSEN) project is an example of nurses taking the responsibility for improving quality and safety outcomes (Cronenwett et al., 2007; Cronenwett et al., 2009). Nurses prepared with the six competencies (patient-centered care, teamwork and collaboration, evidence-based practice, quality improvement, safety, and informatics), have the tools and resources to impact policy at the local, state, and national levels (Textbox 2.1; also see Appendixes A and B; Sherwood, 2011). Improving quality

---

Textbox 2.1   Nurses' engagement in policy at every level of the system

To impact **institutional** policy, every nurse, regardless of setting or specialty, has expertise to contribute to the discussions focused on health care improvement. Nurses can:

- Take the opportunity to question practices that lack a base of evidence, or seek literature that informs practice questions.
- Collect data and utilize National Database of Nursing Quality Indicators to inform and lead better practices that will improve fall assessments or reduce falls, or improve one's own assessment skills regarding stages of decubiti.
- Devise local studies with the assistance of more senior experts, to explore or establish the evidence that either supports or disproves care practices.
- Teach colleagues what has been learned and review institutional or specialty policies about ineffective practices employed.

(Continued)

- Publish findings, experiential learning, and literature reviews to influence policy changes in others.
- Engage with others in the institution to review proposed rules and regulations that impact them and offer public comment on professional organizations' position statements, local or state proposed rules, or CMS (Centers for Medicare and Medicaid Services)-proposed rules.

To **impact local or community** policies, nurses can:

- Assess community needs or practices that perpetuate risks for falls, whether due to poor sidewalks, potholes in grocery parking lots, or cluttered hallways and aisles in stores, schools, or churches.
- Advocate for community consensus on policies or regulations to reduce danger to children and elderly pedestrians.
- Provide education about reducing falls, improving medication adherence, or increasing patient engagement in making care decisions or choices about end-of-life care.
- Volunteer to serve on local YMCA boards, hospital boards, or other local service organizations that may be able to effect changes in services, access to better nutrition, or safer alternatives for exercise.

To impact **state** policy nurses can:

- Demand greater clarity and compliance with CMS guidance regarding Medicaid services for children who are not receiving the supplies they need for their chronic illness, or who lack the services to keep them safe in schools or after school.
- Engage with local or state chapters of professional nursing associations to coordinate advocacy for change, for modifications to practice acts, or improved services for at-risk populations.
- Actively engage in political campaigns around platforms on health care, agree to serve on state licensing boards, or attend state legislative hearings and meetings.

To impact **national** policy nurses must:

- First keep themselves and their colleagues informed of the issues.
- Develop their skills and expertise at representing their specialty.
- Engage in leadership roles within their preferred professional national nursing association.
- Take action to contact congressmen or senators regarding passage of bills that affect their state and community.
- Share stories with their representatives that highlight the need for changes in health care.
- Work with their institutions to invite a congressman or senator to walk a day in the shoes of a nurse, in order to better understand the challenges of short staffing, limited resources, or other needs of the community.

and safety requires the dedicated work of all, and with the work of the QSEN project, nurses will be able to participate in all levels of policy making.

Summary

The improvement of nursing and health care quality is the responsibility of every nurse. It can and needs to occur at every level, from the direct one-on-one interaction with a patient or family to the advocacy for changes in rules or regulations at every level of government, within an institution or in the local community. It takes many forms, but at its most basic level, it requires being unwilling to accept the status quo, and taking the risk to challenge practice behavior. It requires moral courage to stand up to nursing peers or physician colleagues and dissent when something begins to occur that violates basic principles of quality and safety. While many are working on the national level to effect policy change, at the end of the day, all health care is local. It comes back to the individual nurse providing care and living in a community, to articulate when a policy is being crafted, how its implementation will improve or hinder quality of care or the safety of patients. It comes back to each nurse understanding the intent of that policy and implementing it on behalf of patients. Only then, when every patient is provided the same care we would want for our parent, or sister, or best friend, or child, will high-quality health care be achieved.

References

American Nurses Association. (2011). ANA Immunize: Bringing immunity to every community. Retrieved July 8, 2011, from http://www.anaimmunize.org

Cronenwett, L., Sherwood, G., Barnsteiner, J., Disch, J., Johnson, J., Mitchell, P., et al. (2007). Quality and safety education for nurses. *Nursing Outlook, 55*(3), 122–131.

Cronenwett, L., Sherwood, G., Pohl, J., Barnsteiner, J., Moore, S., Taylor Sullivan, D., et al. (2009). Quality and safety education for advanced practice nursing practice. *Nursing Outlook, 57*(6), 338–348.

Deming, W. E. (1986). *Out of crisis*. Cambridge, MA: MIT Press.

Institute of Medicine (2000). *To err is human: Building a safer health system*. Washington, DC: National Academy Press.

Institute of Medicine (2001). *Crossing the quality chasm: A new health system for the 21st century*. Washington, DC: National Academy Press.

Juran, J. M. (1998). *Juran's quality handbook*. New York: McGraw-Hill.

Kingdon, J.W. (2003). *Agendas, alternatives and public policies*, 2nd ed. New York: Addison-Wesley.

Montalvo, I & Dunton, N. (2007). *Transforming nursing data into quality care: Profiles of quality Improvement in US healthcare facilities*. Silver Spring, MD: Nursebooks.org.

Sherwood, G. (2011). Integrating quality and safety science in nursing education and practice. *Journal of Research in Nursing, 16*(3), 226–240.

Simon H. (1966). Political research: the decision-making framework. In D. Easton (Ed.), *Varieties of political theory* (p 19). Englewood Cliffs, NJ: Prentice-Hall.

Warren, J. (2012). Informatics. In G. Sherwood & J. Barnsteiner (Eds.), *Quality and safety in nursing: A competency approach to improving outcomes*. Hoboken, NJ: Wiley-Blackwell.

Resources

Agency for Healthcare Research and Quality (AHRQ) at a Glance. Accessed May 2011. http://www.ahrq.gov/about/ataglance.htm

Alliance for Home Health Quality Innovation. http://www.ahhqi.org/

Alliance for Pediatric Quality. http://improvecarenow.org/care-providers/our-supporters/31-our-supporters-apq

Ambulatory Care Quality Alliance. http://www.ambulatoryqualityalliance.org/

Centers for Medicare and Medicaid Services. http://www.cms.gov/

Hospital Quality Alliance. http://www.hospitalqualityalliance.org/

Institute for Healthcare Improvement. http://www.ihi.org/ihi

Institute of Pediatric Nursing. http://www.ipedsnursing.org/ptisite/control/index

Kidney Care Quality Alliance. http://kidneycarepartners.com/kcp_creating.html

Long-Term Quality Alliance. http://www.ltqa.org/

Measure Applications Partnership. http://www.qualityforum.org/setting_priorities/partnership/map_coordinating_committee.aspx

National Committee for Quality Assurance. http://ncqa.org/

National Database of Nursing Quality Indicators. https://www.nursingquality.org/

National Priorities Partnership. http://www.nationalprioritiespartnership.org/aboutnpp.aspx

National Quality Forum. http://www.qualityforum.org/about/

National Quality Strategy. http://www.healthcare.gov/center/reports/quality03212011a.html

Nursing Alliance for Quality Care. http://nursingaqc.org

Partnership for Patients. www.healthcare.gov/center/programs/partnership

Pharmacy Quality Alliance. http://www.pqaalliance.org/

Quality Alliance Steering Committee. http://www.healthqualityalliance.org/about-qasc

Stand For Quality in Health Care. http://www.standforquality.org/sfq_report_3_19_09.pdf

Technology Informatics Guiding Education Reform (TIGER Initiative). http://tigersummit.com/summit.html

The Joint Commission. http://www.jointcommission.org/about_us/about_the_joint_commission_main.aspx

Utilization Review Accreditation Commission. http://www.urac.org/docs/programs/urac_annual_publication_2010.pdf

Chapter 3

A National Initiative: Quality and Safety Education for Nurses (QSEN)

Linda R. Cronenwett, PhD, RN, FAAN

As I was writing this chapter, a colleague sent an e-mail saying, "I've been doing grant reviews for HRSA [U.S. Health Resources and Services Administration], and half or more of the applications cite QSEN competencies or QSEN work as part of their justification." Two textbook authors inquired about permission to reprint QSEN materials. A visiting scholar from Sweden reported that QSEN is being used as the framework for action for nursing in Sweden this year. Medical colleagues set up a conference call to talk about what they could learn from QSEN to apply to a national initiative on interprofessional education. Almost 400 people have registered for the 2011 QSEN National Forum, and the conference is yet a month away. The number of forum paper and poster presentations has doubled since last year.

Quality and Safety Education for Nurses is an initiative that has been funded since 2005 by the Robert Wood Johnson Foundation (RWJF). The purpose of this chapter will be to posit answers to the questions often asked of those of us who have been involved in leading QSEN, namely, how did QSEN come to be and what do you think accounts for the extent of its spread and impact? A summary of aims and activities for the first three QSEN grants are provided in Figures 3.1 and 3.2, and further information about QSEN outcomes are reported elsewhere, for example, for QSEN Phase I (Cronenwett et al., 2007; Smith, Cronenwett, & Sherwood, 2007), Phase II (Cronenwett, Sherwood, & Gelmon, 2009; Cronenwett et al., 2009), and initial activities of Phase III (Sherwood, 2011). What follows in this chapter is one person's view of the QSEN story, a story that is not yet over. Future historians will evaluate QSEN's outcomes using data that will emerge during the decade to come.

The title *Quality and Safety Education for Nurses* emerged one summer afternoon in 2005 when I spent many hours on my screened porch generating

Quality and Safety in Nursing: A Competency Approach to Improving Outcomes,
First Edition. Edited by Gwen Sherwood and Jane Barnsteiner.
© 2012 John Wiley & Sons, Inc. Published 2012 by John Wiley & Sons, Inc.

an endless list of ideas for what to call a grant proposal that was due to the Robert Wood Johnson Foundation offices within the month. But of course, QSEN began long before that day.

QSEN origins: 2000–2005

Any initiative of the magnitude of QSEN depends on two groups of leaders– thought leaders in the field and thought leaders within a funding organization. Within the professional community, the seeds for what became QSEN were sown in a series of annual summer week-long conferences initiated and led by Paul Batalden, a pediatrician and one of the earliest health care quality thought leaders (Kenny, 2008). Started in 1995, these Dartmouth Summer Symposia (DSS) were invitational meetings for 60-70 participants, about 12-20 of whom were nurses in any given year. The nurse, physician, and hospital administrator educators who attended DSS described themselves as *an interprofessional community of educators devoted to building knowledge for leading improvement in health care*. Linda Norman, Associate Dean at Vanderbilt, was the first nursing leader who worked with Dr. Batalden to attract nursing deans and faculty members to this work.

I had worked with Dr. Batalden during my years at Dartmouth-Hitchcock Medical Center (1984–1998), participated in Quality Improvement Camp training, attended one summer symposium and worked on a number of quality improvement projects. After I became a faculty member at the University of North Carolina (UNC) at Chapel Hill in 1998, I was invited to DSS regularly and subsequently served as the second representative of nursing in the leadership of the DSS community.

From 1997 to 2002, the DSS topics involved work underway within the physician community to alter educational objectives, curricula, and residency training accreditation and certification standards to include requirements for competency development related to the continuous improvement of health care. Leaders of the professional organizations responsible for these initiatives participated with us as we created and advanced ideas about content and learning opportunities that would, as was the stated DSS goal, "change the world." Many subsequently participated in the Institute of Medicine (IOM) conference that resulted in the 2003 IOM publication *Health Professions Education: A Bridge to Quality*, wherein the charge was issued that all health professionals should be educated to deliver *patient-centered care* as members of an *interdisciplinary team*, emphasizing *evidence-based practice*, *quality improvement approaches*, and *informatics*. It was fascinating and exciting work.

Each summer, Dr. Batalden would ask who was going to lead this work for nursing. We nurses would plot strategies for finding funding to advance this agenda and agreed that if anyone could secure funding, the rest of us would help. Each took away an assignment, and, for a couple of years, we came back empty-handed. I presented proposal ideas to RWJF and one other foundation without results. Yet we persisted.

During this same period, seeds were being sown for QSEN on the RWJF leadership side as well. When I first unsuccessfully proposed the idea for a nursing faculty development initiative in quality and safety education to RWJF's nursing leader, Susan Hassmiller, she was involved in directing the RWJF initiative Transforming Care at the Bedside (TCAB). She had recognized the importance of linking nursing faculty to the Transforming Care at the Bedside initiative and its quality/safety/cost goals. Beginning in 2002, first I and then Patricia Chiverton, dean of the University of Rochester School of Nursing, initiated attempts to work with the faculty in schools affiliated with the hospitals involved in the initiative. Few successes were achieved, however, primarily because nursing faculty were generally disconnected from the patient safety/quality improvement methods and goals being adopted by hospitals at the time. As Dr. Hassmiller pressed hospital leaders to engage nursing faculty in their projects, she experienced the faculty knowledge gap firsthand, and this evidence of the need for faculty development would eventually provide the strong rationale Dr. Hassmiller used to convince RWJF executive leaders to fund QSEN.

In another development, Rosemary Gibson, a senior program officer for RWJF and coauthor of the book *Wall of Silence: The Untold Story of the Medical Mistakes that Kill and Injure Millions of Americans* (Gibson & Singh, 2003), joined the DSS community in 2003 as a participant who could contribute the patient advocacy perspective to our conversations. She and Dr. Hassmiller were leading efforts that crossed the quality and nursing portfolios at RWJF, and over the course of the next year, we continued in discussions about ideas for an initiative that would improve quality and safety education in nursing.

In 2004, Ms. Gibson and I spent hours during DSS debating the merits of various approaches to an initiative and its proposed products. One consideration was whether this work should be housed in a nursing professional organization, an idea promoted by the American Association of Colleges of Nursing. Nurses in the DSS community argued that we needed to reach *all* of nursing education, which by definition included diploma and associate degree schools as well as faculty in collegiate schools that affiliated with the National League for Nursing. We proposed that the "thought leader" work would be stronger if done by experts in quality and safety rather than appointees of professional organizational task forces who at times are assigned for reasons other than topical expertise. We wanted to involve and share the work with leaders from *all* the organizations that supported nursing licensure, certification, or accreditation of nursing education programs and thought that would more likely occur if the initial grant were housed in a neutral site. In the end, these views prevailed, and we received an official invitation to submit a proposal.

As the RWJF decision-making processes advanced, Ms. Gibson provided guidance about the need to break the initiative into short phases that, if successful, could build on each other. We were charting unknown territory and did not yet have a basis for knowing how open or resistant nursing faculties would be to this paradigm shift. She suggested taking the work one piece at a time so that we could adapt the methods to the needs that emerged. Her experience with other major RWJF initiatives (e.g., palliative care) was invaluable, and the final proposal was a true partnership with a visionary philanthropic leader.

Members of the DSS community responded to proposal drafts and, most importantly, agreed to play key roles as members of the QSEN faculty (Barnsteiner, Disch, Moore, and Mitchell) and advisory board (Batalden and Hall). Ironside's participation in the DSS community began soon thereafter. At the same time, Dr. Gwen Sherwood became the Associate Dean for Academic Affairs at UNC-Chapel Hill. As someone experienced with patient safety initiatives, she was not only a knowledgeable local colleague but someone with whom I could share the responsibilities of project management. We invited the participation of people we thought would be the strongest contributors with respect to each competency, area of pedagogical expertise, and the major nursing organizations associated with licensure and accreditation. Amazingly, every person invited to participate said yes.

Building will: Phase I (October 2005–March 2007)

Funding for Phase I began October 1, 2005, and we held the first faculty/advisory board meeting 30 days later. For 18 months, this group (see Table 3.1) worked intensively to propose competency definitions and learning objectives for the quality and safety domains outlined in the Institute of Medicine (2003) report on health professions education, assess faculty views about the current state of quality and safety education, and develop a website through which we could share teaching strategies, annotated bibliographies, and other quality and safety education resources.

Phase I impact factors

What Phase I factors contributed to QSEN's eventual influence? First, the underlying issue was a major public concern based on documented quality and safety problems (Kohn, Corrigan, & Donaldson, 2000). The need for changes in health professions education had been made, strongly and clearly, by respected leaders (Institute of Medicine, 2003), but the knowledge of the implications of this work by health professional faculties was minimal at best. We needed QSEN thought leaders who had the requisite expertise in the competencies (patient-centered care, teamwork and collaboration, evidence-based practice, quality improvement, safety, and informatics) and teaching pedagogies (clinical, classroom, skills/simulation laboratory, and interprofessional education). But we also needed leaders who had bridged the academic and practice worlds through personal commitments and experiences working to improve the health of populations, health care system performance, and professional development. We needed people who could tell stories about the knowledge, skills, and attitudes needed to fundamentally improve health and health care.

Table 3.1 QSEN faculty, staff, and advisory board members

Project Team	Faculty–Competency Experts	Faculty–Pedagogy Experts	Advisory Board Members
Project Investigators Linda Cronenwett[3,4] UNC–Chapel Hill Gwen Sherwood UNC–Chapel Hill	Jane Barnsteiner[3] University of Pennsylvania	Carol Durham UNC–Chapel Hill	Paul Batalden[3,4] IHI, ACGME
	Joanne Disch[3] University of Minnesota	Lisa Day UC–San Francisco	Geraldine (Polly) Bednash
Librarian Jean Blackwell	Jean Johnson George Washington University	Pamela Ironside[3] Indiana University	AACN Executive Director
Project Managers Elaine Smith Asst: C. Meyers Denise Hirst[2] Asst: D. O'Neal	Pamela Mitchell[1,3] University of Washington	Shirley Moore[3] Case Western Reserve University	Karen Drenkard AONE
			Leslie Hall[3] RWJF ACT Initiative; IHI Health Professions Education Collaborative
Web Manager Steve Segedy[2]	Dori Taylor Sullivan Sacred Heart University, Fairfield, CT, and Duke University		Mary (Polly) Johnson NCSBN Vice President
	Deborah Ward[2] University of Washington and UC–Davis		Maryjoan Ladden Director, RWJF ACT Initiative
	Judith Warren University of Kansas		Audrey Nelson PI, ANA Safe Patient Handling Initiative
			Joanne Pohl[2] NONPF President
			Elaine Tagliareni NLN President-Elect

[1]Phase I only
[2]Phase II only
[3]Dartmouth Summer Symposium community
[4]IHI board members
Note: UNC = University of North Carolina; IHI = Institute for Health Care Improvement; ACGME = Accreditation Council for Graduate Medical Education; UC = University of California; AACN = American Association of Colleges of Nursing; AONE = American Organization of Nurse Executives; RWJF = Robert Wood Johnson Foundation; ACT = Achieving Competence Today; NCSBN = National Council of State Boards of Nursing; PI = principal investigator; ANA = American Nurses Association; NONPF = National Organization of Nurse Practitioner Faculties; NLN = National League for Nursing.

QSEN faculty and advisory board members brought these attributes to the work and deepened their learning in dialogue with each other as the work progressed. For starters, then, QSEN's spread was derived from the importance of the problem and the unique expertise of QSEN leaders whose collective experiences with improving *both* patient care and health professions education provided a strong platform for new ways of thinking about quality and safety education in nursing.

Second, eight faculty and advisory board members were members of the Dartmouth Summer Symposium community, and thus they were familiar with how to use group processes to generate new ideas. These QSEN leaders had witnessed change in the world of health care improvement and health professions education as a result of DSS community work and were experienced at "thinking big" in attempts to improve health, health care, and health professions education. We were also imbued with the philosophy of community work expressed annually by Dr. Batalden, namely:

- Practice hospitality that invites open sharing. Help keep the space open for exploration.
- Practice your own trustworthiness and enhance the trustworthiness of the commons.
- Share generously, but no stealing. Protect each other's futures.
- Practice listening and dialogue, more than telling and discussion.
- Reflect into the gift of silence when it occurs, rather than rushing to obliterate it with words.

QSEN leaders easily adopted DSS values and methods for generating ideas and making decisions. As a result, people from multiple professional organizations were able to take QSEN work, yet unpublished, into organizational deliberations regarding standards for licensure, accreditation, and certification. They invited QSEN faculty to provide special sessions at annual meetings to build will for proposed changes. They provided in-kind support for announcements of QSEN activities and products. They envisioned the parts of the work that could best be done by their own organizations. Beyond anyone's hopes or expectations, the work was spread, as it was envisioned, as a product of the profession itself.

Another impact factor was the QSEN decision to forge a path slightly different from medicine's response to the IOM (2003) report. Physician leaders who had worked to create alignment on descriptions of system-level competencies for undergraduate, graduate, and continuing medical education chose not to outline learning objectives for the competencies, believing that being overly prescriptive would lessen their ability to attract faculty to the goal of improving quality and safety education. With hundreds of community college, diploma, and university-based nursing education programs, and with the need to develop *thousands* of nursing faculty who taught in classroom, clinical, and simulation/skills laboratory teaching roles, QSEN leaders decided we could not assume everyone would be attracted, willing, and able to independently invent their own objectives and teaching strategies. In fact, QSEN's explicit goal was to make it as easy as possible for nursing faculty to envision their roles in supporting quality and safety education.

As we embarked on the iterative work to outline knowledge, skills, and attitude (KSA) objectives for each of the six QSEN competencies, we completed an initial assessment of undergraduate program leader views of how well nursing was doing currently in each domain. As reported by Smith, Cronenwett, & Sherwood (2007), when QSEN competency definitions were the *sole* reference point, survey respondents from 195 schools reported that they were already teaching to these competencies, albeit with room for some improvement, and that students were generally leaving their programs having developed competencies in patient-centered care, teamwork and collaboration, evidence-based practice, quality improvement, safety, and informatics.

QSEN leaders clearly needed to outline the gap in professional development they knew existed. Collectively, the KSAs provided a template against which schools could identify gaps between current curricular content and the desired future. The intensive group work to define learning objectives, therefore, turned out to be an essential element in the process of building the will to change.

Generating and sharing ideas: Phase II (April 2007–October 2008)

Phase I ended with a burst of national presentations, the publication of a special issue of *Nursing Outlook* (2007), and the launch of the QSEN website, each activity aimed at stimulating the will to change through sharing of initial ideas about competency definitions, learning objectives, and annotated bibliographies. The QSEN faculty/advisory board debated logical next steps and decided the field was not ready for a widespread faculty development initiative. We needed a robust package of teaching ideas to move to a train-the-trainer initiative comparable to the End-of-Life Nursing Education Consortium (Malloy, Paice, Viraini, Ferrell, & Bednash, 2008). Phase II objectives, therefore, were to develop, seek feedback, and build consensus for KSAs applicable to *graduate* education and widen the network of QSEN experts and advocates by attracting prelicensure faculty innovators to develop, test, and disseminate teaching strategies for QSEN competency development (see Figure 3.1).

QSEN leaders were familiar with the Institute for Healthcare Improvement's use of learning collaboratives to inspire innovation and quality improvement (Institute for Healthcare Improvement, 2003) and decided to test the use of that model to accomplish Phase II goals for prelicensure education. Proposals to participate in the QSEN Pilot School Collaborative required that applicants describe curricular changes, faculty development strategies, and other activities that they would conduct within their specific nursing education programs. Cross-collaborative learning was an expectation as well, with attendance at two meetings required of all school teams, which comprised clinical, classroom,

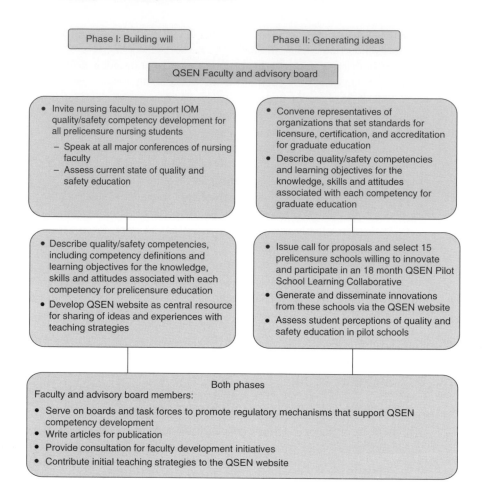

Figure 3.1 QSEN Phases I and II: aims and actions (IOM = Institute of Medicine).

and simulation lab faculty members plus a clinical partner (Cronenwett, Sherwood, & Gelmon, 2009).

For the work related to education for advanced practice registered nurse (APRN) roles, we added APRN leaders to both the QSEN faculty (Ward) and advisory board (Pohl) and invited the input of multiple organizations involved in setting standards for licensure, certification, or accreditation of APRN education programs. Representatives of 13 organizations (see Table 3.2) participated in the generation and organizational reviews of KSA learning objectives for graduate education (Cronenwett et al., 2009).

Phase II impact factors

As in Phase I, linking QSEN with professional organizations potentiated the ideas generated by thought leaders and early innovators. Advisory board members participated fully in both the Pilot School Collaborative and APRN

Table 3.2 Participants in April 2007 workshop to generate graduate-level QSEN competencies and associated knowledge, skills, and attitude learning objectives

Professional organizations	Number of representatives
American Association of Colleges of Nursing[1]	1
American Association of Critical Care Nurses Certification Board	1
American College of Nurse Midwives	1
American Nurses Association	2
American Nurses Credentialing Center	2
American Psychiatric Nurses Association	1
Council on Accreditation of Certified Registered Nurse Anesthetists	1
Commission on Collegiate Nursing Education	2
National Association of Clinical Nurse Specialists	2
National League for Nursing[1]	1
National Organization of Nurse Practitioner Faculties	2
Oncology Nursing Certification Corporation	1
Pediatric Nursing Certification Board	2

[1] Members of QSEN Advisory Board

education work and built on this work from the perspectives of their own organizations. For example, the National Council of State Boards of Nursing (2011) began building a *Transition to Practice* model (QSEN link–Jane Barnsteiner) that required attention to QSEN competency development (now in its pilot phase in three states). The American Association of Colleges of Nursing (QSEN links–Polly Bednash and MaryJoan Ladden) created new standards for accreditation of baccalaureate (American Association of Colleges of Nursing [AACN], 2008) and clinical doctoral education (AACN, 2006) that included quality and safety competencies. The National League for Nursing (2010; QSEN link–Gwen Sherwood and Elaine Tagliareni) developed its education competencies model with a quality and safety thread. The National Organization of Nurse Practitioner Faculties NONPF (QSEN links–Linda Cronenwett and Joanne Pohl) engaged in analyses of core and practice doctorate competencies for evidence of inclusion of the QSEN graduate KSA's (Pohl et al., 2009). The 12 QSEN faculty experts had wide professional networks and were invited to speak at numerous professional conferences, but the efforts of these few alone could not have produced the spread of QSEN-related work throughout the profession. As the major professional organizations associated with licensure and accreditation standards demonstrated the need for and will to change, the momentum for innovation grew.

With that momentum came a need for growing the pool of nursing faculty who could provide consultation among peers in classroom, clinical, and simulation/skills laboratory teaching. A total of 53 schools applied for membership in the QSEN collaborative, and we suspect that the act of applying stimulated attention to improving quality and safety education, even though only 15 schools could be funded. Once again, we used DSS values and methods with 45 expert teachers, and they exceeded our expectations in terms of the breadth and quality of the innovative teaching strategies they developed.

We achieved our goal to end Phase II with at least 40 people who could join the QSEN faculty ranks and provide consultation for associate degree, diploma, and university programs in geographical areas around the country. In addition, a group of collaborative members conducted and published a Delphi study to assist faculties with determining the logical progression of quality and safety competency development across curricula (Barton, Armstrong, Preheim, Gelmon, & Andrus, 2009). We also populated the QSEN website with teaching strategies that became available for faculty throughout the world to use, and QSEN leader Pamela Ironside served as coeditor for a special edition (December 2009) of the *Journal of Nursing Education*, where numerous innovative ideas for developing QSEN competencies (many from collaborative members) were published.

Another influential factor in this phase was our commitment to linking QSEN to practice. Pilot schools were expected to bring clinical partners to the QSEN meetings, and those participants enriched the discussions of both the problem and potential solutions. Many of the teaching innovations required access to root cause analyses, quality improvement project data, methods of error reporting, or electronic health records. Without the common goal of improving quality and safety education for the next generation of nursing graduates, clinical settings often prevented faculty and student access to these learning opportunities. In evaluating their participation in the QSEN Collaborative, faculty participants often commented that a valuable and important outcome had been the extent to which their work on QSEN had strengthened academic-clinical partnerships.

Another potential explanation is that clinical partners helped keep nursing faculty aware of the rationale for the need to change our approaches to nursing professional identity formation. Batalden and Foster proposed that creating an environment in which people generate never-ending improvement of the quality-safety-value of health care requires a commitment that holds three aims together: (1) better outcomes of care, (2) better system performance, and (3) better professional formation and development (personal communication–forthcoming book published by Radcliffe). Indeed, QSEN leaders noted that faculty responded with energy and commitment when it was clear how the work we were asking them to do was linked to the needs of patients, families, and communities. Apart from this link, the call for curricular change to accommodate a paradigm shift in thinking about quality and safety may not have found fertile ground.

Embedding new competencies: Phase III

(November 2008–November 2011 [UNC]; February 2009–February 2012 [AACN])

As Phase II entered its final months, QSEN relationships shifted in preparation for a major faculty development initiative. Our program manager, Rosemary Gibson, resigned her position at RWJF, and we worried about the impact the loss of this long-term partner would have on QSEN work. By some good fortune, QSEN advisory board member MaryJoan Ladden was hired by RWJF shortly thereafter and was appointed our new program manager and spokesperson within the foundation. Her intimate knowledge and support for the work of QSEN was crucial during the downturn in the economy (and foundation resources) that occurred as Phase III began.

In another shift in relationship, Geraldine (Polly) Bednash, the executive director of the American Association of Colleges of Nursing (AACN), moved from QSEN advisory board member to principal investigator of the train-the-trainer faculty development initiative portion of Phase III. Three QSEN faculty members (Barnsteiner, Disch, and Johnson) joined Dr. Bednash to develop the resources and lead the teaching of the regional conferences sponsored by the AACN Phase III grant. Three other QSEN faculty members (Ironside, Moore, and Coinvestigator Sherwood) worked with me on UNC-based initiatives. Collectively, we made up the Steering Committee, which oversaw the incredible investment that RWJF made (see Textbox 3.1 and Figure 3.2).

Finally, Paul Batalden and Mark Splaine, another DSS community member and head of the Veterans Administration Quality Scholars (VAQS) program, suggested that we explore the possibility of making VAQS, until then a program for physicians only, into an interprofessional program that would include nursing pre- and postdoctoral scholars. The VA had mechanisms for paying nursing scholars, but since nursing faculties were not employed by the VA in the way medical faculties were, they had no way to pay faculty members for mentoring VAQS nursing scholars. I met with Dr. Hassmiller to explore the

---

Textbox 3.1   QSEN Phase III: Three aims

1. Promote continued *innovation* in the development and evaluation of methods to elicit and assess student learning of the knowledge, skills, and attitudes of the six IOM/QSEN competencies and the widespread *sharing* of those innovations.
2. Develop the *faculty expertise* necessary to assist the learning and assessment of achievement of quality and safety competencies in all types of nursing programs.
3. Create *mechanisms to sustain the will to change* among all programs through the content of textbooks, accreditation and certification standards, licensure exams, and continued competence requirements.

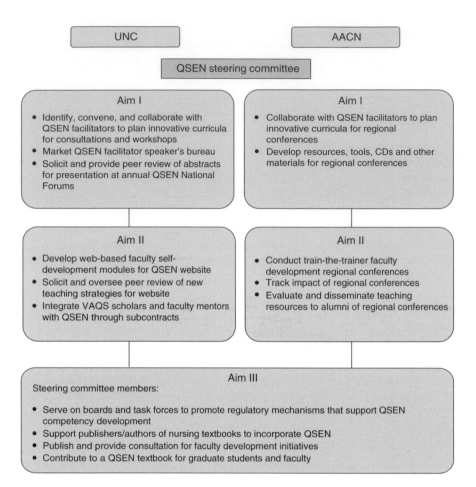

Figure 3.2 QSEN Phase III: embedding new competencies (UNC = University of North Carolina–Chapel Hill; AACN = American Association of Colleges of Nursing; VAQS = Veterans Administration Quality Scholars Program).

possibility of additional RWJF support for this purpose, and she was enthusiastic about the possibility of partnering with the VA to educate the first quality improvement scholars in nursing. Shirley Moore, a QSEN faculty member, proceeded to work with Dr. Splaine to codirect this new interprofessional VAQS program.

Thus began a three-year intensive effort (still underway at the time of writing) to develop faculty expertise for integrating QSEN competency development in curricula throughout the country.

Phase III impact factors

One of the Phase III factors that we believe assisted forward progress in faculty development was the multimodal approach that was taken across two major grants using one steering committee.

- For prospective faculty (pre- and postdoctoral scholars) with an interest in quality improvement science, the VAQS initiative provided a unique opportunity for interprofessional learning and development of scholars in an area of science that was new to nursing.
- Faculty members worldwide could seek their own self-development opportunities on the QSEN website, through teaching strategies submitted from the field at large and through learning modules developed with expert editorial support from Pamela Ironside.
- For schools that wanted to contract with one or more consultants to conduct faculty development activities with entire faculties on their own campuses, descriptions of QSEN facilitators were accessible through the QSEN website.
- For schools that wished to send QSEN champions to train-the-trainer opportunities, nine conferences were held in regions across the country (sold out for each one held to date). These early adopters received extensive resources for themselves and for educating colleagues at home.
- For innovator faculty members who were experimenting with new curricula, pedagogies, and clinical and simulation teaching, the opportunity to submit their work for peer review and presentation at QSEN national forums was provided.

In sum, a faculty development opportunity was in reach of anyone, anywhere. Furthermore, the impact of each faculty development method was potentiated by others. Website learning opportunities were mentioned at conferences, and conferences were advertised on the website. QSEN facilitators presented and moderated panels at the national forums, thus increasing their visibility and subsequent solicitation as consultants. Through the generosity of RWJF, this multimodal, multigrant approach was possible. Add to that the 2009 special issues of *Nursing Outlook* and *Journal of Nursing Education*, and QSEN *was* everywhere.

Another important factor was a conscious focus on what would be needed to support the execution phase of improving quality and safety education for faculty, regardless of whether they were innovators, early adopters, or late adopters. Innovators needed to be able to get together and stimulate each other's creativity and motivation to persist in innovating for the field. The QSEN Pilot School Collaborative, QSEN facilitators group, VAQS program, and QSEN National Forums were designed for these purposes.

Early adopters needed faculty development and consultation opportunities that could bring QSEN ideas to them and their schools without requiring everyone to "reinvent the wheel" from KSA learning objectives alone. QSEN website resources, train-the-trainer regional conferences, and QSEN facilitators, along with this group's publications and presentations, all served to support early adopters.

In spite of the enthusiasm of innovators and early adopters, there remains a large group of faculties who either have never heard of the QSEN competencies (in IOM or QSEN terms) or do not appreciate the fact that accomplishing improvements in this domain requires the knowledgeable support of every faculty member in every school. For those faculty members not innately attracted to or unaware of the work, changing standards for licensure and certification (and continuing competence in both domains) and changing standards for accreditation of nursing education programs are important tools for encouraging continuous improvement.

Another strategy for late adopters was changing the content of the textbooks used in courses. We had expected to have to *push* in this area. Instead we were (and still are) being *pulled* into the processes of change. Textbook authors, working on next editions of more than 20 textbooks, have requested assistance or authorship of sections related to QSEN competency development. Others are undoubtedly making these changes without our knowledge or assistance. One major publisher of nursing textbooks currently requires authors to document the manner in which they are addressing each QSEN competency. Finally, after many calls for a "QSEN Textbook," Drs. Sherwood and Barnsteiner agreed to coedit the book in which this chapter appears.

QSEN and beyond

In May 2011, our RWJF program manager, MaryJoan Ladden, invited Dr. Bednash and me to submit proposals for one final QSEN phase, so the end of this story and the eventual impact on professional identity formation and continuing competency development of nurses is not yet clear. IPEC (the Interprofessional Education Collaborative sponsored by six professional organizations that represent those who educate allopathic and osteopathic physicians, nurses, pharmacists, dentists, and public health) recently published (2011) a monograph that calls upon the health professions to prepare graduates with interprofessional team and team-based care competencies. The four competencies (values/ethics for interprofessional practice, roles/responsibilities for collaborative practice, interprofessional communicaton, and interprofessional teamwork and team-based care) and their learning objectives overlap significantly with QSEN competency definitions and KSAs. We hope that QSEN has prepared nursing faculty with ideas and resources that will increase the quality of their contributions to this important initiative.

What should we expect to see over time if QSEN's impact, along with other national initiatives, "changes the world"? Initially, curricula have to change so that students develop their professional identity assuming that to be a good nurse means being competent in patient-centered care, teamwork and collaboration, evidence-based practice, quality improvement, safety, and informatics. Using a sample of new nurses who graduated August 2004–July 2005, Kovner, Brewer, Yingrengreung, and Fairchild (2010) reported analyses of data from a 2008 survey where 39% of the nurses thought they were "poorly" or "very poorly" prepared about or had "never heard of" quality improvement. Fortunately, Drs. Kovner & Brewer, also funded by RWJF, will follow more recent cohorts of newly licensed nurses during their 10-year study, enriching the assessments and analyses of outcomes pertaining to development of quality and safety competencies. We hope that over time we will be able to answer the question posed in Gregory, Guse, Dick, and Russell's (2007) research brief "Patient Safety: Where is Nursing Education?"

In the end, however, returning to Batalden and Foster's (forthcoming) triangle, we will hopefully find health professionals who, as part of their daily work, care for individual patients while simultaneously improving population health, system performance, and professional development. To be successful, we will need to discover ways to support nursing faculty as key contributors to the interprofessional work of continuous quality improvement, so that they are role models as well as guides for what it means to be a good nurse. If we succeed in reaching these lofty aims and QSEN has been one of the optimistic catalysts for this magnitude of change, it will be a legacy of which to be proud.

References

American Association of Colleges of Nursing. (2006). *The essentials of doctoral education for advanced nursing practice*. Retrieved April 21, from http://www.aacn.nche.edu/dnp/pdf/essentials.pdf

American Association of Colleges of Nursing. (2008). *The essentials of baccalaureate education for professional nursing practice*. Retrieved April 21, 2011, from http://www.aacn.nche.edu/education/bacessn.htm

Barton, A. J., Armstrong, G., Preheim, G., Gelmon, S. B., & Andrus, L. C. (2009). A national Delphi to determine developmental progression of quality and safety competencies in nursing education. *Nursing Outlook, 57*(6), 313-322.

Batalden, P., & Foster, T. C. (forthcoming). [Untitled work]. London: Radcliffe.

Cronenwett, L., Sherwood, G., Barnsteiner, J., Disch, J., Johnson, J., Mitchell, P., et al. (2007). Quality and safety education for nurses. *Nursing Outlook, 55*(3), 122-131.

Cronenwett, L., Sherwood, G., & Gelmon, S. B. (2009). Improving quality and safety education: The QSEN Learning Collaborative. *Nursing Outlook, 57*(6), 304-312.

Cronenwett, L., Sherwood, G., Pohl, J., Barnsteiner, J., Moore, S., Sullivan, D. T., et al. (2009). Quality and safety education for advanced nursing practice. *Nursing Outlook, 57*(6), 338-348.

Gibson, R., & Singh, J. P. (2003). *Wall of silence: The untold story of the medical mistakes that kill and injure millions of Americans*. Washington, DC: Lifeline Press.

Gregory, D. M., Guse, L. W., Dick, D. D., & Russell, C. K. (2007). Patient safety: Where is nursing education? *Journal of Nursing Education, 46*(2), 79-82.

Institute for Healthcare Improvement. (2003). *The breakthrough series: IHI's collaborative model for achieving breakthrough improvement*. Boston: Author.

Institute of Medicine. (2003). *Health professions education: A bridge to quality*. Washington, DC: National Academies Press.

Interprofessional Education Collaborative. (2011). *Core competencies for interprofessional collaborative practice: Report of an expert panel*. Retrieved June 24, 2011, http://www.aacn.nche.edu/Education/pdf/IPECReport.pdf

Kenny, C. (2008). *The best practice: How the new quality movement is transforming medicine*. New York: Public Affairs Perseus Books Group.

Kohn, L. T., Corrigan, J. M., & Donaldson, M. S. (Eds.). (2000). To err is human: Building a safer health system. Washington, DC: National Academies Press.

Kovner, C. T., Brewer, C. S., Yingrengreung, S., & Fairchild, S. (2010). New nurses' views of quality improvement education. *The Joint Commission Journal on Quality and Patient Safety, 36*(1), 29–35.

Malloy, P., Paice, J., Virani, R., Ferrell B. R., & Bednash, G. (2008). End-of-life nursing education consortium: 5 years of educating graduate nursing faculty in excellent palliative care. *Journal of Professional Nursing, 24*(6), 352–357.

National Council of State Boards of Nursing. *Transition to practice*. Retrieved April 21, 2011, from https://www.ncsbn.org/363.htm

National League for Nursing (NLN) Nursing Education Advisory Council for Competency Development. (2010). *The NLN Education Competencies Model*. Retrieved April 21, 2011, from http://www.nln.org/facultydevelopment/competencies/index.htm

Pohl, J. M., Savrin, C., Fiandt, K., Beauchesne, M., Drayton-Brooks, S., Scheibmeir, et al. (2009). Quality and safety in graduate nursing education: Cross-mapping QSEN graduate competencies with NONPF's NP core and practice doctorate competencies. *Nursing Outlook, 57*(6), 349–354.

Sherwood, G. (2011). Integrating quality and safety science in nursing education and practice. *Journal of Research in Nursing, 16,* 226–240.

Smith, E. L., Cronenwett, L., & Sherwood, G. (2007). Current assessments of quality and safety education in nursing. *Nursing Outlook, 55*(3), 132–137.

Section 2

Quality and Safety Competencies: The QSEN Project

Chapter 4

Patient-Centered Care

Mary K. Walton, MSN, MBE, RN
Jane Barnsteiner, PhD, RN, FAAN

The relationship between patients and nurses has always revolved around care, but the nature of the relationship has varied greatly, ranging from totally caring *for* patients—and the health care professionals making all health care decisions, to a full partnership *with* the patient and the family if that is the patient's wish, in identifying the problem, developing a plan, and evaluating the plan's success. For reasons of quality, safety, and consumer preference over the past decade, this relationship is shifting toward one of active involvement, even control, by the patient and family which is requiring cultural and organization change across the health care arena (Disch, 2010). Although this Quality and Safety Education for Nurses (QSEN) competency (see Appendixes A and B) reads "patient-centered care," the term *patient- and family-centered care* (PFCC) is more representative of the concept and acknowledges the significant role that family plays in the health care experience. Here, "family" are those individuals the patient chooses to call family, rather than those defined by providers.

Patient- and family-centered care is a culture, and as such, demands reflection on deeply held values and meaningful life experiences. Uncovering and exploring these values and experiences may be uncomfortable or even threatening to learners. Teaching PFCC requires didactic approaches and engagement through exercises that prompt critical thinking, coupled with demonstration of knowledge and skill acquisition. Learners must be prompted to identify what they experienced through guided reflection connecting them to the didactic content and application to practice. Reflections on personal values and beliefs and their influence on practice should enable learners to explore and grasp the culture of PFCC and contrast it with provider-centered approaches to care. As the learner comes to recognize the relationship of personal values to practice and acquire skill in communication and eliciting patient values, the goal of care reflecting the patient's values and beliefs can be achieved.

Quality and Safety in Nursing: A Competency Approach to Improving Outcomes,
First Edition. Edited by Gwen Sherwood and Jane Barnsteiner.
© 2012 John Wiley & Sons, Inc. Published 2012 by John Wiley & Sons, Inc.

Recalling the personal experiences with health care, illness, and death that shaped the learner's values may evoke memories of mistreatment, suffering, loss, grief, and unresolved relationship issues. Reflections on both personal and professional experiences may prompt distress, anger, and the uncovering of painful life events. Teachers need to be attentive to the range of emotional responses generated through this work and prepared to respond (Brien, Legault, & Tremblay, 2008). The full engagement of the "hearts and minds" of care providers through respectful partnerships and a commitment to shared values of PFCC is identified as one of the primary drivers for an exceptional inpatient hospital experience (Balik, Conway, Zipperer, & Watson, 2011).

The creation of partnerships in learning, rather than the traditional hierarchy of education, is recognized as essential to meeting the needs of today's student. This shift is reflected in the needs of patient care where the move from provider-centered care to one of partnership among patients, their loved ones, and nurses is recognized as essential for quality and safety in today's complex arena of health care. These learner-teacher partnerships mirror the partnerships of PFCC, ranging from a focus on an individual's care to that of a health care organization's systems and structures.

Definitions

The Institute of Medicine (IOM), in its landmark book *Crossing the Quality Chasm* (2001), defined patient-centered as "providing care that is respectful of and responsive to individual patient preferences, needs, and values and ensuring that patient values guide all clinical decisions" (p. 40). Thus, the IOM boldly redirected the orientation of the health care industry to one in which full patient engagement is an essential precursor to quality and safety rather than merely an option (Disch, 2010). Patient-centered care is one of the six dimensions of quality espoused by the IOM (safe, timely, effective, efficient, equitable, and patient-centered; 2001, pp. 39–40).

An important variation of patient-centered care is family-centered care. Henneman and Cardin (2002) suggest that family-centered care is an extension of patient-centered care, "widening the circle of concern to include those persons who are important in a patient's life" (p. 13). They go on to note that family-centered care does not negate the patient's rights to privacy or control but rather recognizes that this is a choice that can be made by the patient. Family-centered care is a philosophy that considers the patient as the unit of attention within the patient's network of relationships. It should not be equated with any one intervention, such as open visiting hours or the family having equal say in the decision making.

Patient- and family-centered care is a term describing a philosophy and culture that emphasizes partnerships between patients, family members, and health care providers. There are several definitions of PFCC offered by three organizations that have studied and influenced the shift in culture from provider-centered to that of patient-centered care. Although they vary slightly, the definitions offered by the Picker Institute, the Institute for Patient- and Family-Centered Care, and Planetree share common elements (Balik et al., 2011, p. 4) (refer to Textbox 4.1).

The Joint Commission (TJC) adopts the definition of PFCC established by the Institute for Patient- and Family-Centered Care. Described as "an innovative approach to plan, deliver, and evaluate health care that is grounded in

---

Textbox 4.1 Definitions of patient- and family-centered care

Note. From *Achieving an exceptional patient and family experience of inpatient hospital care* (IHI Innovation Series white paper), by B. Balik, J. Conway, L. Zipperer, and J. Watson, 2011. Cambridge, MA: Institute for Healthcare Improvement (available on www.IHI.org). Reprinted with permission.

The Picker Institute
Patient- and family-centered care is defined as "improving health care through the eyes of the patient." All patients deserve high-quality health care and patient views and experiences are integral to improvement efforts.

Patient-centered care includes the following principles:

- Effective treatment delivered by staff you can trust;
- Involvement in decisions and respect for patients' preferences;
- Fast access to reliable health care advice;
- Clear, comprehensive information and support for self-care;
- Physical comfort and a clean, safe environment;
- Empathy and emotional support;
- Involvement of family and friends; and
- Continuity of care and smooth transitions.

Institute for Patient- and Family- Centered Care
Patient-and family- centered care has these characteristics:

- People are treated with dignity and respect;
- Health care providers communicate and share complete and unbiased information with patients and families in ways that are affirming and useful;
- Patients and family members build on their strengths by participating in experiences that enhance control and independence; and
- Collaboration among patients, family members, and providers occurs in policy and program development and professional education, as well as in the delivery of care.

(Continued)

> **Textbox 4. 1** *(Continued)*
>
> **Planetree**
> Patient- and family-centered care includes the following components:
>
> - Human interaction;
> - Family, friends, and social support;
> - Information and education;
> - Nutritional and nurturing aspects of food;
> - Architectural and interior design;
> - Arts and entertainment;
> - Spirituality;
> - Human touch;
> - Complementary therapies; and
> - Healthy communities

mutually beneficial partnerships among health care providers, patients, and families. Patient- and family-centered care applies to patients of all ages, and it may be practiced in any health care setting" (2010, p. 92).

Establishing partnerships with patients and their families is an essential element of PFCC including partnerships beyond the individual patient level. Patients and family members as advisors involved in all operations of the organization, from task forces to governing boards, can transform the health care organization to one centered on the patient and family experience of care rather than that of the providers. PFCC is *not* conceptually similar to patient-*focused* care. In this form of care, although the patient/family may be involved, the health care provider retains control over decision making, Patient needs and preferences may or may not be sought and rarely drive care decisions.

The QSEN competencies support the concept of PFCC (Cronenwett et al., 2007, 2009). It is the most inclusive option, underscoring the philosophy that both the patient and family, as defined by the patient, are recipients of care by nurses. This holistic focus on the family unit is a distinguishing characteristic of nursing (Disch, 2010).

Balint (1969) contrasted patient-centered medicine with illness-centered medicine and described positive patient outcomes when physicians "allow their patients to tell them what they want in their own time and in their own way" (p. 276). Over the ensuing years, researchers and clinicians as well as consumers have examined the outcomes of shifting from provider- or illness-focused care to one that engages the patient and provider in a partnership where patient preferences and values direct care. The recent IOM report *The Future of Nursing: Leading Change, Advancing Health* notes the need for patient-centered care to improve quality, access, and value yet recognizes that "practice still is usually organized around what is most convenient for the provider, the payer, or the health care organization and not the patient" (2011, p. 51).

A growing body of evidence shows that improving the patient experience and developing partnerships with patients are linked to improved health outcomes. For example, evidence shows that patients who are more involved in their care are better able to manage complex chronic conditions, seek appropriate assistance, have reduced anxiety and stress, and have shorter lengths of stay in hospital (Balik et al., 2011, p. 6).

A philosophical exploration of the moral nature of patient-centeredness using three ethical schools of thought concludes that it can be justified on moral grounds. The authors believe that patient-centeredness can be advanced by encouraging students to reflect on the reasons that patient-centered care is the right thing to do (Duggan, Geller, Cooper, & Beach, 2006). A business case for hospital redesign reflecting patient-centered principles includes both evidence-based design innovations and experience-based innovations that result in outcomes such as fewer patient falls, reduced adverse drug events, fewer health care-acquired infections, and reduced length of stay (Sadler et al., 2011).

Key concepts

The Institute for Patient- and Family-Centered Care identifies four core concepts: dignity and respect, information sharing, participation, and collaboration (www.ipfcc.org). The foundation for PFCC is the special relationship between the patient/family and the caregivers. In relationship-based care,

> the care provider-patient relationship is one in which the care provider consistently maintains the patient and family as his or her central focus. The care provider knows that each person's unique life story determines how he or she will experience an illness. The care provider conveys an unwavering respect and personal concern for the patient, strives to understand what is most important to this particular patient and family, safeguards their dignity and well-being, and actively engages them in all aspects of the patient's care (Koloroutis, 2004, p. 5).

Gerteis, Edgman-Levitan, Daley, and Delbanco (1993) identified several dimensions of patient-centered care. These include the following:

- *Respect for patients' values, preferences, and expressed needs.* Respect is evident in the sharing of desired information with the patients and families; the active partnering with them to determine care priorities and a plan; tailoring their level of involvement according to their preferences, not those of the care providers; and reformulating the plan as the situation changes.
- *Coordination and integration of care.* As care becomes more complex due to the coexistence of multiple chronic conditions, an increasing number of

care providers, numerous care sites, and shorter episodes of care, the need for creating smooth transitions across the episodes of care becomes even more vital.

- *Information, communication, and education.* Some individuals prefer comprehensive explanations, while others prefer none. Some people learn best visually, while others favor the personal experience. Adjusting the message and its delivery according to the individual patient's preferences is a major challenge yet a cornerstone to patient-centered care. What is common to all situations is that patients want to be able to trust what they are being told, and to receive it in a manner that makes sense to them, at a level they can understand.
- *Physical comfort.* Assuring that patients will be comfortable, and free from pain, is such a basic expectation of patient-centered care. However, for a variety of reasons, this is often not adequately addressed and must form the basis for any personalized plan of care.
- *Emotional support.* Similarly, patients and their families may experience anxiety and distress from a number of sources, and the underlying factors need to be identified and dealt with. This is nursing's work and what enables us to make unique contributions to the patient/family experience.
- *Involvement of family and friends.* For more than 40 years, research has indicated that children need their parents nearby. Patient-centered care requires that visiting hours, and engagement of family and friends in all aspects of the process as defined by the family, are structured to meet the patients' needs, regardless of the age of the patient.

Background: what do patients and families want?

For more than 30 years, research has examined what patients and families want from the care experience, particularly in the critical care environment (Daley, 1984; Hickey & Leske, 1992; Leske, 1986; Mundy, 2010). The results have been fairly consistent with those identified by Molter (1979) in her classic study of relatives of intensive care unit patients, that is, the need for information, to be near the patient, and for reassurance and support. Despite this extensive body of evidence, many critical care units continue to struggle with finding ways to implement patient-centered policies (Davidson, 2007). In 2001, the IOM issued its call for patient-centered care and, in 2006, the IOM report *Preventing Medication Errors* outlined patients' expectations. These include "being listened to and respected as a care partner, being told the truth, having care and information sharing coordinated with all members of the team, and partnering with staff who are able to provide both technically and emotionally supportive care" (Spath, 2008, p. 133). Nurses lack consensus as to what constitutes "appropriate" patient-family involvement. This is witnessed in the disagreements about visiting hours and presence of family members during resuscitation, among other examples. A qualitative study examining the experience of nurse family members of critically ill patients highlights the tension and conflict that can develop when care is not individualized and reflects the values and beliefs of providers over those of the family member (Salmond, 2011). Spath (2008, p. 73) offers a Patient/Family Engagement Self-Assessment tool assessing whether staff are "personally ready to engage patients and families in improving safety." The *American Journal of Nursing*'s "Putting Patients First" series offers examples of patient-centered approaches to the provision of nursing care developed by the Planetree group (Frampton, 2009; Frampton & Guastello, 2010; Frampton, Wohl, & Cappiello, 2010; Michalak et al., 2010).

Patients and families have been engaged for decades in various activities that have equipped them to be partners in their care. Examples include receiving preoperative and home instructions, learning to take medications and perform treatments, monitoring vital signs, and watching for complications. More recently, however, patients and family members are being invited to actively participate on health system boards, committees, and task forces. For example, hospitals are now including patients and/or families as members of patient safety committees, interview teams, and participants in new employee orientation. The growing body of literature describing the benefits of family members' presence at the resuscitation of their loved ones (Emergency Nurses Association, 2009; Halm, 2005; Howlett, Alexander, & Tsuchiya, 2010; MacLean et al., 2003; Mangurten et al., 2005) reflects the increasing inclusion of family throughout the care process. Inclusion of family members in the process for disclosing adverse events to patients and, in some organizations, inviting them to participate in root cause analysis of adverse events is more controversial (Cantor et al., 2005). This form of inclusion requires clear policies, consumer preparation, and close monitoring of the process. Planetree, established in 1978 as a "non-profit organization that provides education and information in a collaborative community of healthcare organizations, facilitating efforts to create patient centered care in healing environments," is another example of an organization that has whole-heartedly embraced the concept of patient-centered care and become an international leader in promoting it (www.planetree.org/about/html). This is accomplished through conferences, publications, networks, and consultations.

National standards and regulations

Over the past few years, the stakes have been raised as more knowledgeable consumers actively select where they will receive care, and patient's evaluation of their experience of care begins to have an effect on payment patterns. National regulatory agencies are weighing in on the issue of PFCC. For example, the Joint Commission, the National Committee for Quality Assurance, and the Centers for Medicare and Medicaid Services (CMS) are increasingly becoming involved in stipulating expectations and monitoring performance. The federal government uses its Hospital Consumer Assessment of Healthcare Providers and Systems (HCAHPS) survey to measure patients' perceptions of their hospital experience and posts public results (www.hospitalcompare.hhs. gov). It is the first tool to help consumers compare hospitals nationally on key variables that include communication, responsiveness, cleanliness, noise, and pain management. Of particular importance to nursing is that some questions specifically relate to nursing performance, which allows for comparisons across organizations. CMS has designed an incentive program to reward facilities that use the tool and, more importantly, report their data (www.cms.gov).

Another example of a national organization using its influence to promote patient and family involvement is the National Quality Forum, a voluntary consensus standards-setting body that has endorsed more than 500 measures of quality and safety. Recently, the National Quality Forum, through its National Priorities Partnership (2008), identified six priorities with the greatest potential for improving care, reducing disparities, and eliminating waste. One priority is patient and family engagement. The group is working to ensure that all patients:

- will be asked for feedback on their experience of care, which health care organizations and their staff will then use to improve care;
- will have access to tools and support systems that enable them to effectively navigate and manage their care; and
- will have access to information and assistance that enables them to make informed decisions about their treatment options.

The National Priorities Partnership (2010) issued a synthesis report with a patient and family engagement action plan.

New accreditation standards and federal regulations for hospitals provide a powerful stimulus toward a culture of patient- and family-centered care. TJC issued *Advancing Effective Communication, Cultural Competence and Patient- and Family-Centered Care: A Roadmap for Hospitals* (2010) to provide specific methods to improve quality and safety initiatives and implement new accreditation standards. This document details many strategies and practices for care improvement with a summary checklist focused on points along the care continuum: admission processes, assessment, treatment, end-of-life care, discharge, and transfer, as well as organizational readiness (TJC, 2010, pp. 5-6). Specific recommendations on assessment and approaches to elicit and understand the patient's values and perspectives are included (TJC, 2010, pp. 13-16).

TJC standards now include the patient's right to identify a support person and have access to that person throughout an inpatient admission. Surveyors will examine the process for notifying patients of this right and identifying the support person. This individual, based on the patient's preference, may be involved in patient care rounds, education, and discharge planning. Patients in intensive care units are particularly vulnerable, with complex communication needs. "These patients must have unrestricted access to their chosen support person while in the ICU to provide emotional and social support" (TJC, 2010, p. 22).

A presidential memorandum focused on hospital visitation and specifically noting the issues of lesbian, gay, bisexual, and transgender patients and their families directed CMS to establish federal regulations for patient rights (White

House, 2010). Effective in January 2011, CMS issued a new condition of participation standard, requiring hospitals to inform patients of visitation rights and the patient's right to receive visitors whom he or she designates, including a spouse, domestic partner, family member, or friend. Thus, these new TJC and CMS requirements recognize the vulnerability of hospitalized individuals and formally establish the role of a "support person" in the hospital setting (DHHS/CMS, 2010). Now patients may choose to have an ally at their bedside to ensure that their preferences, needs, and values are respected and guide clinical decision making.

Teaching the competencies

Recognizing the patient as the source of control and full partner in providing compassionate and coordinated care is a challenge for any health care professional given the hierarchical nature of Western medical care. Furthermore, most practice settings have long been established as provider centered, although some organizations have successfully embedded a philosophy of PFCC and instituted the processes and systems to make this a permanent change (Balik et al., 2011; Frampton, Wohl, & Cappiello, 2010; Reid-Ponte et al., 2003; Wasson, Godfrey, Nelson, Mohr, & Batalden, 2003; Zarubi, Reiley, & McCarter, 2008). Clinical experiences in PFCC organizations offer exposure to a physical environment and a culture of partnership among clinicians, patients, and loved ones in all aspects of operations. Until all care settings reflect PFCC, prelicensure nursing students need to develop competency in providing patient-centered care without necessarily experiencing it. Education to gain competency in PFCC demands a curriculum that is participatory, active, and experiential. Providing patient-centered care reflects a nurse's values and attitudes, arises from a deep knowledge base, and requires skill to practice. Below are teaching strategies for the classroom, simulation, and clinical settings to engage students in learning the knowledge, skills, and attitudes necessary to engage the patient as a full partner in providing compassionate and coordinated nursing care based on the patient's preferences, values, and needs.

Didactic strategies

Narrative pedagogy

Fictional and autobiographical literature is particularly suited to teaching PFCC. Autobiographical stories told by patients about their experiences of illness rather than about the disease process express the truth of personal experience in the patient's own voice (Sakalys, 2003). Illness narratives have evolved into a major literary genre and are increasingly used as an effective teaching strategy (Brown, Kirkpatrick, Mangum, & Avery, 2008; Diekelmann, 2005; Ewing & Hayden-Miles, 2011; Gazarian, 2010; Kumagai, 2008; Sakalys, 2002; Sakalys, 2003; Shattell, 2007; Wall & Rossen, 2004).

The depictions of illness, disease, and caring found in fiction, poetry, drama, film, and paintings are far more powerful and sensitive than the explanations contained in textbooks. Engaging students in reading/viewing, interpreting, and critiquing promotes reflective thinking and the consideration of alternate perspectives and meanings in situations. Students change from reading for information, key points, main ideas, or answers and take authority for their own learning by reading reflectively, observing both their own reactions and the questions the work evokes and actively creating meaning. They gain an understanding of the human experiences and the capacity to adopt another's perspective (Sakalys, 2002). Teachers and students challenge assumptions and interpret situations from multiple perspectives. "Narratives offer an opportunity for discourse that opens up new possibilities for student-centered learning" (Ewing & Hayden-Miles, 2011, p. 212). Incorporating narrative strategies promotes critical thinking, reasoning, and analytical skills along with introspection and self-reflection to facilitate the students' shifting their view from their personal and professional lens to the patient's perspective. There are an infinite variety of ways that patient narratives can be used to develop the knowledge, skills, and attitudes for competency in PFCC. Sakalys (2002) offers numerous strategies to engage students in careful reading and reflections on illness narratives. It is the opportunity to be creative and engage students in identifying published narratives, films, and artwork for class study. Examples of suggested learning strategies are offered below.

Evaluating the hospital experience through the patient's eyes

Illness narratives by patients offer the reader the opportunities to see the patient's experience without a clinical lens. Discuss their stories and compare and contrast to the definitions of PFCC. Introduce the HCAHPS tool. Direct the students to complete the survey based on a published narrative, thus engaging them in reading for context and meaning as well as learning the evaluation process. Students will vary in how they "see," appreciate, and evaluate the patient narrative. Explore these variations in classroom discussion.

Narratives of health care experiences published in the professional literature provide first-person narratives by nurses and physicians and offer the reader the opportunity to "see" a patient's experience through the dual lens of professional and patient. Read, discuss, and evaluate the specific examples in terms of patient-centered care. Was the patient the source of control? Was the care compassionate and coordinated and reflective of the patient's preferences, values, and needs? How was the experience and narrative shaped by the author's professional perspective? Prompt the identification of both patient-directed and provider-directed aspects of care. Where were the missed opportunities to meet patients' needs? What promoted the PFCC aspects of the care experience? What thwarted it? Was nursing visible in the narrative?

Art interpretation

The visual arts offer nonverbal narratives that can prompt reflection on the artist's perspective and help learners develop insight and empathy. Art calls for viewers to listen attentively and think about what is openly expressed or hidden from view and to bring this knowledge to spoken language, providing information about values, conflicts, and beliefs (Ewing & Hayden-Miles, 2011). Because learners differ in their cultural, social, and historical backgrounds, multiple interpretations will be generated through the study of a single image. Many of artist Frida Kahlo's works reflect her life experiences of trauma, surgery, hospitalization, suffering, pain, and loss; one example for study is "Henry Ford Hospital." Viewing, discussing, and journaling about art provides a "refreshing way to enlighten students to gain access to others, make connections, and gain a deeper understanding and appreciation for multiple perspectives and levels of knowledge" (Ewing & Hayden-Miles, 2011, p. 215). This serves to reinforce the need to recognize the variety of perspectives and to elicit the patient's perspective in the provision of care.

Films

Films tell stories. Film is used successfully in both health professions and ethics education (Alexander, Lenahan, & Pavlov, 2005; Ber & Alroy, 2001; Volandes, 2007). Film provides context and can serve to illustrate the patient's perspective. Selecting and using complete films or short clips is a recognized approach to foster the learner's reflection and improve education in the affective domains (Blasco, Moreto, Roncoletta, Levites, & Janaudis, 2006; Wall & Rossen, 2004). As one example, the HBO movie *Wit*, based on the Pulitzer Prize–winning play, is a first-person, fictional narrative of a woman treated for stage IV ovarian cancer. The patient speaks directly to the viewer when narrating her hospital experience. One theme to explore is how the specialty and organizational values influence the patient's experience of care. Clinical research and physician education goals continually override patient care considerations. Other themes to explore are the nurse's partnership with the patient, value conflicts, and moral distress.

Classroom forums for patient/family advisors or student health care narratives

Organizations that embrace the philosophy of PFCC establish formal roles for patient and family advisors. In these organizations, patient/family advisors share their experiences in orientations, grand rounds, and in-service programs. These forums are considered essential to a PFCC organizational culture. Local health care organizations may have advisors interested in classroom presentations. If this is not feasible, an alternate approach would be to engage learners in developing and sharing a first-person account of a health care encounter to illustrate PFCC. The learner can embrace the principles of PFCC, including roles of advisors, offering the class a range of experiences for reflection and critique.

Value identification exercises

Recognition of personal and professional values is a fundamental component to competency in PFCC. Life experiences shape and inform personal values, beliefs, and practice. A variety of personal experiences and values lead each student to select nursing. Published exercises can help; for example, *Toward Culturally Competent Care: A Toolbox for Teaching Communication Strategies* from the Center for the Health Professions, University of California–San Francisco contains exercises to promote introspection and identification of personal as well as professional values and beliefs (Mutha, Allen, & Welch, 2002). This lays the groundwork for approaches to eliciting and understanding the patient's perspective and experience of illness. Two examples follow:

- *Exercise: Family Healing Traditions* (UCSF Toolbox Exercise IB): The purpose is to create an atmosphere where each individual's experiences are valued and to begin to examine cultural differences in healing practices. Participants are asked to write down some of the health beliefs and practices instilled by their families. First in pairs and then in the group, participants share and discuss them. Personal traditions are compared and contrasted with Western biomedical approaches. The use of complementary and alternative medicine approaches and effectiveness in their personal experience can be explored. Learners reflect on how they would feel sharing a personal healing tradition that is not consistent with evidence-based medicine with their own provider. How might this healing tradition be received? How could it be incorporated into a treatment plan?
- *Exercise: What Do We Need to Know About Ourselves to Provide Culturally Competent Care?* (UCSF Toolbox Exercise VIA): The purpose of this exercise is to help participants understand their own norms and preferences and to explore strategies for working with patients who have different norms. Relating these cultural values to the concepts of PFCC can highlight the potential for conflict between the provider and the patient. Refer to Figure 4.1.

Review each value and prompt students to mark where they fall on the continuum. Discuss and compare how these values reflect the four core concepts of PFCC as identified by the Institute for Patient- and Family- Centered Care (www.ipfcc.org; see Table 4.1). Lead a facilitated discussion of how one's personal values might prevent seeing the care situation through the patient's eyes. An individual who values privacy and independent decision making may fail to recognize a need for or even reject a request for family presence in a meeting to discuss an elective surgical procedure for a patient who values family decision making.

Identify organizational values. Values shape health care settings, professional and specialty practices, and therefore the patient experience (Baggs et al., 2007). Academic practice settings place value on the generation of new knowledge and education. Staff may be comfortable promoting participation in clinical research and working with students, and may be challenged when patient care priorities conflict. In contrast, in community-based settings where the primary focus may center on the patient care experience, education and research efforts may not be as highly valued. Values may differ between for-profit and not-for-profit organizations. Ensuring that employees understand

HANDOUT VIA.1

YOUR CULTURAL VALUES

Directions: On each continuum below, place an X indicating where you believe you fall as an individual. Put parentheses around the area on the continuum that reflects your comfort zone when interacting with other people.

SOCIAL STATUS

Inherited . . . .   Earned

PRIVACY

Guarded . . . .   Open/Shared

FATALISM

Fate determined by   . . . .   Fate determined by self
outside influence

GROUP/INDIVIDUAL

Health care decisions   · · · · · · · · · · · · · ·   Health care decisions
made by family/group   made by individual

ACCESS TO INFORMATION

Information withhold. . . . .   Right to know

Figure 4.1 Your cultural values.
Note. From *Toward Culturally Competent Care: A Toolbox for Teaching Communication Strategies*, by S. Mutha, C. Allen, and M. Welch, 2002, San Francisco: Center for the Health Professions, University of California–San Francisco, as adapted from *Managing Diversity in Health Care*, by L. Gardenswartz and A. Rowe, 1999, San Francisco: Jossey-Bass. Reprinted with permission.

and reflect organizational values in their practice is challenging (Neumann & Forsyth, 2008). Engage students in identifying organizational values. An exercise might include a review of health organizations' public websites for values expressed though content as well as the presentation of information.

Identify professional values. Consider the professional values of nursing as articulated by the American Nurses Association and specialty organizations such as the American Association of Critical Care Nurses. Discuss how these values shape both the individual and their practice setting and therefore influence the patient and family experience. Discuss the interpretations and applications of the ANA Code of Ethics for Nurses in light of partnership- or patient-directed care. Where do values converge and where is there risk of conflict? Examples for consideration are the ANA Position Statements on Ethics and Human Rights. Discuss how consistent personal values and beliefs may be with ANA positions on capital punishment or withholding nutrition and hydration.

Nurses may adopt the values of a specialty practice, which in turn may hinder the ability to recognize a patient's alternative value. The promotion of hope in oncology and the use of do-not-resuscitate orders are values reflected

Table 4.1 Cultural values aligned with core concepts of patient/family-centered care

Cultural Values	Patient/Family-Centered Care Concepts
Social status: inherited or earned	Dignity and respect
Privacy: guarded-open/sharing	Information sharing
Fatalism	
Group/individual: How decisions are made	Participation and independence
Access to information	Collaboration

in specialty literature. The fields of organ transplantation and neonatology reflect specialty beliefs and values. How can practitioners ensure that the patient's values are respected in light of these well established specialty values? How does a nurse honor personal values if the patient's values create conflict? How have minority group values shaped or influenced health care in the United States? Topics such as the debate over childhood immunizations or mandatory influenza vaccination for health care workers can be used to illustrate the impact of values on practice. Consider how the rejection of blood transfusions based on spiritual beliefs prompted the development of bloodless surgery. Pain management is another area where values shape practice. How does the nurse concerned about relief of pain honor a patient or family spiritual belief that suffering is part of the human experience and should not be mitigated?

Care at the end of life is guided by deeply held values concerning the meaning of life, duties to family and friends, beliefs about the significance of pain and suffering, and spiritual considerations. The primacy of patient's values is well recognized in end of life care; yet conflict among providers, patients, and loved ones is evident in public debate and professional literature. Advances in knowledge and technology, such as ventricular assist devices, extracorporeal membrane oxygenation, and hypothermia therapy, make the determination of actual death challenging. Less complex therapies such as placement of gastrostomy tubes for enteral nutrition still prompt conflict over values among all stakeholders. Identifying and communicating individual values and care preferences at the end of life is challenging. Review a website developed by lay people: www.engagewithgrace.org. Each of the five questions on "the one slide" offers a discussion guide and stories illustrating a variety of values and preferences (Figure 4.2).

The phenomenon of moral distress resulting from value conflicts is increasingly recognized in the profession. An assignment to share preferences for end of life care with the person identified as a surrogate decision maker can help to clarify personal values that will influence their feelings in practice. The focus is communicating preferences and values to another rather than preparing a legal document such as an advance directive. Learners will experience the difficulty of articulating and sharing their values. The website

Can you and your loved ones answer these questions?

1. On a scale of 1 to 5, where do you fall on this continuum?

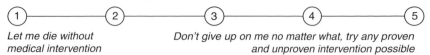

Let me die without
medical intervention

Don't give up on me no matter what, try any proven
and unproven intervention possible

2. If there were a choice, would you prefer to die at home, or in a hospital?

3. Could a loved one correctly describe how you'd like to be treated in the case of a terminal illness?

4. Is there someone you trust whom you've appointed to advocate on your behalf when the time is near?

5. Have you completed any of the following: written a living will, appointed a healthcare power of attorney, or completed an advance directive?

Figure 4.2 The One Slide Project.
Note. From Engage with Grace (www.engagewithgrace.org). Reprinted with permission.

developed for National Health Care Decisions Day offers a range of materials and links to resources to promote discussion (www.nhdd.org).

Teaching what PFCC looks like in action: examples of patient–family engagement

Engage learners in examining the philosophy and concepts of PFCC as well as what the experience of care in a PFCC organization looks like by introducing them to the myriad resources available in the public domain. Most of them are accessible via organizational websites.

● The Joint Commission Roadmap (2010) provides many clinical strategies and prescribes actions (pp. 5–6). This document can be used in a variety of ways to teach the standards as well as how hospitals will be evaluated to determine organizational enculturation during an accreditation survey.

● The Planetree and Picker Institute websites offer many resources, including the jointly developed *Patient-Centered Care Improvement Guide* (Frampton et al., 2008). This document includes self-assessment tools and practical approaches to building a patient-centered culture. The appendices include examples of materials from organizations around the country, including tools to promote patient participation in clinical rounding, bedside posters for patients to tell their story, and implementation strategies for patient-directed visitation. This document offers many opportunities for classroom activities.

● The Institute for Patient- and Family-Centered Care has materials to develop an understanding of PFCC, for example, *Partnering with Patients and Families to Enhance Safety and Quality: A Mini Toolkit* (2011).

● The 2011 CMS Regulations on Patient Visitation Rights (DHHS/CMS, 2010) were prompted by an egregious care situation in a Florida hospital. Learners may research the origin of the regulations and how the media and public have varied in the portrayal of the regulations. Facilitate student discussion on how relevant and significant regulations influence the clinical encounter.

Exercise: simulate a family meeting

Direct learners to plan a family meeting where information is shared and difficult treatment decisions are discussed. Curtis and White (2008) offer approaches for evidence-based ICU conferences and include a communication component to "explore and focus on patient values and treatment preferences" (p. 839). The Planetree/Picker *Patient-Centered Care Improvement Guide* provides a "Patient Care Conference Form" with nine topics ranging from the hospital's culture of safety to wishes concerning resuscitation (Frampton et al., 2008, p. 132). Learners can compare and contrast the quality of communication and influence of patient values with two approaches to a family meeting: (1) starting with a medical overview and offering of information from the provider's perspective, versus (2) starting with the patient/family expressed goals for the meeting and summarizing their current understanding of patient condition/prognosis.

Communication between the patient and the health care team is essential if patients are the source of control and care is based on their preferences, values, and needs. The Joint Commission's SPEAK UP initiative, launched in 2002, offers a variety of materials to promote communication for patients, including videos, for example, "Speak Up: Prevent Errors in Your Care" (www.jointcommission.org/speakup.aspx). Videos focused on engaging individuals in promoting safety are posted on Facebook by the Joint Commission and can be reviewed and discussed for content as well as technique.

Use of technology to support PFCC

Barton (2010) examines how technology can enhance patient-centered care and provides two examples that use the computer and equipment alarms. The nurse can place and use the computer in relation to the patient and structure the flow of assessment to allow the patient to tell their story rather than answer a series of questions. Equipment alarms prompt a nurse to respond to the patient, providing an opportunity for meaningful contact and explanation.

Simulation

Simulation training is an effective strategy to teach clinical practice. McKeon, Norris, Cardell, and Britt (2009) report a pilot study to compare required resources and learning outcomes for prelicensure, intermediate-level nursing students. Faculty developed a pretest-posttest case study design to compare simulation learning methods for achievement of the six QSEN patient-centered care competences. Many of the exercises in this chapter would be considered low fidelity and could be used in the classroom or learning laboratory.

Clinical strategies

Evaluation of a clinical environment

Significant attention has turned toward the importance of the physical environment itself and its impact on health and healing as a component of patient-centered care. Reiling, Hughes, and Murphy (2008) provide a comprehensive review of the impact of facility design on patient safety. The Green Guidelines for Health Care (2010) offer a premier resource for health care leaders as they build new and remodel old facilities. Planetree and the Picker Institute (2008) offer guidelines for designing this environment:

> A patient-centered environment of care is one that is safe and clean, and that guards patient privacy. It also engages all the human senses with color, texture, artwork, music, aromatherapy, views of nature, and comfortable lighting, and considers the experience of the body, mind, and spirit of all who use the facility. Space is provided for loved ones to congregate, as well as for peaceful contemplation, meditation, or prayer, and patients, families, and staff have access to a variety of arts and entertainment that serve as positive diversions. At the heart of the environment of care, however, are the human interactions that occur within the physical structure to calm, comfort, and support those who inhabit it. Together the design, aesthetics, and these interactions can transform an institutional, impersonal, and alien setting into one that is truly healing (Environment of Care section, para. 2)

The Picker Institute and Planetree offer tools to assess the patient centeredness of organizations and recommend their use to select one's care setting. Direct students to evaluate a practice setting in their community. Entry into the building provides an opportunity to simulate the patient experience through way finding and access to language services. Facilitate discussion of the learner's perceptions and compare to the principles of PFCC. If evaluations of the same practice setting vary, discuss the differing perceptions. Prompt reflection on the impact of environment-patient interaction on the nurse-patient encounter. For example, might a patient's initial interaction with a nurse reflect the experiences in the parking lot, lobby, or admission's office prior to an encounter with the clinician? How does the milieu affect the quality of the patient experience? What opportunities can be identified to improve the environment? How do they support the patient and family engaging in a partnership for care with clinicians?

Patient-centered clinical rounds/change of shift report

In the inpatient setting, practice patterns are well established for care, provider transitions, and physician education. These patterns may present challenges to patient and family participation. Surgical team rounds are held based on operating room schedules. Medical rounds may focus on education in addition to care review. Meaningful participation of patients and families in interdisciplinary rounds and change of shift report will promote PFCC. Discuss practices in clinical sites. Are there innovative approaches to fostering partnerships in the acute care setting if participation in rounds is not feasible?

Reframing constructive criticism using reflection based on the QSEN competencies

Language used in the clinical setting matters and shapes meaning and perspectives. Consider the these two examples reflecting family presence: "We allow 24-hour visitation" versus "We welcome you throughout the hospitalization." On the QSEN website, Altmiller posted examples of reframing constructive criticism based on the QSEN competencies (2010). Consider the shift in perspective from "Your patient needs attention now. You cannot leave him like that" to "If you were that patient lying in that bed, what would be the most important thing the nurse could do for you at this minute?"

When work is challenging, the problem may be identified as with the patient and family rather than a deficiency or gaps in the provider or system/organization (Neal, Twibell, Osborne, & Harris, 2010). A difficult IV placement may be communicated to a patient as "you have bad veins" versus "I am not skilled enough to place your IV." When family members fill a patient room, a nurse may say, "This is a crowd—too many people here" rather than "This room is too small to accommodate all those who care about you." Close examination of nursing language may reflect a provider rather than a patient perspective. Analysis and discussion of common language and the perspective it highlights can illustrate PFCC concepts.

Eliciting patient preferences and values

Nurses need to develop skill in listening and eliciting patient's values in order to ensure they are reflected in care. Elements of individual variation in communication styles include language fluency, health literacy, degree of directness, use of facial expressions and eye contact, touch, and use of silence. For oral communication: use of plain language; speak slowly; provide small amounts; reinforce with written materials with key points circled. A collaborative style builds from the patient perspective using an "Ask, Tell, Ask" and "Tell Me More" approach (Back et al., 2005).

Eight questions developed by Arthur Kleinman, a Harvard psychiatrist/anthropologist, offer an effective approach for nurses to elicit a patient's illness experience and beliefs. Known as "Kleinman's Questions," they are included in the TJC Roadmap (Kleinman, Eisenberg, & Good, 1978; TJC, 2010; see Textbox 4.2).

In Fadiman's (1997) book *The Spirit Catches You and You Fall Down*, in which a Hmong child is cared for in Western society with disastrous results, the questions are used to illustrate how eliciting the family's explanatory framework would have changed the patient outcome. If care is to reflect a patient's health beliefs and values, the ability to elicit those values is an essential competency for nurses.

Textbox 4.2   Kleinman's questions

Note. From "Culture, illness and care," by A. Kleinman, L. Eisenberg, and B. Good, 1978, *Annals of Internal Medicine, 88*, pp. 251-258.

1. What do you think has caused your problem?
2. Why do you think it started when it did?
3. What do you think your sickness does to you? How does it work?
4. How severe is your sickness? Will it have a short or a long course?
5. What kind of treatment do you think you should receive?
6. What are the most important results you hope to receive from this treatment?
7. What are the chief problems your sickness has caused for you?
8. What do you most fear from your sickness?

Conclusion

Patient-centered care is supported by many individuals, groups, and organizations, but it requires a paradigm shift. The care delivery system in the United States has been largely based on the premise that the health care provider is responsible for providing the care and knows best what works in each situation. There is momentum and support from many. Achievement requires all health care providers, administrators, and policy makers to recognize the patient-centered value of "nothing about me without me" and act accordingly (Delbanco et al., 2001).

References

Alexander, M., Lenahan, P. A., & Pavlov, A. (2005). *Cinemeducation: A comprehensive guide to using film in medical education.* Oxford: Radcliffe. 2005.

Altmiller, G. (2010). *Reframing constructive criticism using reflection based on QSEN competencies.* Retrieved from www.qsen.org

Back, A. I., Arnold, R. M., Baile, W. F., Tulsky, J. A., & Fryer-Edwards, K. (2005). Approaching difficult communication tasks in oncology. *CA: A Cancer Journal of Clinicians, 55,* 164-177.

Baggs, J. G., Norton, S. A., Schmitt, M. H., Dombeck, M. T., Sellers, C. R., & Quinn, J. R. (2007). Intensive care unit cultures and end-of-life decision making. *Journal of Critical Care, 22,* 159-168.

Balik, B., Conway, J., Zipperer, L., & Watson, J. (2011) *Achieving an exceptional patient and family experience of inpatient hospital care.* IHI Innovation Series white paper. Cambridge, Massachusetts: Institute for Healthcare Improvement (available on www.IHI.org).

Balint, E. (1969). The possibilities of patient-centered medicine. *Journal of Royal College of General Practitioners, 1,* 269-276.

Barton, A. J. (2010). Patient-centeredness and technology-enhanced care. *Clinical Nurse Specialist, 24,* 121-122.

Ber, R., & Alroy, G. (2001). Twenty years of experience using trigger films as a teaching tool. *Academic Medicine, 76,* 656-658.

Blasco, P. G., Moreto, G., Roncoletta, A., Levites, M. R., & Janaudis M. A. (2006). Using movie clips to foster learners' reflection: Improving education in the affective domain. *Family Medicine, 38,* 94-96.

Brien, L., Legault, A., & Tremblay, N. (2008). Affective learning in end-of-life care education: The experience of nurse educators and students. *The International Journal of Palliative Nursing, 14,* 610-614.

Brown, S. T., Kirkpatrick, M. K., Mangum, D., & Avery, J. (2008). A review of narrative pedagogy strategies to transform traditional nursing education. *Journal of Nursing Education, 47,* 283-286.

Cantor, M.D., Barach, P., Derse, A., Maklan, C. W., Wlody, G. S., & Fox, E. (2005). Disclosing adverse events to patients. *The Joint Commission Journal on Quality and Patient Safety, 31*(1), 5-12.

Cronenwett, L., Sherwood, G., Barnsteiner, J., Disch, J., Johnson, J., Mitchell, P., et al. (2007). Quality and safety education for nurses. *Nursing Outlook, 55,* 122-131.

Cronenwett, L., Sherwood, G., Pohl, J., Barnsteiner, Moore, S., Sullivan, D. T., et al. (2009). Quality and safety education for advanced practice nurses. *Nursing Outlook, 57,* 338-348.

Curtis, J. R., & White, D. B. (2008) Practical guidance for evidence-based ICU family conferences. *Chest, 134*(4), 835-843.

Daley, L. (1984). The perceived immediate needs of families with relatives in the intensive care setting. *Heart & Lung, 13,* 231-237.

Davidson, J. E., Powers, K., Hedayat, K. M., Tieszen, M., Kon, A. A., Shepard, E., et al. (2007). Clinical practice guidelines for support of the family in the patient-centered intensive care unit: American College of Critical Care Medicine Task Force 2004-2005. *Critical Care Medicine, 35*(2), 605-622.

Delbanco, T., Berwick, D. M., Boudfford, J. I., Edgman-Levitan, S., Ollenschlager, G., Plamping, D., & Rockefeller, R. G. (2001). Healthcare in a land called PeoplePower: Nothing about me without me. *Health Expectations, 4,* 144-150.

Department of Health and Human Services, Centers for Medicare and Medicaid Services. (2010, Nov. 19). Changes to the hospital and critical access hospital conditions of participation to ensure visitation rights for all patients (42 CFR Parts 482, 485). *Federal Register, 75*(223), 70831-70844.

Diekelmann, N. (2005). Engaging the students and the teacher: Co-creating substantive reform with narrative pedagogy. *Journal of Nursing Education, 44,* 249-252.

Disch, J. (2010). Patient-centered care. Enhancing quality and safety in nursing education: Preparing nurse faculty to lead curricular change (Vol. 1, Version 7A) [CDROM]. Quality and Safety Education for Nurses/American Association of Colleges of Nursing.

Duggan, P. S., Geller, G., Cooper, L. A., & Beach, M. C. (2006). The moral nature of patient-centeredness: Is it "just the right thing to do"? *Patient Education and Counseling, 62,* 271-276.

Emergency Nurses Association. (2009). *Emergency nursing resource: Family presence during invasive procedures and resuscitation in the emergency department.* Des Plaines, IL: Author. Retrieved from http://www.ena.org/Research/ENR/Documents/FamilyPresence.pdf

Ewing B., & Hayden-Miles, M. (2011). Narrative pedagogy and art interpretation. *Journal of Nursing Education, 50,* 211-215.

Fadiman, A. (1997). *The spirit catches you and you fall down*. New York: Farrar, Straus and Giroux.

Frampton, S. B. (2009). Creating a patient-centered system. *American Journal of Nursing, 109*, 30–33.

Frampton, S. B., & Guastello, S. (2010). Patient centered care: More than the sum of its parts. *American Journal of Nursing, 110*, 49–53.

Frampton, S., Guastello, S., Brady, C., Hale, M., Horowitz, S., Bennett Smith, S., & Stone S. (2008). *Patient-centered care improvement guide*. Derby, CT: Planetree; Camden, ME: Picker Institute. Available at http://www.patient-centeredcare.org/inside/practical.html#enviornment

Frampton, S. B., Wohl, C., & Cappiello, G. (2010). Partnering with patients' families: Three ways hospitals can enhance family members' involvement in health care. *American Journal of Nursing, 110*, 53–56.

Gazarian, P. K. (2010). Digital stories: Incorporating narrative pedagogy. *Journal of Nursing Education, 49*, 287–290.

Gerteis, M., Edgman-Levitan, S., Daley, J., & Delbanco, T. L. (1993). *Through the patient's eyes: Understanding and promoting patient-centered care*. San Francisco: Jossey-Bass.

Green Guidelines for Health Care. (2010). http://www.gghc.org

Halm, M. (2005). Family presence during resuscitation: A critical review of the literature. *American Journal of Critical Care, 14*(6), 494–511.

Henneman, E. A., & Cardin, S. (2002). Family-centered critical care: A practical approach to making it happen. *Critical Care Nurse, 22*(6), 12–19.

Hickey, M. L., & Leske, J. S. (1992). Needs of families of critically ill patients: State of the science and future directions. *Critical Care Nursing Clinics of North America, 4*, 645–649.

Howlett, M. S., Alexander, G. A., & Tsuchiya, B. (2010). Health care providers' attitudes regarding family presence during resuscitation of adults: An integrated review of the literature. *Clinical Nurse Specialist, 24*, 161–174.

Institute of Medicine. (2001). *Crossing the quality chasm: A new health system for the 21st century*. Washington, DC: National Academies Press.

Institute of Medicine. (2006). *Preventing medication errors*. Washington, DC: National Academies Press.

Institute of Medicine. (2011). *The future of nursing: Leading change, advancing health*. Washington, DC: National Academies Press.

Institute for Patient- and Family-Centered Care. (2010). *Changing hospital "visiting" policies and practices: Supporting family presence and participation*. Retrieved from www.ipfcc.org

Institute for Patient- and Family-Centered Care. (2011). *Partnering with patients and families to enhance safety and quality: A mini toolkit*. Retrieved from http://www.ipfcc.org/tools/Patient-Safety-Toolkit-04.pdf

Joint Commission. (2010). *Advancing effective communication, cultural competence, and patient-and family-centered care: A roadmap for hospitals*. Oakbrook Terrace, IL: Author.

Kleinman, A., Eisenberg, L., & Good, B. (1978). Culture, illness and care. *Annals of Internal Medicine, 88*, 251–258.

Koloroutis, M. (2004). Introduction. In M. Koloroutis (Ed.), *Relationship-based care: A model for transforming practice* (2nd ed.). Minneapolis, MN: Creative Health Care Management.

Kumagai, A. K. (2008). A conceptual framework for the use of illness narratives in medical education. *Academic Medicine, 83*(7), 653–658.

Leske, J. S. (1986). Needs of relatives of critically ill patients: A follow-up. *Heart & Lung, 15,* 189-193.

MacLean, S. L., Guzzetta, C. E., White, C., Fontaine, D., Eichhorn, D. J., Meyers, T. A., & Désy, P. (2003). Family presence during cardiopulmonary resuscitation and invasive procedures: Practices of critical care and emergency nurses. *American Journal of Critical Care, 12*(3), 246-257.

Mangurten, J. A., Scott, S. H., Guzzetta, C. E., Sperry, J. S., Vinson, L. A., Hicks, B. A., et al. (2005). Family presence: Making room. *American Journal of Nursing, 105*(5), 40-47.

McKeon, L. M, Norris, T., Cardell, B., & Britt, T. (2009). Developing patient-centered competencies among prelicensure nursing students using simulation. *Journal of Nursing Education, 48*(12), 711-715.

Michalak, J., Schreiner, N. J., Tennis, W., Szekely, L., Hale, M., & Guastello, S. (2010). The patient will see you now. *American Journal of Nursing, 110,* 61-63.

Molter, N. C. (1979). Needs of relatives of critically ill patients: A descriptive study. *Heart & Lung, 8,* 332-339.

Mundy, C. A. (2010). Assessment of family needs in neonatal intensive care units. *American Journal of Critical Care, 19*(2), 156-163.

Mutha, S., Allen, C., & Welch, M. (2002). *Toward culturally competent care: A toolbox for teaching communication skills.* San Francisco: Center for the Health Professions, University of California. Available at http://futurehealth.ucsf.edu/Public/Leadership-Programs/Program-Details.aspx?pid=155&pcid=88

National Priorities Partnership. (2008). *National priorities and goals: Aligning our efforts to transform America's healthcare.* Washington, DC: National Quality Forum.

National Priorities Partnership. (2010). *Patient & family engagement convening meeting synthesis report.* Retrieved from http://www.nationalprioritiespartnership.org/PriorityDetails.aspx?id=596

Neal, A., Twibell, R., Osborne, K. E., & Harris, D. (2010). Providing family-friendly care—even when stress is high and time is short. *American Nurse Today,* November.

Neumann, J. A., & Forsyth, D. (2008). Teaching in the affective domain for institutional values. *Journal of Continuing Education in Nursing, 39,* 248-254.

Planetree and the Picker Institute. (2008). *Patient-centered care improvement guide.* Retrieved from http://www.patient-centeredcare.org/inside/practical.html#environment.

Reid-Ponte, P. R., Conlin, G., Conway, J. B., Grant, S., Medeiros, C, Nies, J., et al. (2003). Making patient-centered care come alive: Achieving full integration of the patient's perspective. *Journal of Nursing Administration, 33*(2), 82-90.

Reiling, J., Hughes, R. G., & Murphy, M. R. (2008). The impact of facility design on patient safety. In *Patient safety and quality: An evidence-based handbook for nurses* (Prepared with support from the Robert Wood Johnson Foundation, AHRQ publication No. 08-0043). Rockville, MD: AHRQ.

Rossen, E. K. (2004). Media as a teaching tool in psychiatric nursing education. *Nurse Educator, 29*(1), 36-40.

Sadler, B. L., Berry, L. L., Guenther, R., Hamilton D. K., Hessler, A., Merritt, C., & Parker D. (2011). Fable hospital 2.0: The business care for building better health care facilities. *Hastings Center Report, 41,* 13-23.

Sakalys, J. A. (2002). Literary pedagogy in nursing: A theory-based perspective. *Journal of Nursing Education, 41,* 386-392.

Sakalys, J. A. (2003). Restoring the patient's voice: The therapeutics of illness narratives. *Journal of Holistic Nursing, 21,* 228-241.

Salmond, S. W. (2011). When a family member is a nurse: The role and needs of nurse family members during critical illness of a loved one. *Intensive and Critical Care Nursing, 27*10–2718.

Shattell, M. M. (2007) Engaging students and faculty with diverse first-person experiences: Use of an interpretive research group. *Journal of Nursing Education, 46*(12), 572–575.

Spath, P. L. (2008). *Engaging patients as safety partners*. Chicago: Health Forum.

Volandes, A. (2007). Medical ethics on film: toward the reconstruction of the teaching of healthcare professionals. *Journal of Medical Ethics, 33*, 678–680.

Wall, B. M., & Rossen, E. K. (2004) Media as a teaching tool in psychiatric nursing education. *Nurse Educator, 29*, 36–40.

Wasson, J. H., Godfrey, M. M., Nelson, E. C., Mohr, J. J., & Batalden, P.B. (2003). Microsystems in health care. Part 4: Planning patient-centered care. *The Joint Commission Journal on Quality and Patient Safety, 29*(5), 227–237.

White House Office of the Press Secretary. (2010, April 15). *Presidential memorandum for the Secretary of Health and Human Services: Hospital visitation*. Retrieved from http://www.whitehouse.gov/the-press-office/presidential-memorandum-hospital-visitation

Zarubi, K., Reiley, P., & McCarter, B. (2008). Putting patients and families at the center of care. *Journal of Nursing Administration, 38*(6), 275–281.

Resources

Centers for Medicare and Medicaid. www.cms.gov

Institute for Patient- and Family-Centered Care. www.ipfcc.org

Planetree. www.plantree.org

Picker Institute www.picker.org

Chapter 5

Teamwork and Collaboration

Joanne Disch, PhD, RN, FAAN

In 1998, the Institute of Medicine (IOM, 1998) alerted the public that 98,000 deaths were occurring annually, needlessly. In 2001, the IOM in its Ten New Rules for delivering safe, effective care stipulated that cooperation among clinicians is essential and, more specifically: "Clinicians and institutions should actively collaborate and communicate to ensure an appropriate exchange of information and coordination of care" (p. 9). As a result, in 2003, the IOM identified the five core competencies that are required for all health care professionals' education. Among them is the ability to work in interdisciplinary teams. This chapter will explore the competency on teamwork and collaboration, with the state of the science in this complex area, and offer suggestions for helping students and clinicians learn the knowledge, skills, and attitudes to prepare them for interprofessional practice.

Collaboration

Collaboration is the "process of joint decision making among independent parties involving joint ownership of decisions and collective responsibility for outcomes. The essence of collaboration involves working across professional boundaries" (Liedtka & Whitten, 1998, p. 185). The parties bring individual areas of expertise to a particular situation, as well as diverse perspectives that are influenced by professional orientation, experience, age, gender, education, and socioeconomic status. Conditions that enhance collaboration include shared goals, an understanding of the other's roles and responsibilities, mutual respect, clear communication, an openness to learning, and an ability to change one's viewpoint, given new information. Barriers to collaboration include persistent worldview differences (Baggs & Schmidt, 1997), professional autonomy (Shine, 2002) and inequitable power gradients (Roberts, 1997).

Quality and Safety in Nursing: A Competency Approach to Improving Outcomes, First Edition. Edited by Gwen Sherwood and Jane Barnsteiner.
© 2012 John Wiley & Sons, Inc. Published 2012 by John Wiley & Sons, Inc.

Nurse-physician collaboration

Nurse-physician collaboration is a historically important form of collaboration in health care. Baldwin (2007) asserts that the focus of nurse-physician collaboration started in World War II with multidisciplinary medical and surgical teams and expanded in the late President Lyndon B. Johnson's Great Society with the idea that the poor and underserved would be cared for by teams.

Fairman and Lynaugh (1998) in their landmark book on the early days of critical care noted the impact that each profession exerted on the development of the other:

> To gain expertise about the care of complex patients, nurses learned through experience and from physicians. Although many physicians were equally unskilled in the care of physically unstable patients, physicians provided much of nurses' postgraduate education through formal lectures and informal conversations. Nurses learned through slow periods in the intensive care area. During these times, residents (usually) and nurses in the intensive care unit discussed patients in detail, each learning from the other. When cardiac monitors were introduced at one hospital, a nurse remembered nurses and physicians grouped informally around the monitor screen in "pick-up" sessions. ... Unusually close camaraderie developed between nurses and physicians in the units because of the small areas, shared sense of adventure in the new setting, and the selection of the "expert nurses," usually young and "energetic," to staff the unit. "We [nurses and physicians] were all in this together," one nurse noted. "We all learned from each other" (p. 85).

While most health care professionals strongly believe in the merits of collaboration, relatively little definitive research has been done to connect interprofessional collaborative interventions with improved outcomes. For example, in the most recent Cochrane Review (Zwarenstein, Goldman, & Reeves, 2009), five studies were found that evaluated the effects of practice-based interventions occurring as a result of interprofessional collaboration. One is a study by Curley, McEachern, and Speroff (1998) retained from the first review (Zwarenstein & Bryant, 2000), while four are newly included (Schmidt, Claesson, Westerholm, Nilsson, & Svarstad, 1998; Wild, Nawaz, Chan, & Katz, 2004; Wilson, Marks, Collins, Warner, & Frick, 2004; Cheater, Hearnshaw, Baker, & Keane, 2005). The interventions were categorized as interprofessional rounds, interprofessional meetings, and an externally facilitated interprofessional audit. Three of the studies found improvements in key patient care outcomes, for example, drug use, length of stay and total hospital charges. One study described mixed outcomes and one showed no impact.

Although only five studies met the Cochrane criteria, hundreds of narratives and reports are available that examine the presence and impact of collaboration. Comprehensive reviews of the current status of research on collaboration between nurses and physicians (Jennings, Disch, & Senn, 2008), and team collaboration (O'Daniel & Rosenstein, 2008) can be found in the first edition of *Patient Safety and Quality: An Evidence-Based Handbook for Nurses* (Hughes, 2008).

The benefits of collaboration

Over the past 25 years, a growing body of research has been generated, supporting the belief that collaboration offers numerous benefits to patients (Baggs et al., 1992, 1999; Estabrooks, Midodzi, Cummings, Ricker, & Giovannetti, 2005; Knaus, Draper, Wagner, & Zimmerman, 1986), care providers (Boyle & Kochinda, 2004; Messmer, 2008), and the organizations in which care is provided (Cowan et al., 2006; Mohr, Burgess, & Young, 2008).

However, as important as most health care professionals believe collaboration to be, nurses and physicians do not similarly define it. For example, Makary and colleagues (2006) noted that nurses in the operating room described collaboration as having input into decision making, while physicians described it as having their needs anticipated and directions followed. Fletcher, Baker, Copeland, Reeves, and Lowery (2007) examined nurse practitioner and physician perceptions of the role of NPs as providers of primary care, noting that NPs saw their role as one of autonomous practice while physicians saw the role similar to a physician extender. Casanova and colleagues (2007, p. 69) noted that "physicians perceive themselves as the dominant authority in patient care while perceiving nursing's main function as carrying out orders" and that "collaboration is sometimes seen as undermining their [physicians] authoritarian role." Interestingly, in almost every study asking physicians and nurses of their perceptions about collaboration, physicians routinely report the perception of greater levels of collaboration than nurses (Carney, West, Neily, Mills, & Bagian, 2010; King & Lee, 1994; Mills, Neily, & Dunn, 2008; O'Leary et al., 2010; Rosenstein, 2002; Thomas, Sexton, & Helmreich, 2003).

It is predictable that nurses and physicians would approach collaboration from different viewpoints. They come from different cultures, use specialized languages, face different societal expectations, hold differing viewpoints and goals, and often define success very differently. Increasingly, intergenerational differences about motivation, work ethic, learning styles, authority relationships, and communication patterns are affecting the harmony of work teams. To some extent, the different views of collaboration occur because the concept is closely linked to a number of other concepts that share certain characteristics, for example, communication and teamwork, both of which are described below; collegiality (Feiger & Schmitt, 1979; Schmalenberg et al., 2005); trust (Liedtka & Whitten, 1998; Succi, Lee, & Alexander, 1998); and coordination (Knaus et al., 1986).

Communication

Communcation is "a process by which information is exchanged between individuals through a common system of symbols, signs, or behavior" (Merriam-Webster, 2009). While communication can occur verbally or nonverbally, it is widely accepted that effective communication is a precursor to collaboration. Disch (2009) identified 10 qualities or abilities of effective communicators: They are interested, open, purposeful, passionate, connect the dots, succinct, use compelling evidence, deliver a clear message, put themselves in the others' situations, and listen carefully (pick up cues) while they are communicating with their audiences.

Barriers to communication in health care are plentiful and arise from the different languages that professionals use among themselves and with patients and families; across gender, age, cultural and ethnic boundaries; and under conditions of stress that can be experienced by patients, families, and care providers. With the escalating pace of society today, forms of communication such as e-mail and text messaging add complexity and potential confusion to the exchange of vital information.

Poor communication has been identified as a major contributor to patient error: The Joint Commission (TJC; 2008) cited communication failures as the most frequently identified root cause of sentinel events reported to TJC between 1995 and 2008. In 2010, TJC noted that communication played a role in 661 of 802 sentinel events (TJC, 2011).

Teamwork

A particular form of collaboration occurs through teams. "Teamwork is a joint action by two or more people, in which each person contributes with different skills and expresses his or her individual interests and opinions to the unity and efficiency of the group in order to achieve common goals." (Wikipedia, 2011). For teamwork to be effective, all members must work toward a common goal and contribute their particular skills and abilities to its accomplishment.

Teams are the functional groups through which much of health care is delivered. However, Katzenbach and Smith (2005, p. 165) note that "people use the word 'team' so loosely that it gets in the way of learning and applying the discipline that leads to good performance." Teams differ in terms of their purpose, size, membership, experience, level of authority, history, and chemistry.

Interprofessional teams

For the most part, interdisciplinary teams are defined as individuals from at least two different disciplines who coordinate their expertise to deliver care to patients (Farrell, Schmitt, & Heinemann, 2001). Drinka and Clark (2000) extend this definition to note that interdisciplinary teams work together as an identified unit or system. Nelson and colleagues (2002) call this a *microsystem*:

[the] small, functional, front-line units that provide most health care to most people. They are the essential building blocks of larger organizations and of the health system. They are the place where patients and providers

meet. The quality and value of care produced by a large health system can be no better than the services generated by the small systems of which it is composed. (p. 473)

The terms *multidisciplinary* and *interdisciplinary* are often used interchangeably when two or more disciplines are involved. Schofield and Amodeo (1999) suggest that interdisciplinary infers interaction or collaboration. However, within academic health centers, *interdisciplinary* often refers to physicians who are from different specialties or disciplines within the profession of medicine, for example, cardiologists versus nephrologists. Internationally and in many parts of the United States, the term *interprofessional* is increasingly being used to emphasize the inclusion of individuals from different professions (Horder, 2004).

Four challenges in working as a member of a team in health care today are: (1) there are so many individuals involved; (2) each has a different scope of practice, which can result in overlap across the professions; (3) the composition of the team can often change due to factors such as 12-hour shifts, float staff, intern/resident/attending physician rotations; and (4) new roles are emerging at a fast pace. Ingersoll and Schmitt (2004) published a comprehensive summary of the linkages between interdisciplinary collaboration, team functioning, and patient safety.

The research on teams in health care

In *Keeping Patients Safe: Transforming the Work Environment of Nurses* (IOM, 2004), six integrative reviews of the literature regarding interdisciplinary teams and care delivery outcomes are highlighted. Studies that were incorporated into these reviews used different methods, examined different types of outcomes, and found mixed assessments of team effectiveness. In spite of the massive amount of work represented in these reviews, Schofield and Amodeo (1999) aptly sum up a conclusion drawn by many of the researchers: The team model is roundly endorsed but with little ability to evaluate its impact. Perhaps the wrong outcomes are being examined. A comprehensive project undertaken by the Rand Corporation, in collaboration with the Department of Defense and the Agency for Healthcare Research and Quality (AHRQ), identified patient safety or quality of care process and outcomes measures that are expected to be affected by health care team effectiveness (Sorbero, Farley, Mattke, & Lovejoy, 2008). Work is underway to test the relationships.

Building team performance

A number of success factors have been identified to enhance team performance (O'Daniel & Rosenstein, 2008). They include the following:

- Open communication
- Nonpunitive environment
- Clear direction

- Clear and known roles and tasks for team members
- Respectful atmosphere
- Shared responsibility for team success
- Appropriate balance of member participation in the task at hand
- Acknowledgement and processing of conflict
- Clear specifications regarding authority and accountability
- Clear and known decision-making procedures
- Regular and routine communication and information sharing
- Enabling environment, including access to needed resources
- Mechanism to evaluate outcomes and adjust accordingly

Salas and colleagues (2006, p. 440) suggest that we should be focusing on preparing expert teams rather than teams of experts, which has been the paradigm within the professions and across professions. They define an expert team as a "set of interdependent team members, each of whom possesses unique and expert-level knowledge, skills, and experience related to task performance, and who adapt, coordinate, and cooperate as a team, thereby producing sustainable and repeatable team functioning at superior or at least near-optimal levels of performance." Expert teams possess high levels of team and task outcomes, attained by using team member task-related expertise and skill with team processes.

Factors that compromise effective team performance

Several factors compromise the ability of a well-intentioned group of individuals to form an effective team, for example, *groupthink* (Janis, 1972), *excessive authority gradients* and *excessive professional courtesy* (Sasou & Reason, 1999), and *performance-shaping factors* (Sasou & Reason, 1999). These latter factors can be internal or personal to the individual (high stress, excessive fatigue, deficiencies in knowledge and skill), or external related to the work environment, and have drawn greater scrutiny with the growing body of evidence that is confirming their significant influence on the safety of patient care (Rogers, Hwang, Scott, Aiken, & Dinges, 2004; Samaha, Lal, Samaha, & Wyndham, 2007; Trinkoff, Geiger-Brown, Brady, Lipscomb, & Muntaner, 2006).

Disruptive behavior can also disrupt team performance (Barnsteiner, 2012; Rosenstein & O'Daniel, 2005; Rosenstein & O'Daniel, 2006) According to Porto (2009), disruptive behavior is

behavior that interferes with the ability of everyone on the team to provide safe and effective care; undermines the confidence of any member of the healthcare team in effectively caring for patients; undermines patients' confidence in the healthcare team or organization; causes concern for anyone's physical safety, and undermines effective teamwork.

It can take the form of verbal abuse (e.g., profane or disrespectful language, name-calling, failure to respond to concerns about safety, outbursts of anger) and physical (e.g., throwing objects, pushing). It can also be seen as intimidation and retaliation. Unfortunately, it's fairly common. Rosenstein (2002) noted that it was reported by 96% of nurses. However, nurses are not the only recipients of abusive behavior. Health care professionals in other professions also experience abusive behavior (Speedie, personal communication, 2006; Porto, 2009), and nurses can actually be the agents of abusive behavior with physicians, other nurses, and nursing students.

The Joint Commission has identified disruptive behavior as a major cause for concern and has issued a new leadership standard:

- EP 4–The hospital/organization has a code of conduct that defines acceptable and disruptive and inappropriate behaviors.
- EP 5–Leaders create and implement a process for managing disruptive and inappropriate behaviors.

Along with these standard statements, the Joint Commission (2008) has issued a number of suggested actions, including to educate all team members, establish a zero tolerance approach, and develop organizational processes for monitoring and reporting. In total, there are 11 recommendations, which can be accessed at http://www.jointcommission.org/sentinel_event_alert_issue_40_ behaviors_that_undermine_a_culture_of_safety/.

Increasingly, health care organizations and professional organizations are developing policies to address this issue, for example, Barnsteiner, Madigan, & Spray (2001) instituted a Disruptive Physician Conduct policy at the Children's Hospital of Philadelphia, and the American Association of Critical-Care Nurses (2005) issued its set of Standards for Establishing and Sustaining Healthy Work Environments.

Examples of programs for improving interprofessional team performance

One specific model for strengthening team effectiveness among professionals is Crew Resource Management (O'Daniel & Rosenstein, 2008). Used for years in the aviation and nuclear power industries, the concepts have been applied over the past few years to the health sector as a means of improving patient safety. Both the IOM and AHRQ have asserted that patient safety can be enhanced with this approach, although evidence has not been fully generated regarding its effectiveness. The training emphasizes six key areas: managing fatigue, creating and managing teams, recognizing adverse situations (red flags), cross-checking and communication, decision making, and performance feedback.

Two programs that have been particularly helpful within health care are TeamSTEPPS and Achieving Competence Today (Institute for Healthcare Improvement, 2011). Originally developed for work in the military, the TeamSTEPPS (Team Strategies and Tools to Enhance Performance and Patient Safety; Agency for Healthcare Research and Quality, 2011) principles have been adapted for use with physicians, nurses, and other health care providers to reduce clinical errors and improve patient outcomes and patient and staff satisfaction. Four key skill areas form the basis for training: leadership, situation monitoring, mutual support, and communication.

Achieving Competence Today (ACT)

This interdisciplinary teaching program focuses on quality, safety, and health systems improvement (Ladden, Bednash, Stevens, & Moore, 2006). The program is a self-directed, web-facilitated, action-learning curriculum for graduate students in the health care professions. It consists of four modules: the structure of health care and its impact on care delivery; payment of health care; quality improvement of individuals, populations, and practices; and improving personal and system performance.

While there is much support for this kind of training, evidence regarding its impact is mixed. One randomized trial of teamwork training in obstetrics wards did not demonstrate positive outcomes (a reduction in errors, or improved clinical outcomes; Nielsen et al., 2007), but a separate study, however, at a single institution with a similar intervention, was associated with a decrease in the frequency and severity of errors (Pratt et al., 2007). Weaver and colleagues (2010) found that a multilevel evaluation of the TeamSTEPPS training program in the OR demonstrated positive results with all levels. Salas and colleagues (2009) have identified several critical success factors for team training in health care:

1. Align team training objectives and safety aims with organizational goals
2. Provide organizational support for the team training initiative
3. Get frontline care leaders on board
4. Prepare the environment and trainees for team training
5. Determine required resources and time commitment and ensure their availability
6. Facilitate application of trained teamwork skills on the job
7. Measure the effectiveness of the team training program

The patient/family as a member of the team

While the competency of patient- and family- centered care is covered elsewhere in this text, (Walton & Barnsteiner, 2012), its linkage to teamwork and collaboration has to be asserted here. The relationship between patients and health care professionals is changing from totally caring *for* patients—and the health care professional making all health care decisions—to a full partnership *with* the patient, and family if that is the patient's wish, in identifying the problem, developing a plan, and evaluating the plan's success. For reasons of quality, safety, and consumer preference over the past 10 years, this relationship is shifting toward one of active involvement, even control, by the patient and family, which is requiring significant cultural and organizational change. The IOM in *Crossing the Quality Chasm* (2001, p. 40) defined patient-centered as "providing care that is respectful of and responsive to individual patient preferences, needs, and values and ensuring that patient values guide all clinical decisions." Thus, the IOM boldly redirected the orientation of the health care industry to one in which full patient engagement is an essential precursor to quality and safety, rather than merely an option.

The QSEN competency on teamwork and collaboration

In a survey of 629 schools of nursing from prelicensure programs, Smith, Cronenwett, and Sherwood (2007) found that 82% of programs indicated that they had content related to teamwork and collaboration (TWC), with 15% indicating that they had dedicated courses on the topic. Seventy-five percent of educators felt they were "expert/very comfortable" in teaching the content. However, once educator focus groups were asked to critique the knowledge, skills, and attitudes (KSAs) for TWC developed as part of the Quality and Safety Education for Nurses (QSEN) project, their reactions were markedly different:

> Although the faculty agreed that they should be teaching these competencies and, in fact, had thought they were, focus group participants did not understand fundamental concepts related to the competencies and could not identify pedagogical strategies in use for teaching the KSAs. An advisory board member led a focus group of new graduates. Not only did the nurses report that they did not have the learning experiences related to the KSAs, they did not believe their faculties had the expertise to teach the content. (Cronenwett et al., 2007, p. 122)

This finding was not isolated to teamwork and collaboration. In a similar vein, educators viewed that they comprehensively covered content on patient-centered care and safety. However, again, the content that had been covered did not reflect that identified with the QSEN competencies.

The prelicensure KSAs that were then developed for the competency on TWC as part of the QSEN project are listed in Appendix A. They reflect a progression from simple to complex, and from the individual to the team. Perhaps this competency more than the others requires joint experiential learning for successfully demonstrating certain KSAs. They are an excellent example of the need for a "both/and" approach: There are KSAs that must be addressed within the nursing curriculum, *and also* there are KSAs that require interprofessional effort and integrated learning.

Sequencing the content

Barton and colleagues from the University of Colorado (2009) conducted a web-based Delphi study to recommend sequencing of the KSAs for all six of the competencies when taught within prelicensure programs. Appendix C includes a recommended sequencing for the TWC KSAs.

Sequencing of the KSAs for TWC can also proceed from KSAs an individual must develop to those achieved through group learning. A precursor to becoming an effective team member and collaborating with others is possessing emotional intelligence, or the ability to identify, assess, and manage one's own emotions and the responses to them, as well as to assess and manage our relationships with others. Gardner (1993), one of the early thought leaders in this phenomenon, described *inter*personal intelligence as the ability to understand other people: "what motivates them, how they work, how to work cooperatively with them" and "*intra*personal intelligence … [as] a correlative ability, turned inward. It is a capacity to form an accurate, veridical model of oneself and to be able to use that model to operate effectively in life" (p. 9). More recently, Goleman (2001) offers a simpler definition: "The ability to recognize and regulate emotions in self and others" (p. 14). Kooker, Shoultz, and Codier (2007) assert that incorporating emotional intelligence concepts strengthens nurses' professional identify and may improve nurse retention and patient/client outcomes.

KSAs for TWC that could be developed through individual work include the following:

- Describe own strengths, limitations, and values in functioning as a member of a team
- Demonstrate awareness of own strengths and limitations as a team member
- Initiate plan for self-development as a team member
- Acknowledge own potential to contribute to effective team functioning
- Describe scopes of practice and roles of health care team members

Learning strategies for these KSAs could be enhanced through journaling, use of learning portfolios, dyadic feedback, and personal reflection (Disch, 2010).

Some of the learning can occur within *intra*professional groups, such as with other students or nurses. These KSAs include the following:

- Initiate requests for help when appropriate to the situation
- Describe impact of own communication style on others
- Discuss effective strategies for communicating and resolving conflict
- Initiate actions to resolve conflict

Conflict resolution

Conflict resolution is a good example of an activity that has both individual and group implications. Conflict can exist within a person, occur between two or more people, or within a large group of people who may or may not know each other. There can be actual confrontation, verbal expression, or a conflict that is unexpressed yet apparent through avoidance, denial, or nonverbal signs.

An inability to resolve disagreements among team members is a major impediment of effective team performance. Disagreements can involve minor disputes about an aspect of a particular plan or major conflicts related to the group's direction, performance, or functioning. Disagreements can also arise from different worldviews, or misperceptions. Given the differences cited earlier about characteristics of various health professionals, it is not surprising that one's health profession or role may be associated with a particular response to conflict. For example, Valentine (2001) found that nurses (staff nurses, nurse managers, and educators) used avoidance most often, with staff nurses accommodating, and nurse managers and educators compromising as their back-up responses. In a study by Hendel, Fish, and Berger (2007) of 75 physicians and 54 head nurses in five hospitals, they found that there was no difference between nurses and physicians in their choice of the most frequently used approach, the compromising mode. Collaboration was frequently used next by nurses, while least frequently by physicians.

Conflict can be addressed through avoidance, diffusion, or confrontation. *Conflict resolution* is a term that has evolved over the past 50 years, referring to a set of strategies employed to diffuse the conflict and, hopefully, satisfy the wishes of all parties involved. Formal negotiation processes to resolve the conflict are available, but in reality, since conflict or disagreements occur so frequently, this is impractical for daily use. In these situations, a simple process for handling conflict is necessary. Patterson, Grenny, McMillan, and Switzler (2005) and Grenny (2009) suggest that a framework of *crucial conversations* is helpful for "talking when the stakes are high." Crucial conversations are discussions that occur when (1) opinions vary, (2) the stakes are high, and/or (3) emotions run strong. Individual responsibility requires that the individual assesses his/her own comfort with conflict, what he/she might have contributed to the situation, and develop a respectful approach for addressing the conflict. The group work requires respectful communication, an openness to exploring differences, development of an acceptable plan of action, and turning conversation into action.

As part of the Joint Commission's most recent leadership standards, they have included the following: "The hospital manages conflict between leadership groups to protect the quality and safety of care" (Schyve, 2009). Scott and Gerardi (2011a, 2011b) describe the importance of transitioning from an approach of conflict avoidance to one of conflict engagement. To assist organizations in doing this, they outline the steps in developing a strategic approach to conflict management among boards of directors, senior management, and the leaders of the medical staff. They describe how this approach will have "ripple effects throughout the institution. Creating a process that models the type of conflict engagement that is supportive of safe patient care is a powerful means of improving conflict management at all levels of the organization" (2011b, p. 79).

Interprofessional education and practice

Given the importance of interprofessional collaboration in the health care delivery site, the need for educating tomorrow's professionals in this competency in new ways is tremendously important. For the most part, health care professionals have been educated in professional silos, although this is slowly changing. TWC was verbally advocated but rarely practiced. The IOM (2003) accelerated the pace of change when it declared that five competencies should be demonstrated by graduates of all health professions' schools, among them the ability to function effectively in interdisciplinary teams. Where formerly the goal for teamwork and collaboration was to work effectively with other health care professionals while performing nursing skills, the new definition offers a more dynamic vision: *To function effectively within nursing and interprofessional teams, fostering open communication, mutual respect, and shared decision making to achieve quality patient care.* The IOM report shaped the work of the nursing profession in its development of competencies for teamwork and collaboration for the prelicensure student (Cronenwett et al., 2007), as well as the graduate student (Cronenwett et al., 2009).

Interprofessional competencies

In May 2011, the Interprofessional Education Collaborative released an important complementary document: *Core Competencies for Interprofessional Collaborative Practice.* The Interprofessional Education Collaborative is a group of leaders from the American Association of Colleges of Nursing, the American Association of Colleges of Osteopathic Medicine, the American Association of Colleges of Pharmacy, the American Dental Education Association, the Association of American Medical Colleges, and the Association of Schools of Public Health. The document introduces a set of interprofessional collaborative competencies, with the intent of building on the strengths of the *intra*disciplinary work and creating a paradigm shift toward *interprofessional* education whereby students from different professions would learn with and from each other. The document also highlights the concept of *interprofessionality* drawn from the work of D'Amour and Oandasan (2005), who define interprofessionality as follows:

> The process by which professionals reflect on and develop ways of practicing that provides an integrated and cohesive answer to the needs of the client/family/population. ... It involves continuous interaction and knowledge sharing between professionals, organized to solve or explore a variety of education and care issues all while seeking to optimize the patient's participation. ... Interprofessionality requires a paradigm shift, since interprofessional practice has unique characteristics in terms of values, codes of conduct, and ways of working. (p. 9)

This concept clearly extends the intended outcome of interprofessional education to incorporate professional socialization.

Interprofessional education

Barnsteiner, Disch, Hall, Mayer, and Moore (2007) provide a comprehensive review of the history of interprofessional education and suggest six criteria for effective interprofessional education. These criteria are listed in Textbox 5.1.

For interprofessional education to be successful, educators from the schools or colleges involved must be jointly involved in planning and executing the learning; students must be experiencing the learning together; and the learning experiences must be embedded in the formal curricula, not voluntary or above their normal course loads. Offering opportunities for effective interprofessional education is challenging because of a number of very real factors: conflicting schedules among the schools, differing levels of clinical knowledge, preconceived ideas about other health professions, and educator priorities. However, when successfully offered, they can be transformative to the students' learning and professional socialization.

One misconception about interprofessional education is that it should involve, at a minimum, nursing and medical students. That may not be feasible if a university or college doesn't have a medical school. The important thing is to engage nursing students in learning with and about students from other disciplines and professions. For example, currently at the University of Minnesota School of Nursing, the collaborative venture with the largest scope (a grant totaling more than $50 million) is with the College of Veterinary Medicine where researchers from both entities, and with educators from other universities, are working together to examine the transmission of infectious diseases between humans and animals.

Textbox 5.1 Criteria for full engagement of interprofessional education (IPE)

1. Explicit philosophy of IPE that permeates the organization. The philosophy will be well-known, observable, measurable
2. Educators from the different professions cocreating the learning experiences
3. Students having integrated and experiential opportunities to learn collaboration, teamwork, and how it relates to the delivery of safe, quality care delivery
4. IPE learning experiences embedded in the curricula and part of the required caseload for students
5. Demonstrated competence by students with a single set of interprofessional competencies such as those promoted by the Institute of Medicine
6. Organizational infrastructure that fosters IPE, such as support for educator time to develop IPE options, incentive systems for educators to engage in IPE, and integrated activities across schools and professions for students and educators

From "Promoting Interprofessional Collaboration," by J. H. Barnsteiner, J. M. Disch, L. Hall, D. Mayer, and S. Moore, S., 2007, *Nursing Outlook*, *55*, pp. 144-150. Reprinted with permission from Elsevier Ltd.

Thoughts about the best time for introducing the interprofessional content vary. On the one hand, there is some evidence that students enter medical school with preconceived ideas about nurses and physicians, so that introducing interprofessional education early and acknowledging the stereotypes may be helpful (Rudland & Mires, 2005). On the other hand, some educators are concerned that socialization to one's own profession has to be sufficiently underway so that students are able to contribute effectively as a member of an interprofessional team.

Strategies for learning TWC

Participating in shared learning experiences

- Educators can assign an interprofessional cohort of students throughout the length of their educational programs to a multigenerational family to follow their changes in health status and experiences with the health care system.
- Educators in two or more schools or colleges can jointly develop and conduct a course by educators in at least two health professions' schools on a topic of mutual relevance, for example, ethics or health economics. Nursing educators at Grand Valley State University are taking the lead, working with educators from physical therapy, occupational therapy, speech, and the physician assistants' program, in developing a course titled Building Relationships Across Interprofessional Domains (BRAID).
- Les Hall, MD, and colleagues at the University of Missouri, offer a course designed to be used with health professional students of all types who are brought together to review a health care incident in which an adverse event occurred. After one introductory session, all further work in this curriculum is conducted in interprofessional small groups.
- Students can be offered the choice of reading a book about health care, such as *The Spirit Catches You and You Fall Down* (Fadiman, 1997) and conducting a book review and reflection with an interprofessional group of students.
- CLARION is a student organization that originated at the University of Minnesota through its Center for Health Interprofessional Programs (2010), and is dedicated to improving health care through interprofessional collaboration. A national organization since 2005, it promotes local student case competitions for health professional students, enabling them to achieve a 360-degree perspective on patient safety in today's health care system and how it might be improved. Student teams, consisting of four students, comprising at least two disciplines, are given a case and are charged with creating a root cause analysis. The team presents their analysis to a panel of interprofessional judges that evaluates their analysis in the context of real world standards of practice. Local winners advance to the national competition. The center's website also offers numerous other suggestions for engaging students in interprofessional activities (www.chip.umn.edu).

Participating in shared service experiences

- The Philips Neighborhood Clinic (www.phillips.neighborhoodclinic.com) is a student-run community clinic that provides accessible, culturally appropriate, interdisciplincary health care services and education to health professional students on the skills they need to effectively and compassionately serve people who are underinsured and/or unstably housed.
- The Immunization Tour is a partnership between the nursing and pharmacy schools at the University of Minnesota to plan and implement a mass immunization clinic for the campus during flu season. Engaging approximately 60 students in four interprofessional teams, they administer approximately 4,500 doses of vaccine. Students learn leadership principles, organization, giving injections, teamwork, and collaboration (Univ. of Minnesota Office of Student Affairs, 2011).

Practicing communication

- *SBAR (situation, background, assessment, and recommendation)*. This tool offers a framework for clearly, consistently, and succinctly communicating pertinent information among health care professionals. Developed at Kaiser Permanente in Denver (Leonard, Graham, & Bonacum, 2004), the tool structures communication and helps clinicians respond to situations with a shared mental model. Haig, Sutton, and Whittington (2006) describe its implementation at OSF St. Joseph Medical Center in Bloomington, Illinois, providing helpful tools and a handoff form to assist in its use.
- *Practicing a handoff*. This is a time when information is transferred, along with authority and responsibility, during transitions in care across the continuum and includes an opportunity to ask questions, clarify, and confirm responses. Examples include shift changes, physicians transferring off from a patient's care, and patient transfers to other facilities; or a *call-out* to communicate important or critical information, for example, during resuscitations; or a *check-back*, using closed-loop communication to ensure that information conveyed by the sender is understood by the receiver as intended. Verbal orders are a situation when check-backs are helpful.
- *Role-playing actual situations that have occurred or simulating new ones*. The increasing use of high-fidelity simulation offers extremely rich learning experiences, but the lack of expensive equipment doesn't preclude this from being an effective tool. According to Ironside, Jeffries, and Martin (2009), what's needed is active and diverse learning, feedback, student/educator interaction, collaboration, and high expectations. Role-playing shouldn't be reserved only for use with patients and families. Helping students effectively communicate with physicians and nurses in simulated work encounters is critically important. An exercise used at the University of Missouri by Hall (2007) takes the learner through a simulated conversation between a nurse and a physician regarding a patient who is deteriorating. The nurse is challenged to find effective means of assertively yet

professionally escalating the dialogue on behalf of a patient whose condition does not allow for delay.

The QSEN website (www.qsen.org) offers dozens of learning experiences that relate to teamwork, collaboration, and the other competencies. Similarly, the AHRQ website provides several guides and a resource kit for the TeamSTEPPS program, and the Institute for Healthcare Improvement website offers modules for interprofessional learning (http://www.ihi.org/IHI/Programs/IHIOpenSchool/). Also, Finkelman and Kenner (2009) have developed a very helpful resource text, *Teaching IOM*.

Conclusion

Serving as a member of a dynamic, effective team is a rewarding experience that can enrich one's own personal and professional life, as well as enhance the work of a group and, in the case of health care, save lives. Given the complexity of the health care environment and the threats to patient safety and quality care, collaboration with other members of the health care team is vital. Cooke, Salas, Cannon-Bowers, and Stout (2000, p. 151) pointed out the obvious: "The growing complexity of tasks frequently surpasses the cognitive capabilities of individuals and, thus, necessitates a team approach."

In addition to the numerous national organizations promoting teamwork and collaboration today, international organizations are also developing initiatives to advance interprofessional education, among them the Centre for the Advancement of Interprofessional Education, the Health Resources and Services Administration, and the World Health Organization (Newhouse & Spring, 2010). The direction is clear: Interprofessional practice and education form the basis for safe, quality patient care for all.

References

Agency for Healthcare Research and Quality. (2009). *TeamSTEPPS*. Retrieved from http://teamstepps.ahrq.gov/

American Association of Critical-Care Nurses. (2005). *AACN standards for establishing and sustaining healthy work environments: A journey to excellence*. Aliso Viejo, CA: Author.

Baggs, J. G., Ryan, S. A., Phelps, C. E., Richeson, J. F., & Johnson, J. E. (1992). The association between interdisciplinary collaboration and patient outcomes in medical intensive care. *Heart & Lung, 21*, 18-24.

Baggs, J. G., & Schmitt, M. H. (1997). Nurses' and resident physicians' perceptions of the process of collaboration in a MICU. *Research in Nursing & Health, 20*, 71-80.

Baggs, J. G., Schmitt, M. H., Mushlin, A. I., Mitchell, P. H., Eldredge, D. H., Oakes, D., et al. Hutson, A. D. (1999). Association between nurse-physician collaboration and patient outcomes in three intensive care units. *Critical Care Medicine, 27*(9), 1991-1998.

Baldwin, D. C. (2007). Some historical notes on interdisciplinary and interprofessional education and practice in health care in the USA. *Journal of Interprofessional Care, 21*(SI), 23-37.

Barnsteiner, J. H., Disch, J. M., Hall, L., Mayer D, & Moore, S. (2007). Promoting interprofessional collaboration. *Nursing Outlook*, *55*(3), 144-150.

Barnsteiner, J. H., Madigan, K., & Spray, T. L. (2001). Instituting a disruptive conduct policy for medical staff. *AACN Clinical Issues*, *12*, 378-382.

Barnsteiner, J. (2012). Workplace abuse in nursing: Policy strategies. In D. Mason, J. K. Leavitt, & M. W. Chafee (Eds), *Politics and policy in nursing and health care*, 6th ed., St. Louis, MO: Elsevier.

Barton, A., Armstrong, G., Preheim, G., Gelman, S. B., & Andrus, L. C. (2009). A national Delphi to determine developmental progression of quality and safety competencies in nursing education. *Nursing Outlook*, *57*, 313-322.

Boyle, D., & Kochinda, C. (2004). Enhancing collaborative communication of nurse and physician leadership in two intensive care units. *Journal of Nursing Administration*, 34(2), 60-70.

Carney, B. T., West, P., Neily, J., Mills, P. D., & Bagian, J. P. (2010). Differences in nurse and surgeon perceptions of teamwork: Implications for use of a briefing checklist in the OR. *AORN Journal*, *91*(6), 722-729.

Casanova, J., Day, K., Dorpat, D., Hendricks, B., Theis, L., & Weisman, S. (2007). Nurse-physician relations and role expectations. *Journal of Nursing Administration*, *37*(2), 68-70.

Center for Health Interprofessional Programs. (2010). Retrieved from http://www.chip.umn.edu/clarion/home.html

Cheater, F. M., Hearnshaw, H., Baker, R., & Keane, M. (2005). Can a facilitated programme promote effective multidisciplinary audit in secondary care teams? An exploratory trial. *International Journal of Nursing Studies*, *42*, 779-791.

Cooke, N. J., Salas, E., Cannon-Bowers, J. A., & Stout, R. J. (2000). Measuring team knowledge. *Human Factors*, *42*, 151-173.

Cowan, M. J., Shapiro, M., Hays, R. D., Afifi, A., Vazirani, S.,Ward, C. R., et al. (2006). The effect of a multidisciplinary hospitalist/physician and advanced practice nurse collaboration on hospital costs. *Journal of Nursing Administration*, *36*(2), 79-85.

Cronenwett, L., Sherwood, G., Barnsteiner, J., Disch, J., Johnson, J., Mitchel, P., et al. (2007). Quality and safety education for nurses. *Nursing Outlook*, *55*(3), 122-131.

Cronenwett, L., Sherwood, G., Pohl, J., Barnsteiner, J., Moore, S., Sullivan, D. T., et al. (2009). Quality and safety education for advanced nursing practice. *Nursing Outlook*, *57*(6), 338-348.

Curley, C., McEachern, J. E., Speroff, T. (1998). A firm trial of interdisciplinary rounds on the inpatient medical wards. *Medical Care*, *36*(8, Supplement), AS4-AS12.

D'Amour, D., & Oandasan, I. (2005). Interprofessionality as the field of interprofessional practice and interprofessional education: An emerging concept. *Journal of Interprofessional Care*, *19* (Supplement 1), 8-20.

Disch, J. (2009). Developing leadership skills for today. AJN Advancing Excellence in Nursing Practice Conference October 4. Chicago, IL: American Journal of Nursing.

Disch, J. (2010). Teamwork and collaboration. Enhancing quality and safety in nursing education: Preparing nurse faculty to lead curricular change (Vol. 1, Version 7A) [CDROM]. Quality and Safety Education for Nurses/American Association of Colleges of Nursing.

Drinka, T., Clark, P. J. (2000). *Healthcare teamwork: Interdisciplinary practice and teaching*. Westport, CT: Auburn House.

Estabrooks, C. A., Midodzi, W. K., Cummings, G. G., Ricker, K. L., & Giovannetti P. (2005). The impact of hospital nursing characteristics on 30-day mortality. *Nursing Research, 54*(2), 74–84.

Fadiman, A. (1997). *The spirit catches you and you fall down*. New York: Farrar, Straus and Giroux.

Fairman, J., & Lynaugh, J. (1998). *Critical care nursing: A history*. Philadelphia: University of Pennsylvania Press.

Farrell, M., Schmitt, M., & Heinemann, G. D. (2001). Informal roles and the stages of interdisciplinary team development. *Journal of Interprofessional Care, 15*, 281–293.

Feiger, S. M., & Schmitt, M. H. (1979). Collegiality in interdisciplinary health teams: Its measurement and its effects. *Social Science and Medicine, 31A*, 217–229.

Finkelman, A., & Kenner, C. (2009). *Teaching IOM*. Silver Spring, MD: American Nurses Association.

Fletcher, C. E., Baker, S. J., Copeland, L. A., Reeves, P. J., & Lowery, J. C. (2007). Nurse practitioners and physicians' views of NPs as providers of primary care to veterans. *Journal of Nursing Scholarship, 39*(4), 358–362.

Gardner, H. (1993). *Multiple intelligences: The theory in practice*. New York: Basic Books.

Goleman, D. (2001). Issues in paradigm building. In C. Cherniss & D. Goleman (Eds.), *The emotionally intelligent workplace: How to select for, measure, and improve emotional intelligence in individuals, groups, and organizations*. San Francisco: Jossey-Bass.

Grenny, J. (2009). Crucial conversations: The most potent force for eliminating disruptive behavior. *Health Care Manager, 28*(3), 240–245.

Haig, K. M., Sutton, S., & Whittington, J. (2006). SBAR: A shared mental model for improving communication between clinicians. *Journal on Quality & Patient Safety, 32*(3), 167–175.

Hall L. (2007). Nurse-physician communication exercise. Retrieved from http://www.qsen.org/search_strategies.php?id=50)

Hendel, T., Fish, M., & Berger, O. (2007). Nurse/physician conflict management mode choices: Implications for improved collaborative practice. *Nursing Administration Quarterly, 31*(3), 244–254.

Horder, J. (2004). Interprofessional collaboration and interprofessional education. *British Journal of General Practice, 54*, 243–245.

Hughes, R. G. (Ed.). (2008). *Patient safety and quality: An evidence-based handbook for nurses* (Prepared with support from the Robert Wood Johnson Foundation). AHRQ Publication No. 08-0043. Rockville, MD: Agency for Healthcare Research and Quality.

Ingersoll, G. L., & Schmitt, M. (2004). Interdisciplinary collaboration, team functioning and patient safety. In IOM's *Keeping patients safe: Transforming the work environment of nurses* (pp. 341–383). Washington, DC: National Academies Press.

Interprofessional Education Collaborative Expert Panel. (2011). *Core competencies for interprofessional collaborative practice: Report of an expert panel*. Washington, DC: Interprofessional Education Collaborative.

Institute for Healthcare Improvement. (2011). *Achieving competence today*. Retrieved from http://www.ihi.org/IHI/Programs/IHIOpenSchool/TeachingResourceACT.htm?tabId=0

Institute of Medicine. (1998). *To err is human*. Washington, DC: National Academies Press.

Institute of Medicine. (2001). *Crossing the quality chasm: A new health system for the 21st century*. Washington, DC: National Academies Press.

Institute of Medicine. (2003). *Health professions education: A bridge to quality*. Washington, DC: National Academies Press.

Institute of Medicine. (2004). *Keeping patients safe: Transforming the work environment of nurses*. Washington, DC: National Academies Press.

Ironside, P., Jeffries, P. R., & Martin, A. (2009). Fostering patient safety competencies using multiple-patient simulation experiences. *Nursing Outlook, 6*, 332–337.

Janis, I. L. (1982). *Groupthink* (2nd ed.). Boston: Houghton-Mifflin.

Jennings, B. M., Disch, J., & Senn, L. (2008). Leadership. In R. Hughes (Ed.), *Patient safety and quality: An evidence-based handbook for nurses* (Prepared with support from the Robert Wood Johnson Foundation). AHRQ Publication No. 08-0043. Rockville, MD: Agency for Healthcare Research and Quality.

Joint Commission. (2008). Causes of errors and sentinel events. Retrieved from http://www.jointcommission.org/SentinelEventsData

Joint Commission. (2011). Retrieved from http://www.jointcommission.org/Sentinel_Event_Statistics/

Katzenbach, J. R., & Smith, D. K. (2005, July/August). The discipline of teams. *Harvard Business Review*, 162–171.

King, L., & Lee, J. L. (1994). Perceptions of collaborative practice between Navy nurses and physicians in the ICU setting. *American Journal of Critical Care, 3*(5), 331–336.

Knaus, W. A., Draper, E. A., Wagner, D. P., & Zimmerman, J. E. (1986). An evaluation of outcomes from intensive care in major medical centers. *Annals of Internal Medicine, 104*, 410–418.

Kooker, B. M., Shoultz, J., & Codier, E. E. (2007). Identifying emotional intelligence in professional nursing practice. *Journal of Professional Nursing, 23*(1), 30–36.

Ladden, M., Bednash, G., Stevens, D., & Moore, G. T. (2006). Educating interprofessional learners for quality, safety, and systems improvement. *Journal of Interprofessional Care, 20*(5), 497–505.

Leonard, M., Graham, S., & Bonacum, D. (2004). The human factor: The critical importance of effective teamwork and communication in providing safe care. *Quality and Safety in Health Care, 13*(Supp. 1), 185–190.

Liedtka, J. M., & Whitten E. (1998). Enhancing care delivery through cross-disciplinary collaboration: A case study. *Journal of Healthcare Management, 43*(2), 185–205.

Makary, M. A., Sexton, J. B., Freischlag, J. A., Holzmueller, C. G., Millman, E. A., Rowen, L., et al. (2006). Operating room teamwork among physicians and nurses: Teamwork in the eye of the beholder. *Journal of the American College of Surgeons, 202*(5), 746–752.

Merriam-Webster (2009). Communication. Retrieved from http://www.merriam-webster.com/dictionary/communication

Messmer, P. R. (2008). Enhancing nurse-physician collaboration using pediatric simulation. *Journal of Continuing Education in Nursing, 39*(7), 319–327.

Mills, P., Neily, J., & Dunn, E. (2008). Teamwork and collaboration in surgical teams: Implications for patient safety. *Journal of the American College of Surgeons, 206*(1), 107–112.

Mohr, D. C., Burgess, J. F., & Young, G. J. (2008). The influence of teamwork culture on physician and nurse resignation rates in hospitals. *Health Services Management Research, 21*(1), 23–31.

Nelson, E. N., Batalden, P. B., Huber, T. P., Mohr, J. J., Godfrey, M. M., Headrick, L. A., et al. Wasson, J. H. (2002). Microsystems in health care: Part I. Learning from high-performing front-line clinical units. *Joint Commission Journal on Quality Improvement, 28*(9), 472–497.

Newhouse, R. P., & Spring, B. (2010). Interdisciplinary evidence-based practice: Moving from silos to synergy. *Nursing Outlook, 58*(6), 309–317.

Nielsen, P. E., Goldman, M. B., Mann, S., Shapiro, D. E., Marcus, R. G., Pratt, S. D., et al. (2007). Effects of teamwork training on adverse outcomes and process of care in labor and delivery: A randomized control trial. *Obstetrics and Gynecology, 109*, 48–55.

O'Daniel, M., & Rosenstein, A. H. (2008). Professional communication and team collaboration. In R. Hughes (Ed.), *Patient safety and quality: An evidence-based handbook for nurses* (Prepared with support from the Robert Wood Johnson Foundation). AHRQ Publication No. 08-0043. Rockville, MD: Agency for Healthcare Research and Quality.

O'Leary, K. J., Ritter, C. D., Wheeler, H., Szekendi, M. K., Brinton, T. S., & Williams, M. V. (2010). Teamwork on inpatient medical units: Assessing attitudes and barriers. *Quality and Safety in Health Care, 19*, 117–121.

Patterson, K., Grenny, J., McMillan, R., & Switzler, A. (2005). *Crucial confrontations: Tools for resolving broken promises, violated expectations, and bad behavior.* New York: McGraw Hill.

Porto, G. (2009). *Disruptive clinician behavior: How it affects your patients and you.* Presentation at the 6th National Patient Safety Conference. Philadelphia: University of Pennsylvania School of Nursing.

Pratt, S. D., Mann, S., Salisbury, M., Greenberg, P., Marcus, R., Stabile, B., et al. (2007). Impact of CRM-based team training on obstetric outcomes and clinicians' patient safety attitudes. *Joint Commission Journal on Quality and Patient Safety, 33*, 720–725.

Roberts, K. H. (1997). The Challenger launch decision: Risky technology, culture and deviance at NASA. *Administrative Science Quarterly, 42*, 405–410.

Rogers, A. E., Hwang, W., Scott, L. D., Aiken, L. H., & Dinges, D. F. (2004). The working hours of hospital staff nurses and patient safety. *Health Affairs, 23*(4), 202–212.

Rosenstein, A. H. (2002). Nurse-physician relationships: Impact on nurse satisfaction and retention. *American Journal of Nursing, 102*(6), 26–34.

Rosenstein, A. H., & O'Daniel, M. (2005). Disruptive behavior and clinical outcomes: Perceptions of nurses and physicians. *American Journal of Nursing, 105*(1), 54–64.

Rosenstein, A. H., & O'Daniel, M. (2006). Addressing disruptive nurse-physician behaviors: Developing programs and policies to improve outcomes of care. *Harvard Health Policy Review, 7*, 86–91.

Rudland, J. R., & Mires, G. J. (2005). Characteristics of doctors and nurses as perceived by students entering medical school: Implications for shared teaching. *Medical Education, 39*, 448–455.

Salas, E., Almeida, S. A., Salisbury, M., King, H., Lazzara, E. H., Lyons, R., et al. (2009). What are the critical success factors for team training in health care? *Joint Commission Journal on Quality and Patient Safety, 35*(8), 398–405.

Salas, E., Rosen, M. A., Burke, C., Rosen, M. A., Burke, S. C., Goodwin, G. F., & Fiore, S. M. (2006). The making of a dream team: When expert teams do test. In K. A. Ericsson, N. Charness, P. J. Feltovish, & R. R. Hoffman (Eds.), *The Cambridge handbook of expertise and expert performance* (pp. 439–453). New York: Cambridge University Press.

Samaha, E., Lal, S., Samaha, N., & Wyndham, J. (2007). Psychological, lifestyle and coping contributors to chronic fatigue in shift-worker nurses. *Journal of Advanced Nursing, 59*(3), 221–232.

Sasou, K., Reason, J. (1999). Team errors: Definition and taxonomy. *Reliability engineering and system safety*, *65*, 1–9.

Schmalenberg, C., Kramer, M., King, C. R., Krugman, M., Lund, C., Poduska, D., & Rapp, D. (2005). Excellence through evidence: Securing collegial, collaborative nurse-physician relationships, Part 1. *Journal of Nursing Administration, 35*(10), 450–458.

Schmidt, I., Claesson, C. B., Westerholm, B., Nilsson, L. G., & Svarstad, B. L. (1998). The impact of regular multidisciplinary team interventions on psychotropic prescribing in Swedish nursing homes. *Journal of the American Gerontological Society*, *46*(1), 77–82.

Schofield, R. F., & Amodeo M. (1999). Interdisciplinary teams in heath care and human services settings: Are they effective? *Health & Social Work*, *24*, 210–219.

Schyve P (2009). *Leadership in healthcare organizations*: *A guide to Joint Commission leadership standards*. San Diego, CA: Governance Institute. Retrieved from http://www.jointcommission.org/assets/1/18/WP_Leadership_Standards.pdf

Scott, C., & Gerardi, D. (2011a). A strategic approach for managing conflict in hospitals: Responding to the Joint Commission leadership standard, Part 1. *Joint Commission Journal on Quality and Patient Safety, 37*(2), 59–69.

Scott, C., & Gerardi, D. (2011b). A strategic approach for managing conflict in hospitals: Responding to the Joint Commission leadership standard, Part 2. *Joint Commission Journal on Quality and Patient Safety, 37*(2), 70–80.

Shine, K. I. (2002). Health care quality and how to achieve it. *Academic Medicine*, *77*, 91–99.

Smith, E. L., Cronenwett, L., & Sherwood, G. (2007). Current assessments of quality and safety education in nursing. *Nursing Outlook*, *55*(3), 132–137.

Sorbero, M. E., Farley, D. O., Mattke, S., & Lovejoy, S. (2008). Outcome measures for effective teamwork in inpatient care (Project supported by the Agency for Healthcare Research and Quality and the Department of Defense, contract #290-02-0010). Santa Monica, CA: Rand.

Succi, M. J., Lee, S. D., & Alexander, J. A. (1998). Trust between managers and physicians in community hospitals: The effects of power over hospital decisions. *Journal of Healthcare Management; 43*(5), 397–414.

Thomas, E. J., Sexton, J. B., & Helmreich, R. L. (2003). Discrepant attitudes about teamwork among critical care nurses and physicians. *Critical Care Medicine*, *31*(3), 956–959.

Trinkoff, A., Geiger-Brown, J., Brady, B., Lipscomb, J., & Muntaner, C. (2006). How long and how much are nurses now working? *American Journal of Nursing*, *106*(4), 60–71.

University of Minnesota Office of Student Affairs (2011). Immunization Tour. Retrieved from http://www.osa.umn.edu/documents/Issue42.html

Valentine, P.E.B. (2001). A gender perspective on conflict management: Strategies of nurses. *Journal of Nursing Scholarship*, *33*, 69–74.

Walton, M. K., & Barnsteiner, J. (2012). Patient-centered care. In G. Sherwood & J. Barnsteiner (Eds.), *Quality and safety in nursing: A competency approach to improving outcomes*. Hoboken, NJ: Wiley-Blackwell.

Weaver, S. J., Rosen, M. A., DiazGranados, D., Lazzara, E. H., Lyons, R., Salas, E., et al. (2010). Does teamwork improve performance in the operating room? A multilevel evaluation. *Joint Commission Journal on Quality and Patient Safety*, *36*(3), 133–142.

Wikipedia. (2011). Teamwork. Retrieved from http://wiki.answers.com/Q/What_is_the_definition_of_'teamwork'/

Wild, D., Nawaz, H., Chan, W., & Katz, D. L. (2004). Effects of interdisciplinary rounds on length of stay in a telemetry unit. *Journal of Public Health Management and Practice*, *10*(1), 63–69.

Wilson, S. F., Marks, R., Collins, N., Warner, B., & Frick, L. (2004). Benefits of multidisciplinary case conferencing using audiovisual compared with telephone communication: A randomized controlled trial. *Journal of Telemedicine and Telecare*, *10*, 351–354.

Zwarenstein, M., & Bryant, W. (2000). Interventions to promote collaboration between nurses and doctors (Review). *The Cochrane Database of Systematic Reviews*, Issue 2. Art. no. CD000072. doi: 10.1002/14651858.CD000072.

Zwarenstein, M., Goldman, J., & Reeves, S. (2009). Interprofessional collaboration: Effects of practice-based interventions on professional practice and healthcare outcomes. *Cochrane Database of Systematic Reviews*, Issue 3. Art. no. CD000072. doi: 10.1002/14651858.CD000072.

Chapter 6
Quality Improvement
Jean Johnson, PhD, RN, FAAN

Background of quality improvement

The need for quality improvement

As the profession comprising the largest percentage of the health care work-force in the United States, nursing seems the obvious choice when it comes to determining the cornerstone upon which health care quality improvement efforts should be built. Who better to lead the effort to improve health care delivery and outcomes than the professionals delivering the majority of health care in America? However, nurses have not led the charge on improving care during the past 50 years, and as a result, limited progress has been made. A study of hospitals in Colorado finds that from 2006 to 2008, the same number of patients died each year as a result of medical errors, similar to the findings of the Institute of Medicine studies of a decade ago (Institute of Medicine, 1999, 2001; Landrigan et al., 2010). In order to be a major force that makes a difference in the lives of millions of patients, nurses need to have the tools to measure the quality of care that they provide as well as the skills to create and implement change that will make a difference. Providing nurses with these skills and tools will offer new opportunities for success in improving health care quality and outcomes.

Quality improvement as defined by the Quality and Safety Education for Nurses project is the "use of data to monitor the outcomes of care processes and use improvement methods to design and test changes to continuously improve the quality and safety of health care systems" (Cronenwett et al., 2007). To improve care, nurses must first know how well they are doing. Data reflecting the important elements of care is the only credible way of demonstrating the quality of care nurses provide. Thus, it is essential that nurses be taught a systematic process of defining problems, identifying potential causes of those problems, and methods for testing possible solutions to improve care.

Quality and Safety in Nursing: A Competency Approach to Improving Outcomes,
First Edition. Edited by Gwen Sherwood and Jane Barnsteiner.
© 2012 John Wiley & Sons, Inc. Published 2012 by John Wiley & Sons, Inc.

Leadership in quality by Florence Nightingale

To understand the pressing need for nurses to spearhead health care quality improvement efforts, it is important to first understand the historical context surrounding the role of nurses in quality improvement efforts. Quality improvement is a relatively new concept that has its roots in the 1800s. What we now consider to be health care quality improvement grew from seeds initially planted in the nascent years of evidence-based medicine and epidemiology. Pierre-Charles-Alexandre Louis' 1835 research on the effects of bloodletting employed quantitative measures to evaluate the effects of bloodletting on patient outcomes (Morabia, 2006). However, it was Florence Nightingale who first outlined a comprehensive approach to health care quality improvement and called for the collection and analysis of statistical data to ascertain patient outcomes beyond simple mortality. In her seminal work *Notes on Hospitals*, first published in 1859, Nightingale (1863) notes the importance of information beyond mortality to more fully understand the interactions of multiple factors in determining outcomes of care:

> The first step in the way of improvement is to obtain a terse and accurate registration of the elements of the problem. Every well-kept hospital record ought to contain these. But for the sake of uniformity, I enumerate them as follows: 1. Age; 2. Sex; 3. Occupation; 4. Accident or disease leading to operation; 5. Date of accident and of operation, or date of operation if from disease; 6. Nature of operation; 7. Constitution of patient; 8. Complications occurring after operation; 9. Date of recovery or of death; 10. Fatal complication, a. Resulting directly from the accident, b. Occurring after the operation.

Nightingale not only understood the issues related to outcomes of care but also the economics of care as demonstrated in the following excerpt:

> "These methods ... would enable us to ascertain how much of each year of life is wasted by illness—what diseases and ages press most heavily on the resources of particular hospitals. ... The relation of the duration of cases to the general utility of a hospital requires also to be shown, because it must be obvious that if, by any sanitary means or improved treatment, the duration of cases could be reduced to one-half, the utility of the hospital would be doubled, so far as its funds are concerned."

Nightingale's vision was that rigorous data collection would yield a "uniform record of facts from which to deduce statistical results" (1863). Her prescient treatise on the value of collecting and analyzing health care outcomes data is remarkable when one reflects on the social and financial costs incurred as a direct result of her guidance being largely ignored.

The evolution and activities of quality improvement organizations

Since the mid 1990s several independent organizations have been established to focus on quality measurement (Schumann, 2012). The National Committee for Quality Assurance (NCQA) was one of the first with the development of the Healthcare Effectiveness Data and Information System (HEDIS) measures used to assess the quality of health plans. Numerous measures have been added to HEDIS over the years. NCQA has developed many other measurement programs since HEDIS (NCQA, 2011). While the HEDIS measures are not specific to nursing, they are important measures of the quality of care health plans provide and have provided useful information to purchasers of health care such as employers in choosing health plans as well as providing the basis for NCQA accreditation. Other accrediting bodies such as The Joint Commission, which accredits hospitals as well as the state nursing home agencies, all require measures to be monitored and reported for accreditation (Joint Commission, 2011).

The National Quality Forum was chartered in 1999 and became operational in 2000 as the culmination of recommendations by President Clinton's Commission on Consumer Protection and Quality Health Care Industry (National Quality Forum, 2011a). The forum has been established as the endorser of measures and has well over 400 measures that have been endorsed (National Quality Forum, 2011b). The National Quality Forum has a rigorous endorsement process that examines the evidence to support the validity and reliability of measures and acts as the final arbiter of measures being recognized. However, while endorsement of a measure is critical to having that measure considered for public reporting, not every endorsed measure is integrated into a reporting system.

Numerous alliances of health care providers have emerged with an initial mission to review and endorse measures. The first was the Hospital Quality Alliance, which was a partnership of providers, purchasers, Centers for Medicare and Medicaid (CMS), and others that provided the impetus to establishing hospital measures for public reporting. Those measures are now part of the Hospital Compare public reported measures (Hospital Quality Alliance, 2011). Another alliance, the Ambulatory Quality Alliance, was initiated by the American Academy of Family Physicians, the American College of Physicians, America's Health Insurance Plans, and the Agency for Healthcare Research and Quality in 2004 (Ambulatory Quality Alliance, 2011). The focus of this alliance has been on measures related to outpatient care.

Nursing also has an alliance that was started in 2010 with funding from the Robert Wood Johnson Foundation (Nursing Alliance for Quality Care, 2011). The focus of the Nursing Alliance for Quality Care is to ensure that patients get the right care at the right time from the right providers. This alliance differs from others in that its mission is to improve patient care through advocating for use of existing measures, ensuring that nursing has a voice at policy tables, and focusing on improving nursing's impact on care coordination and patient engagement.

In addition, the largest force in moving quality improvement forward is CMS. The Medicare and Medicaid programs are huge federally funded programs (Medicaid partially funded by federal funds), and CMS has a significant interest in making sure that care paid for is effective and efficient. CMS funds a number of different demonstration projects such as the project to have hospitals report specific measures that are in turn reported on the Hospital Compare website (CMS, 2011c). They are also funding a demonstration project related to medical homes that includes a significant component of measure reporting (CMS, 2011d). CMS carries a big carrot and stick in creating change around quality since they can require the reporting of measures as well as create financial incentives for hitting certain benchmarks in those measures.

Value-based purchasing as an impetus for quality improvement

There are several important drivers of quality improvement, including payers and purchasers; regulators, certifiers, and accreditors; professional organizations; and advocates and technical support organizations (Johnson, Dawson, & Acquaviva, 2008). The purchasers and payers have considerable influence on quality and increasingly look at quality measures to make decisions about the selection of health plans to offer. The U.S. health care system is the most expensive in the world without having health outcomes that are as good as other developed countries that spend less. As a result of issues related to the value of health care in the United States, the strongest impetus to quality improvement efforts has been through the concept of value-based purchasing, particularly by the federal government (Conway, 2009; Ferman, 2009; Hazelwood & Cook, 2008; Robinson, 2008).

The precursor to value-based purchasing has been the pay for performance approach in which providers get a financial benefit for first reporting measures and then providing good care. Value-based purchasing is a broader concept that not only combines quality and payment but also incorporates methods to drive purchasers to the high-performing institutions and health plans. Several examples include the CMS policy against paying for specific adverse events that happen to hospitalized patients, such as surgery on the wrong body part and stage III or IV pressure sores. Hospitals will not be paid for the costs of the secondary diagnosis related to a preventable adverse event, and nursing has a significant role to play in the monitoring and preventing of adverse events (Englebright & Perlin, 2008; Kurtzman, Dawson, & Johnson, 2008).

The most recent attempts to add value to the health care system are through the development of accountable care organizations (Berenson, 2010; Devore & Champion, 2011; Fisher & Shortell, 2010; Goldsmith, 2011). According to Devers and Berenson (2009), these organizations would have the following characteristics:

(1) The ability to provide, and manage with patients, the continuum of care across different institutional settings, including at least ambulatory and inpatient hospital care and possibly post acute care;
(2) The capability of prospectively planning budgets and resource needs; and
(3) Sufficient size to support comprehensive, valid, and reliable performance measurement.

A key factor in defining accountable care organizations is that the organizations need to have a robust quality measurement and improvement capacity across settings. If an accountable care organization meets a predetermined set of performance standards, it can then participate in a shared savings plan. Many hospitals, physician groups, and others are trying to position themselves to be an accountable care organization with the belief that funding from Medicare and/or Medicaid will be enhanced for such organizations.

As part of the value-based purchasing movement, there are demonstrations to test the concept of "bundled payments" for specific conditions or treatments (Birkmeyer et al., 2010; Goroll, Berenson, Schoenbaum, & Gardner, 2007; Hackbarth, Reischauer, & Mutti, 2008; Liu, Subramanian, & Cromwell, 2001). Bundled payments require a seamless approach to care, such as that provided through an accountable care organization, that crosses settings. For instance, bundled payment for a person needing hip replacement would include all of the services needed as part of the hip replacement such as presurgery care, surgery, rehabilitation, and physician visits. Bundled payments are considered a middle ground between fee for service payment and capitation.

Quality improvement approaches

There have been numerous quality improvement approaches and philosophies based on measurement of performance that have been embraced over the years by a variety of industries. Well-known approaches include the Deming method, which uses 14 principles to improve quality and reduce costs (Deming, 1986; Neuhauser, 1988). Deming is best known for his work with Japanese industries in the 1950s and is credited with beginning the Total Quality Management approach to quality improvement.

Six Sigma is another approach to quality, focused on reducing variation in order to improve quality. It was developed by Motorola Company in 1981 and widely adapted as a strategy to improve products and customer service (Accountable care organizations in "very early stages" of growth, 2011). The concept of Six Sigma is that 99.99966% of products are free of defects. Individuals can become expert in the approach, with the most accomplished earning a "black belt." Six Sigma has been applied to numerous health care issues, including decreasing Methicillin-resistant Staphylococcus aureus (MRSA) and reducing postsurgical problems (Carboneau, Benge, Jaco, & Robinson, 2010; Glasgow, Scott-Caziewell, & Kaboli, 2010; Kuo, Borycki, Kushniruk, & Lee, 2011; Murphree, Vath, & Daigle, 2011; Sedlack, 2010).

Yet another perspective is the lean production philosophy that is largely based on the Toyota Production approach to quality (Lean Enterprise Institute, 2010). Lean approaches focus on value to the customer; anything that is not of value to the customer is waste and should be eliminated. This approach has also been used to improve system efficiency in health care (Dickson, Anguelov, Vetterick, Eller, & Singh, 2009; Furman & Caplan, 2007; Kim, Spahlinger, Kin, & Billi, 2006; Kim, Spahlinger, Kin, Coffey, & Billi, 2009; Ng, Vail, Thomas, & Schmidt, 2010; Snyder & McDermott, 2009).

While the Deming, Toyota, and Lean approaches have similarities in terms of overall concept, the International Organization for Standardization (ISO) has a strong influence on quality for many different industries as well as health care internationally. It is an organization of 160 national standards institutes from a variety of countries (ISO, 2011). The ISO sets standards for businesses to ensure product quality for customers and also establishes guidelines for how to measure whether businesses have met the standards. The ISO has developed standards for health care.

A common thread for each of these approaches (all of which can be found in health care) is the use of statistical monitoring techniques to monitor variation in production or services in order to identify and then correct problems as quickly as possible.

Measuring nursing care quality

Framework for measuring the Institute of Medicine aims

As part of the Institute of Medicine series of reports on quality, *Crossing the Quality Chasm* (2001) established an "aim" for quality measurement. There are six aims marking high-quality health care: safe, timely, efficient, effective, equitable, and patient-centered care. These six aims define the areas that are important for measurement development. The measurement framework most used in developing and monitoring measures is the structure/process/ outcome framework developed by Avedis Donabedian (1966; see Figure 6.1). The theoretical underpinning of this framework is that the right structure will support the right processes, which will in turn result in the desired patient outcomes. The Donabedian framework can be applied to the Institute of Medicine aims. All measures related to one of the aims fall into structure, process, or outcome measures.

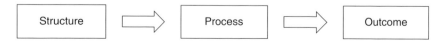

Figure 6.1 Structure, process, outcome framework (Donabedian framework).

Nursing-sensitive quality measures

While there are hundreds of endorsed measures, several sets of quality measures have been developed that relate directly to nursing care. Measures that reflect the impact of nursing care are considered nursing-sensitive measures. There are several sets of nursing-sensitive measures that have been developed for hospital-based care. These measures include the National Database for Nursing Quality Indicators (NDNQI) noted above, Collaborative Alliance for Nursing Outcomes, Military Nurses Outcomes Database, VA Nursing Outcomes Database, and a portion of the Hospital Consumer Assessment of Healthcare Providers and Systems (HCAHPS; American Nurses Association, 2009). Currently the five questions related to nursing in the HCAHPS are the only measures collected uniformly and nationally that are related to nursing (CMS, 2011a). See Textbox 6.1 one for a summary of the nursing-related HCAHPS questions.

Measures need to have scientific data supporting their validity and reliability before going through the rigorous process to be endorsed. Once rigorous studies of a particular measure have been done, they can be submitted to the National Quality Forum, which currently recognizes through endorsement 12 nursing-sensitive measures. See Textbox 6.2 for a listing of nursing-sensitive measures.

Validity, reliability, and risk adjustment of measures

It is important that measures are useful for either internal use to improve care or for public reporting in order for the public to be able to make judgments about the quality of care provided by an institution or specific provider. Public reporting is intended to guide consumers to the best care. In addition, measures need to be reliable so that anyone who measures a particular event, set of events, or phenomenon measures in the same way and uses the same specifications for the measure. For instance, if one facility measures falls based on people who only hit the ground when they fall and another facility counts a fall even if someone caught the patient before he or she hit the ground, falls will

---

Textbox 6.1   Nursing-related HCAHPS (Hospital Consumer Assessment of Healthcare Providers and Systems) survey questions

How often did nurses communicate well with patients?
During this hospital stay …

- how often did nurses treat you with courtesy and respect? (Q1)
- how often did nurses listen carefully to you? (Q2)
- how often did nurses explain things in a way you could understand? (Q3)

Textbox 6.2 National Quality Forum–endorsed nursing-sensitive measures

Patient-centered outcome measures:

● *Death among surgical inpatients with treatable serious complications (failure to rescue):* The percentage of major surgical inpatients who experience a hospital-acquired complication and die.
● *Pressure ulcer prevalence:* Percentage of inpatients who have a hospital-acquired pressure ulcer.
● *Falls prevalence:* Number of inpatient falls per inpatient days.
● *Falls with injury:* Number of inpatient falls with injuries per inpatient days.
● *Restraint prevalence:* Percentage of inpatients who have a vest or limb restraint.
● *Urinary catheter–associated urinary tract infection for intensive care unit (ICU) patients:* Rate of urinary tract infections associated with use of urinary catheters for ICU patients.
● *Central line catheter–associated blood stream infection rate for ICU and high-risk nursery patients:* Rate of blood stream infections associated with use of central line catheters for ICU and high-risk nursery patients.
● *Ventilator-associated pneumonia for ICU and high-risk nursery patients:* Rate of pneumonia associated with use of ventilators for ICU and high-risk nursery patients.

System-centered measures:

● *Skill mix:* Percentage of registered nurse, licensed vocational/practical nurse, unlicensed assistive personnel, and contracted nurse care hours to total nursing care hours.
● *Nursing care hours per patient day:* Number of registered nurses per patient day and number of nursing staff hours (registered nurse, licensed vocational/practical nurse, and unlicensed assistive personnel) per patient day.
● *Practice Environment Scale–Nursing Work Index:* Composite score and scores for five subscales:

  (1) Nurse participation in hospital affairs
  (2) Nursing foundations for quality of care
  (3) Nurse manager ability, leadership, and support of nurses
  (4) Staffing and resource adequacy
  (5) Collegiality of nurse-physician relations.

● *Voluntary turnover:* Number of voluntary uncontrolled separations during the month by category (RNs, APNs, LVN/LPNs, NAs).

be counted in very different ways. Measures also need to be valid and assess the event or phenomena that they are intended to assess. For measures to be useful in measuring quality of care, there has to be variation in the measure, with that variation being influenced by the provision of good or bad care. If there is no variation, there is no way to determine if someone is providing good or bad care because everyone performs the same. Measures also need to be risk adjusted. This means that some institutions or providers will appear to perform worse than others because of factors that are related to the population cared for and not the quality of care provided. For instance, those hospitals that have sicker patients than others will have a higher likelihood of an increased mortality rate than hospitals with less sick patients. The mortality rate needs to be risk adjusted based on the severity of patient conditions in order to compare their mortality rate with hospitals that have less acutely ill patients (Jerant, Iancredl, & Franks, 2011; Joynt, Orav, & Jha, 2011).

Specification of measures

As mentioned previously regarding the need for reliable measures, measures must be clearly specified so that each person and institution involved in reporting an event defines that event in the same way. For instance, a measure related to falls could be defined or specified as any event in which a patient hits the ground. This eliminates any circumstances when someone was in the act of falling but was caught by someone else, or if the patients fell across a bed or chair or some other object. If nurses and others define it differently, then there can be no comparison of a fall rate across units or across institutions. In addition, as part of specifying a measure, there has to be the inclusion of the total population at risk (denominator) and the number of events that occurred in that population (numerator) to determine a rate. The populations have to be defined in the same way as well.

Quality measures and Health Information Technology (HIT)

Until recently, much of the quality improvement data has been collected from either paper records or computerized administrative data. With the investment by the federal government of more than $20 billion, adoption of HIT is beginning to move more quickly (CMS, 2009). Having robust electronic health records will make the collection of patient-level clinical data much easier and will accelerate the use of data to improve care.

To ensure that health care institutions use HIT to improve care, the Office of the Health Information Technology Coordinator (a federal agency that is part of the Department of Health and Human Services) has begun to require institutions to collect data related to specific measures before they receive federal funds for HIT implementation. The required measures are called "meaningful use" measures to reflect that HIT has to be meaningfully used by an institution if it is to receive payment (Department of Health and Human Services, 2010). There will be three stages of implementation of meaningful use, including (1) collection of health information electronically and establishment of basic meaningful use measures for hospitals and ambulatory care, (2) expansion of stage one to include more providers and expand set of measures, and (3) improvement care.

Publically reported measures and benchmarking

Measures have maximum utility when there is a comparison with measures that have been established as standards or best practices measures. This allows an organization to know how their performance compares with others. Common benchmarks are based on national and/or state averages as well as highest scoring and lowest scoring institutions, agencies, or providers. CMS publically reports many measures for hospitals, nursing homes, and home care through a series of websites referred to collectively as the Compare websites. In the Compare websites, each institution is benchmarked against state and national comparisons. CMS has created a website called Hospital Compare for consumers to use in examining hospital measures pertaining to patient surveys, specific medical conditions such as diabetes or congestive heart failure, and surgical procedures such as surgery related to heart, vessels, or female organs (CMS, 2010). Information about specific hospitals compared to the state and national averages for each measure is included in Hospital Compare. An example of benchmarking for the question related to "How well do nurses communicate with patients?" is in Table 6.1.

The Nursing Home Compare website presents information from the state survey process (CMS, 2011e). Every nursing home is reviewed by onsite surveyors on a periodic basis—with no longer than 18 months between surveys. The Compare site has detailed information in several categories including report of deficiencies, self-report with verification on nurse staffing, and quality measures. CMS has a five-star rating for nursing homes based on these categories of information. The best rating is five stars and the worst rating is one star. The Nursing Home Compare website also has benchmarking of state and national data for each measure reported.

Similar to Hospital Care and Nursing Home Compare, the Home Health Compare website reports quality measures for specific home health agencies compared with state and national data. Home Health Compare has several categories of measures that include managing pain and treating

Table 6.1 HCAHPS survey questions example of benchmarking for "How often did nurses communicate well with patients?"

Average of all hospitals in U.S.	76%
Average of hospitals in Illinois (example of a state-level data source)	74%
Hospital A	73%
Hospital B	65%
Hospital C	79%

symptoms, managing daily activities, preventing harm, preventing unplanned hospital care, treating wounds, and preventing pressure sores (CMS, 2011b). As with the other Compare sites, there is benchmarking for state and national measures.

While there are no public reporting sites yet for individual physicians or medical teams, there is a significant amount of attention now being focused in this area. Currently, decisions about the quality of care of individual providers have been made based on where they went to school and if they were board certified. As measures related to the quality of care provided by individual clinicians evolve, advanced practice registered nurses will need to make sure that they are recognized in data collected about quality.

Quality improvement process

Monitoring and improving quality

Monitoring care through the use of valid and reliable measures is foundational to the quality improvement process. The quality improvement process begins with monitoring the specific measures that are part of a care process to identify variations and compare findings with benchmarks. If monitoring indicates that a particular measure is outside of the expected performance level, a problem is identified. Once a problem is noted, the cause(s) of the problem, or root cause, needs to be determined. Once causes are determined, a small test of change using the plan, do, study, act (PDSA) process is then implemented. PDSA is a process used for many different problems worldwide (Boyd, Aggarwal, Davey, Logan, & Nathwani, 2011; Ingraham et al., 2010; Krimsky et al., 2009; Lehman, Simpson, Knight, & Flynn, 2011; Millar, 2009; Nakayama et al., 2010; Wolfenden, Dunn, Holmes, Davies, & Buchan, 2010).

For example, a hospital unit may be monitoring patient falls as part of a required measure. After monitoring falls for months, one week of data indicates that the number of falls far exceeds the unit average, the hospital average, and the national average. A problem is then identified as a fall rate that is too high. A root cause analysis is then done, followed by the PDSA process.

Quality improvement tools

There are several tools that can help to monitor measures. These tools include control charts, histograms, run charts, scatter grams, and ways to visually show frequency of events. Everyone should know how to at least use a control chart and histogram. See Figure 6.2 for an example of a control chart used to monitor nurse-to-patient ratios. The control chart has three lines on it: an upper limit that indicates the upper limit of acceptable variation, a lower limit representing the lowest acceptable limit of variation, a middle line representing the average number of events. The upper and lower limits are calculated statistically. Any time the frequency of errors goes above the upper limit, it

Nurse to patient ratios

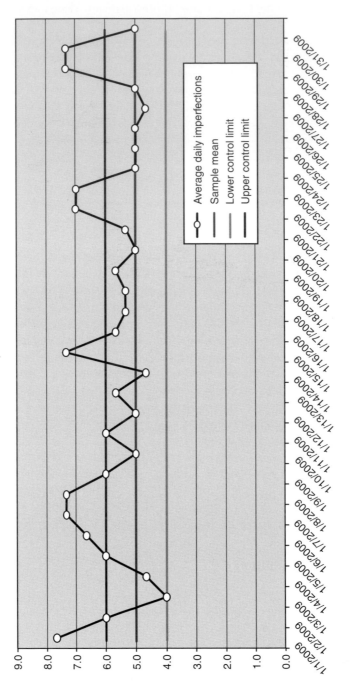

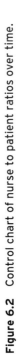

Figure 6.2   Control chart of nurse to patient ratios over time.

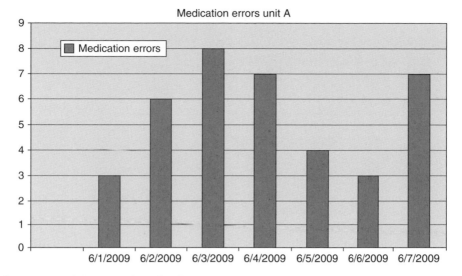

Figure 6.3 Histogram of medication errors.

should trigger an investigation for the reason the frequency has increased above acceptable levels.

A histogram can also be used to show frequencies. A histogram is essentially a bar graph that displays the number of events occurring. Figure 6.3 below shows the number of medication errors each day that occurred on a specific unit.

In identifying the reason for the problem, a root cause analysis is useful. Root cause analysis is a systematic approach to get to the root causes of the problem. The use of a fishbone diagram was originated in the 1960s by Kaoru Ishikawa, a leader in modern quality management. The diagram is used to reflect the results of brainstorming and/or the use of "five whys" to get to the root cause of a problem. The process of five whys is simply to keep asking why for each problem statement related to an overall problem identified. For instance, a problem identified is that residents of a nursing home have more pressure ulcers than the national average. The first why is why do residents of a nursing home have more pressure ulcers than the national average? One possible reason is that pressure ulcer risk assessments are not being done or done correctly. The second why is then focused on why isn't the risk assessment being done or done correctly? The group keeps going through this exercise until they have answered "five whys." After identifying all the possible reasons for a problem, the one or two most likely reasons for the problem are then the presumed root cause.

An example of the fishbone diagram is in Figure 6.4. The problem statement is at the tip of the fishbone. The fishbone usually has several organizing categories that provide a guide to identifying problems. The categories commonly used include people, equipment, processes, environment, materials, and management. All six categories or as few as two categories may be

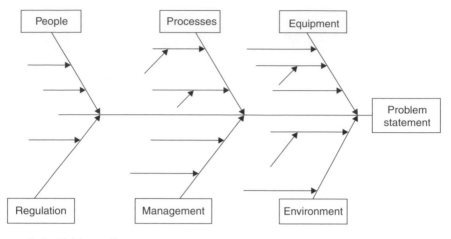

Figure 6.4 Fishbone diagram.

Table 6.2 Questions related to Plan, Do, Study, Act

Plan	Do	Study	Act
What is the objective? What do you think will happen? What is the plan for the test of change (who, what, where, when)?	Conduct the test. Document unexpected observations and problems.	Analyze the data. How do the findings compare with predictions? What was learned from the test?	What modifications should be made? What is the next test?

applicable to a specific problem. For each category, everyone involved in the quality improvement team brainstorms possible reasons for the problem. Brainstorming and/or the five whys are applied to each category used in the fishbone.

After all of the possible causes are considered and the top two are identified, the PDSA is initiated. The PDSA process can be guided by the questions and/or information noted for each phase of the PDSA in Table 6.2.

Figure 6.5 summarizes the complete quality improvement process. The process begins with monitoring. There are specific measures that are required to be monitored. However, monitoring can also include being vigilant about possible problems that are not being measured. The frequency of events that are being measured can be put into a histogram or control chart for ease in tracking the events. If a problem is identified, then a root cause analysis is conducted to determine the most likely root cause of the problem, and then a PDSA to do a small test of change to fix the problem is conducted. Then the process continues.

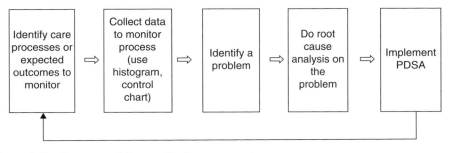

Figure 6.5 Summary of the quality improvement process.
Note: PDSA = plan, do, study, act.

Teaching quality improvement

Educational strategies for the classroom

Strategies for teaching quality improvement include classroom, online, and clinical opportunities. Every student should be able to attain the Quality and Safety Education for Nursing (QSEN) competencies defined for quality improvement (Cronenwett et al., 2007; Cronenwett, Sherwood, & Gelmon, 2009; Johnson, 2010). There are numerous teaching strategies that can help students attain competency in the knowledge, skills, and attitudes defined.

To assist students in learning about public reported measures of care:

• Ask students to review the Medicare Compare websites for all hospital, nursing home, or home care agency clinical assignment prior to beginning their clinical experiences. Have the students focus on the consumer assessment portion of the websites as well as any measure particularly relevant to nursing care. At the end of the clinical experience, have the student write a paper comparing the data in the websites with their personal experience and assessment of the level of quality delivered by the institution. The following questions could be used to structure the comparison:

  o Could you make a decision about choosing where to get care from the Compare site?
  o How did nursing care measures compare to state/national benchmarks? How would you explain the difference?
  o What questions did you have about the Compare websites?
    ▪ Through your observations, would you agree with the rating of the institution/agency by the Compare site? Explain and give examples.
  o Did the institution/agency have quality improvement programs that you observed or participated in? If so, describe.

• Assign students to assess the philosophy of quality improvement at each clinical site. The students should base their assessment on talking with nurses on their assigned unit about the philosophy and observe signs and messages that are in the facility that convey the presence of a commitment to quality and patient safety.

- Use a case study method in which students are asked to do a root cause analysis using a fishbone diagram and five whys. Students then engage in the PDSA process to define a small test of change. A root cause analysis can also be integrated into a simulation lab using the fishbone in which the "patient" develops a central line infection. The student would then be told that the rate of central line infections on that unit is the highest in the hospital and significantly higher than the national average. Students would be expected to apply the PDSA process as above.

Bridging education and clinical practice

Integrating quality improvement into the clinical site is critical for students to understand the real-life application and outcomes of quality improvement. One strategy for integrating quality improvement into clinical experiences is to have students attend a quality improvement meeting. After students have attended the meeting, have them address the following questions:

- Describe the topics discussed in the meeting.
- Did the meeting address issues relevant to the quality of nursing care?
- Do you think that the committee is effective in improving quality of care? If so, describe why. If not, describe why.

Another teaching strategy to bridge education and clinical practice is to have students find out if a hospital they are assigned to participates in the National Database for Nursing Quality Indicators (NDNQI). Students should then assess the benefits to improving nursing care by participating in the NDNQI or the concerns about nursing care quality if they do not participate.

The learning experience with the NDNQI can be extended to having nursing students brainstorm additional measures that could be considered for inclusion in the NDNQI. The students could then be asked to review the literature related to the potential measure to assess whether there is sufficient evidence to support the use of the measure. Students could also be asked to write a specification for the suggested measure in order to understand the complexity of measures. Information related to measure specification could include the following:

- Are there a sufficient number of events to support use of the measure?
- What is the target population that will be assessed for the event to occur?
- What is the event? Describe it in sufficient detail so that different people will interpret the measure in the same way.

Students can also be expected to talk with the nurse in charge of the unit to identify all the measures that are collected related to nursing care and what is then done with the information. It will be important for students to understand how quality measures are used in each clinical unit.

Finally, have students if possible participate in a root cause analysis in the clinical setting. Either they can participate in a quality group with nurses on the unit, or students can create their own quality group and identify a clinical problem to investigate.

Conclusion

Nurses are critical to improving quality of care in all health care settings. Monitoring measures to identify problems, engaging in a root cause analysis, and using the plan, do, study, act process are the fundamentals of quality improvement. To improve care, nurses have to be able to measure important processes and outcomes. Clinical sites expect nurses to know how to apply quality improvement processes to patient care improvement. Pressure from health care payers, particularly the federal government, will financially reward good care and reduce payment for bad care. Nurses will be held accountable for providing good care.

References

Accountable care organizations in "very early stages" of growth. (2011). *Healthcare Benchmarks and Quality Improvement, 18*(1), 1-4.

Ambulatory Quality Alliance. (2011). *About AQA*. Retrieved April 2, 2011, from http://www.aqaalliance.org/about.htm

American Nurses Association. (2009). *The national database*. Retrieved October 13, 2009, from http://www.nursingworld.org/MainMenuCategories/The PracticeofProfessionalNursing/PatientSafetyQuality/Research-Measurement/ The-National-Database.aspx

Berenson, R. A. (2010). Shared savings program for accountable care organizations: A bridge to nowhere? *American Journal of Managed Care, 16*(10), 721-726.

Birkmeyer, J. D., Gust, C., Baser, O., Dimick, J. B., Sutherland, J. M., & Skinner, J. S. (2010). Medicare payments for common inpatient procedures: Implications for episode-based payment bundling. *Health Services Research, 45*(6 Pt. 1), 1783-1795.

Boyd, S., Aggarwal, I., Davey, P., Logan, M., & Nathwani, D. (2011). Peripheral intravenous catheters: The road to quality improvement and safer patient care. *Journal of Hospital Infection, 77*(1), 37-41.

Carboneau, C., Benge, E., Jaco, M. T., & Robinson, M. (2010). A LeFan Six Sigma team increases hand hygiene compliance and reduces hospital-acquired MRSA infections by 51%. *Journal for Healthcare Quality: Official Publication of the National Association for Healthcare Quality, 32*(4), 61-70.

Centers for Medicare and Medicaid. (2009). *Medicare and Medicaid health information technology: Title IV of the American Recovery and Reinvestment Act*. Retrieved August 17, 2009, from http://www.cms.hhs.gov/apps/media/press/ factsheet.asp?Counter=3466&intNumPerPage=10&checkDate=&checkKey=&sr chType=1&numDays=3500&srchOpt=0&srchData=&keywordType=All&chkNews Type=6&intPage=&showAll=&pYear=&year=&desc=&cboOrder=date

Centers for Medicare and Medicaid. (2010). *Medicare hospital compare*. Retrieved March 12, 2011, from http://www.hospitalcompare.hhs.gov/

Centers for Medicare and Medicaid. (2011a). *HCAHPS survey.* Retrieved March 12, 2011, from http://www.cms.gov/HospitalQualityInits/Downloads/HospitalHCAHPSFactSheet201007.pdf

Centers for Medicare and Medicaid. (2011b). *Home health compare.* Retrieved March 12, 2011, from http://www.medicare.gov/HomeHealthCompare/search.aspx

Centers for Medicare and Medicaid. (2011c). *Hospital quality initiatives: Overview.* Retrieved April 2, 2011, from https://www.cms.gov/HospitalQualityInits/01_Overview.asp#TopOfPage

Centers for Medicare and Medicaid. (2011d). *Medicare demonstrations: Details for Medicare medical home demonstration.* Retrieved April 2, 2011, from http://www.cms.gov/demoprojectsevalrpts/md/itemdetail.asp?itemid=cms1199247

Centers for Medicare and Medicaid. (2011e). *Nursing home compare.* Retrieved March 12, 2011, from http://www.medicare.gov/NHCompare/Include/DataSection/Questions/SearchCriteriaNEW.asp?version=default&browser=Firefox|3.5|WinXP&language=English&defaultstatus=0&pagelist=Home&CookiesEnabledStatus=True

Conway, P. H. (2009). Value-driven health care: Implications for hospitals and hospitalists. *Journal of Hospital Medicine: An Official Publication of the Society of Hospital Medicine, 4*(8), 507–511.

Cronenwett, L., Sherwood, G., Barnsteiner, J., Disch, J., Johnson, J., Mitchell, P., et al. (2007). Quality and safety education for nurses. *Nursing Outlook, 55*(3), 122–131.

Cronenwett, L., Sherwood, G., & Gelmon, S. B. (2009). Improving quality and safety education: The QSEN learning collaborative. *Nursing Outlook, 57*(6), 304–312.

Deming, E. (1986). *Out of the crisis.* Cambridge, MA: MIT Press.

Department of Health and Human Services. (2010, July). *42 CFR parts 412, 413, 422 et al. Medicare and Medicaid programs; electronic health record incentive program; final rule.*

Devers, K., & Berenson, R. A. (2009). *Can accountable care organizations improve the value of health care by solving the cost and quality quandaries?* Washington, DC: Urban Institute.

Devore, S., & Champion, R. W. (2011). Driving population health through accountable care organizations. *Health Affairs (Project Hope), 30*(1), 41–50.

Dickson, E. W., Anguelov, Z., Vetterick, D., Eller, A., & Singh, S. (2009). Use of Lean in the emergency department: A case series of 4 hospitals. *Annals of Emergency Medicine, 54*(4), 504–510.

Donabedian, A. (1966). Evaluating the quality of medical care. *Milbank Memorial Fund Quarterly, 44*, 166–206.

Englebright, J., & Perlin, J. (2008). The chief nurse executive role in large healthcare systems. *Nursing Administration Quarterly, 32*(3), 188–194.

Ferman, J. H. (2009). Healthcare reform and a VBP program: Value-based purchasing concepts continue to evolve through the legislative process. *Healthcare Executive, 24*(2), 56–59.

Fisher, E. S., & Shortell, S. M. (2010). Accountable care organizations: Accountable for what, to whom, and how. *Journal of the American Medical Association, 304*(15), 1715–1716.

Furman, C., & Caplan, R. (2007). Applying the Toyota production system: Using a patient safety alert system to reduce error. *Joint Commission Journal on Quality and Patient Safety, 33*(7), 376–386.

Glasgow, J. M., Scott-Caziewell, J. R., & Kaboli, P. J. (2010). Guiding inpatient quality improvement: A systematic review of Lean and Six Sigma. *Joint Commission Journal on Quality and Patient Safety, 36*(12), 533–540.

Goldsmith, J. (2011). Accountable care organizations: The case for flexible partnerships between health plans and providers. *Health Affairs (Project Hope), 30*(1), 32–40.

Goroll, A. H., Berenson, R. A., Schoenbaum, S. C., & Gardner, L. B. (2007). Fundamental reform of payment for adult primary care: Comprehensive payment for comprehensive care. *Journal of General Internal Medicine, 22*(3), 410–415.

Hackbarth, G., Reischauer, R., & Mutti, A. (2008). Collective accountability for medical care: Toward bundled Medicare payments. *New England Journal of Medicine, 359*(1), 3–5.

Hazelwood, A., & Cook, E. D. (2008). Improving quality of health care through pay-for-performance programs. *The Health Care Manager, 27*(2), 104–112.

Hospital Quality Alliance. (2011). *Hospital Quality Alliance: About us*. Retrieved April 2, 2011, from http://www.hospitalqualityalliance.org/hospitalqualityalliance/aboutus/aboutus.html

Ingraham, A. M., Cohen, M. E., Bilimoria, K. Y., Dimick, J. B., Richards, K. E., Raval,M. V., et al. (2010). Association of surgical care improvement project infection-related process measure compliance with risk-adjusted outcomes: Implications for quality measurement. *Journal of the American College of Surgeons, 211*(6), 705–714.

Institute of Medicine. (1999). *To err is human: Building a safer health system*. Washington, DC: National Academy Press.

Institute of Medicine. (2001). *Crossing the quality chasm: A new health system for the 21st century*. Washington, DC: National Academy Press.

International Organization for Standardization. (2011). *About ISO*. Retrieved March 26, 2011, from http://www.iso.org/iso/about.htm

Jerant, A., Tancredi, D. J., & Franks, P. (2011). Mortality prediction by quality-adjusted life year compatible health measures: Findings in a nationally representative US sample. *Medical Care, 49*(5), 443–450.

Johnson, J. (2010). *Quality improvement enhancing quality and safety in nursing education: preparing nurse faculty to lead curricular change*. CDROM, Vol 1, Version 7A. Quality and Safety Education for Nurses/American Association of Colleges of Nursing.

Johnson, J., Dawson, E., & Acquaviva, K. (2008). The quality improvement landscape. In E. R. Ransom, M. Joshi, D. B. Nash, and S. B. Ransom (Eds.), *The quality improvement landscape* (2nd ed.). Chicago: Health Administration Press.

Joint Commission. (2011). *About The Joint Commission*. Retrieved April 2, 2011, from http://www.jointcommission.org/about_us/about_the_joint_commission_main.aspx

Joynt, K. E., Orav, E. J., & Jha, A. K. (2011). The association between hospital volume and processes, outcomes, and costs of care for congestive heart failure. *Annals of Internal Medicine, 154*(2), 94–102.

Kim, C. S., Spahlinger, D. A., Kin, J. M., & Billi, J. E. (2006). Lean health care: What can hospitals learn from a world-class automaker? *Journal of Hospital Medicine: An Official Publication of the Society of Hospital Medicine, 1*(3), 191–199.

Kim, C. S., Spahlinger, D. A., Kin, J. M., Coffey, R. J., & Billi, J. E. (2009). Implementation of lean thinking: One health system's journey. *Joint Commission Journal on Quality and Patient Safety, 35*(8), 406–413.

Krimsky, W. S., Mroz, I. B., McIlwaine, J. K., Surgenor, S. D., Christian, D., Corwin, H. L., et al. (2009). A model for increasing patient safety in the intensive care unit: Increasing the implementation rates of proven safety measures. *Quality & Safety in Health Care, 18*(1), 74–80.

Kuo, A. M., Borycki, E., Kushniruk, A., & Lee, T. S. (2011). A healthcare Lean Six Sigma system for postanesthesia care unit workflow improvement. *Quality Management in Health Care, 20*(1), 4–14.

Kurtzman, E. T., Dawson, E. M., & Johnson, J. E. (2008). The current state of nursing performance measurement, public reporting, and value-based purchasing. *Policy, Politics & Nursing Practice, 9*(3), 181–191.

Landrigan, C. P., Parry, G. J., Bones, C. B., Hackbarth, A. D., Goldmann, D. A., & Sharek, P. J. (2010). Temporal trends in rates of patient harm resulting from medical care. *New England Journal of Medicine, 363*(22), 2124–2134.

Lean Enterprise Institute. (2010). *A brief history of Lean*. Retrieved March 2011 from http://www.lean.org/whatslean/History.cfm

Lehman, W. E., Simpson, D. D., Knight, D. K., & Flynn, P. M. (2011). Integration of treatment innovation planning and implementation: Strategic process models and organizational challenges. *Psychology of Addictive* Behaviors, *25*(2), 252–261.

Liu, C. F., Subramanian, S., & Cromwell, J. (2001). Impact of global bundled payments on hospital costs of coronary artery bypass grafting. *Journal of Health Care Finance, 27*(4), 39–54.

Millar, M. (2009). Are national targets the right way to improve infection control practice? *Journal of Hospital Infection, 73*(4), 408–413.

Morabia, A. (2006). Pierre-Charles-Alexandre Louis and the evaluation of bloodletting. *Journal of the Royal Society of Medicine, 99*(3), 158–160.

Murphree, P., Vath, R. R., & Daigle, L. (2011). Sustaining Lean Six Sigma projects in health care. *Physician Executive, 37*(1), 44–48.

Nakayama, D. K., Bushey, T. N., Hubbard, I., Cole, D., Brown, A., Grant, T. M., et al. (2010). Using a plan-do-study-act cycle to introduce a new or service line. *AORN Journal, 92*(3), 335–343.

National Committee for Quality Assurance. (2011). *HEDIS and quality measurement*. Retrieved March 19, 2011, from http://www.ncqa.org/tabid/59/Default.aspx

National Quality Forum. (2011a). *About NQF*. Retrieved April 2, 2011, from http://www.qualityforum.org/About_NQF/About_NQF.aspx

National Quality Forum. (2011b). *NQF-endorsed® standards*. Retrieved April 2, 2011, from http://www.qualityforum.org/Measures_List.aspx

Neuhauser, D. (1988). The quality of medical care and the 14 points of Edward Deming. *Health Matrix, 6*(2), 7–10.

Ng, D., Vail, G., Thomas, S., & Schmidt, N. (2010). Applying the lean principles of the Toyota production system to reduce wait times in the emergency department. *Canadian Journal of Emergency Medical Care, 12*(1), 50–57.

Nightingale, F. (1863). *Notes on hospitals* (3rd ed.). London: Longman, Green, Longman, Roberts and Green.

Nursing Alliance for Quality Care. (2011). *Nursing Alliance for Quality Care*. Retrieved April 2, 2011, from http://www.gwumc.edu/healthsci/departments/nursing/naqc/index.cfm

Robinson, J. C. (2008). Value-based purchasing for medical devices. *Health Affairs (Project Hope), 27*(6), 1523–1531.

Sedlack, J. D. (2010). The utilization of Six Sigma and statistical process control techniques in surgical quality improvement. *Journal for Healthcare Quality, 32*(6), 18–26.

Schumann, M. J. (2012). Policy implications driving national quality and safety initiatives. In G. Sherwood & J. Barnsteiner (Eds.), *Quality and safety in nursing: A competency approach to improving outcomes.* Hoboken, NJ: Wiley-Blackwell.

Snyder, K. D., & McDermott, M. (2009). A rural hospital takes on lean. *Journal for Healthcare Quality, 31*(3), 23–28.

Wolfenden, J., Dunn, A., Holmes, A., Davies, C., & Buchan, J. (2010). Track and trigger system for use in community hospitals. *Nursing Standard, 24*(45), 35–39.

Chapter 7

Evidence-Based Practice

Mary Fran Tracy, PhD, RN, CCNS, FAAN
Jane Barnsteiner, PhD, RN, FAAN

Health care in the United States is at the brink of unprecedented transformation. The public is concerned with obtaining quality preventive and acute care in the most effective and cost efficient manner at the same time that patients and patient care are becoming increasingly complex. Successful evolution of this health care transformation depends on a variety of factors—one of them being the provision of education that prepares health care providers to optimally function in this new era.

The groundbreaking Institute of Medicine (IOM, 2001) report *Crossing the Quality Chasm* outlined 10 rules to redesign and improve health care. Rule 5 for improving health care in the United States is using evidence-based decision making. However, it is estimated that there is a significant lag of 17 years between the time patient care evidence is generated and the time it is fully embedded into clinical practice (Balas & Boren, 2000). Why does this gap exist? Is it because health care providers are unaware the evidence exists? Are providers unable to critically evaluate the evidence? Is it easier to continue to practice as you were originally taught and tradition is difficult to alter? It would seem that the purpose of the educational setting is to instill the value of using current best evidence to guide practice.

The 2003 report by the Institute of Medicine, *Healthcare Professions Education: A Bridge to Quality*, calls for competencies for all health care professionals in the areas of safe and quality care. Competencies outlined by the IOM call on academic institutions to advance the education of health care professionals in order to have highly functioning interdisciplinary teams focused on patient-centered care. It is essential that this safe care be guided by evidence, continuous quality improvement outcomes, and optimal use of informatics (IOM, 2003).

The Affordable Care Act of 2010 emphasizes evidence-based policies and interventions when making recommendations about health care prevention

Quality and Safety in Nursing: A Competency Approach to Improving Outcomes,
First Edition. Edited by Gwen Sherwood and Jane Barnsteiner.
© 2012 John Wiley & Sons, Inc. Published 2012 by John Wiley & Sons, Inc.

strategies (Department of Health and Human Services [DHHS], 2010b). In addition, the Centers for Medicare and Medicaid Services are increasingly focused on hospitals, nursing homes, home health care agencies, and dialysis facilities to meet standards for providing evidence-based care (DHHS, 2010a) and are adjusting reimbursement accordingly. They are improving consumer access to performance data from agencies and guiding consumers on how to make informed decisions based on that data (DHHS, 2010a). In this way, evidence-based practice becomes an important link to continuous quality improvement.

Since the time of Nightingale, nursing as a profession has been committed to providing safe and quality care for our patients. However, it is clear there is a gap in relation to the IOM recommendations related to performance competencies and competency preparation in nursing education. The Robert Wood Johnson Foundation funded the Quality and Safety Education in Nursing (QSEN) project to initiate dialogue and develop recommendations for closing that gap. The QSEN faculty and advisory board leaders explored the literature and adapted the IOM competencies to fully explicate competency expectations for all registered nurses. These competencies include patient-centered care, teamwork and collaboration, evidence-based practice, quality improvement, safety, and informatics. In addition to defining the competencies, the QSEN group also delineated the knowledge, skills, and attitudes (KSAs) components that are essential for each of the competencies. This work is a foundation for promoting advances in nursing education to address the gap in competency achievement (Cronenwett et al., 2007; Cronenwett et al., 2009; Cronenwett, Sherwood, & Gelmon, 2009).

This chapter will explore the competency related to evidence-based practice (EBP)—what it is, description of the KSAs that make up the competency for EBP, the state of the science, and innovative approaches for teaching strategies to achieve the student EBP competency. The chapter includes application to student learners in academic settings, both prelicensure and graduate, as well as clinicians in clinical settings.

Definition and description of evidence-based practice

Evidence-based practice is defined as practice based on the best available evidence that also incorporates patient values and preferences and clinician judgment and expertise (Sackett, Strauss, Richardson, Rosenberg, & Haynes, 2000; Cronenwett et al., 2007; Cronenwett et al., 2009). As many as 33 different terms have been used to describe EBP and translational research (Tetroe et al., 2008). Over time, the concept of using evidence to guide nursing practice has evolved from simple research utilization to more broad-based and inclusive evidence-based practice.

It has been estimated that approximately 15% of health care is actually research based (McKenna, Cutcliffe, & McKenna, 2000). The remainder of care interventions fall into three other categories: (1) interventions supported by other types of evidence such as expert opinion or quality improvement, (2) interventions based on tradition in which it is not clearly known whether they do more harm or good, and (3) interventions that we know cause more harm than good but practitioners either refuse or are slow to change practice. The goal of EBP should be to advance practice so interventions are based on the best available evidence and eliminate any interventions that we know cause more harm than good (McKenna et al., 2000; Newhouse & Spring, 2010).

While the purpose of research utilization is to disseminate and translate research findings as the basis for sound clinical practice, EBP recognizes the value of the gamut of evidence that can be incorporated into decision making about best care for the individual patient. The randomized, controlled trial has traditionally been considered the gold standard for guiding health care practice, but from an EBP paradigm we should recognize the value that controlled nonrandom, quasi-experimental, and descriptive studies can contribute to decision making along with quality improvement data, program evaluation data, and expert consensus opinions (Ferguson & Day, 2005). Significant skill on the part of the health care provider is required to be able to analyze and synthesize the evidence based on the credibility of the source, while simultaneously exploring and acknowledging the patient's values in relation to that evidence and the clinician's judgment as to the fit of the body of evidence with the particular individual's situation.

The KSAs developed for the six competences as related to prelicensure education were initially drafted by the QSEN group through workshops and e-mail communication (Cronenwett et al., 2007; Cronenwett et al., 2009) to reach consensus. The KSAs for EBP range from basic to increasingly complex and are intended to guide the EBP curriculum (see Appendixes A and B). Critical thinking skills are essential in having an evidence-based practice and developing alternative interventions as needed to achieve the best outcome for the individual patient (Ferguson & Day, 2005). It is these analytical and critical thinking skills that nurse educators are being challenged to develop in nursing students at all educational levels.

Evidence-based practice—models and process

Numerous models have been developed to guide nurses through the EBP process (Mitchell, Fischer, Hastings, Silverman, & Wallen, 2010). The most commonly known models are the Iowa, STAR, Hopkins, and University of Arizona (Melnyk & Fineout-Overholt, 2004; Newhouse, Dearholt, Poe, Pugh, & White, 2005; Rosswurm & Larrabee, 1999; Stetler, 2003; Stevens, 2004; Titler et al., 2001). While models may take slightly different approaches, all essentially guide nurses through the EBP process utilizing the Planned Action theoretical approach (Straus, Tetroe, & Graham, 2009).

There are five basic steps to the EBP process. Each needs to be thoroughly addressed in order to have sound decision making for patient care (Fineout-Overholt, Melnyk, & Schultz, 2005; Johnston & Fineout-Overholt, 2005).

Develop a searchable question

Inquiry is the driving force to questioning why nurses practice as they do. Developing a question that accurately reflects the practice to be evaluated will start the EBP process down a sound path. Students can use the PICOT format to structure the question: **P**atient population; **I**ntervention; **C**omparison intervention or group; **O**utcome; **T**ime (Fineout-Overholt et al., 2005). The more refined and explicit the question, the easier the search to find relevant evidence.

Search for the best evidence available

The PICOT question components will provide guidance for the databases and keywords to search. Performing a database search can require multiple strategies. Since the PICOT question may have already been asked and answered by others, starting with sites that provide systematic reviews (e.g., Cochrane Collaboration) or evidence-based care guidelines (AHRQ National Guideline Clearinghouse) is prudent (see Textbox 7.1). Reviews may also be indexed in databases such as Medline and CINAHL. If no systematic reviews or guidelines are found, then individual articles must be searched and retrieved. The assistance of a medical librarian who is skilled at searching the health care literature can be invaluable.

Critical analysis and synthesis of the evidence

A critical appraisal and synthesis of the evidence is the next step. What are the results of the evidence you've found? How closely does the population and evidence match the question you are asking?

Several models for grading of evidence exist, ranging from four to eight levels of evidence strength. Many of these models originated from medicine and therefore posit that the randomized controlled trial is the gold standard from which all subsequent levels are based. Models differ in what and how evidence is graded. For example, the American Heart Association uses both Level A, B, C and Class I, IIa, IIb, III to describe certainty and size of the treatment effect (Gibbons, Smith, & Antman, 2003). There are nursing grading

---

Textbox 7.1   Systematic reviews and evidence websites

Agency for Healthcare Research and Quality: www.AHRQ.gov
Campbell Collaboration: www.campbellcollaboration.org/Fralibrary.html
Cochrane Collaboration Library: www.cochrane.org
Evidence-Based Medicine Librarian: http://ebmlibrarian.wetpaint.com/ page/3.+Appraising+the+evidence
Joanna Briggs Institute for Evidence-Based Nursing and Midwifery: www. joannabriggs.edu.au/about/home.php
National Guideline Clearinghouse: www.guideline.gov

models as well (Rosswurm & Larrabee, 1999; Stetler, 2001). It is important for nursing students to learn that just because a study is not a randomized controlled trial does not mean it has no value in influencing nursing practice. The clinical question to be answered dictates the research design (Barnsteiner, 2010; Barnsteiner, Palma, Preston, Reeder, & Walton, 2010).

The new paradigm of evidence analysis and synthesis allows for the possibility that the strength of evidence does not need to be an "all or nothing" proposition—in other words, either all of the evidence from one source is strong and can be incorporated into the synthesis or none of it can be utilized. It is rare that evidence has no limitations. We need to critically evaluate all evidence to determine if even minor components of the evidence can contribute to decision making for patient care (Fineout-Overholt et al., 2005).

Develop recommendations for practice

The health care provider will take the synthesis of evidence to determine if there is sufficient validity and strength to incorporate it into practice. The evidence may be applicable to an entire patient population or the provider may incorporate specific clinical judgment and patient preferences to make care decisions for an individual patient. Providers must have the insight to determine whether they alone have adequate expertise to make the patient care decision with the available evidence or whether they need to consult with other experts.

Evaluate the outcome of evidence-based practice changes

The final step in the EBP process is to evaluate the practice change. Evaluation of the change includes impact to patient outcomes, provider practice, and the cost effectiveness of the practice. To effectively evaluate the outcome, one must know the expected outcomes, the baseline performance prior to the change, and how and when to collect the evaluation data (Barnsteiner, 2010). Understanding the outcomes of the changes we make offers opportunities for continual improvement as well as for nurses to own accountability for our evidence-based practice.

These five steps are an overview of the EBP process. Each of these steps is frequently divided into further additional components in order to successfully accomplish the complicated process of implementing and maintaining practice changes.

The extent of knowledge development and level of expert skill attainment expected related to the EBP competency will vary based on the educational level of the student. For instance, the associate degree and baccalaureate prepared nurse can be expected to identify searchable questions, develop beginning analysis and synthesis skills, formulate initial recommendations for practice based on the synthesis, and participate as members of implementation and evaluation teams. Masters and DNP prepared nurses should have more extensive skill at developing practice recommendations, taking into account patient populations, organizational priorities, and stewardship of resources; developing detailed implementation plans for practice changes based on change theory; and developing processes to fully evaluate the impact on patient and organizational outcomes of the evidence-based practice changes (see Appendix B).

The evidence for evidence-based practice

EBP skills in students and new graduates

As the QSEN group delineated the KSAs for the six competencies for prelicensure education, they sought feedback from faculty. Nurse educators initially believed they were teaching to all six of the identified competencies. However, in reviewing the details of the expectations, many agreed that students were not being adequately prepared at the identified competency level (Cronenwett et al., 2007). This was corroborated by perspectives of new graduates who stated they were not receiving significant learning experiences in the competency areas and to some extent that they were not taught by nurse educators with expertise in these areas (Cronenwett et al., 2007). In fact, a survey of all member schools of the American Association of Colleges of Nursing as well as a convenience sample of community college associate degree programs in North Carolina showed that more than 50% of schools reported that nurse educators had only "some" comfort in teaching EBP. Eleven percent of schools considered them "novice" in that area. Schools that had BSN and graduate programs were more likely to rate nurse educators as "expert" in EBP, though that rating was still only 47% of nurse educators (Smith, Cronenwett, & Sherwood, 2007).

Sullivan, Hirst, and Cronenwett (2009) reported that although there has been increasing awareness of EBP terms and the concept of EBP over time, new graduates reported they felt the least prepared/skilled in EBP and quality improvement. In addition, they believed that having an attitude of valuing the competencies was least important in these same two areas when compared with the other four competencies. This brings unique challenges to nurse educators to instill KSAs in these areas that nursing students and new graduates may feel are "optional" competencies rather than "essential" competencies (Moch & Cronje, 2010; Moch, Cronje, & Branson, 2010).

Teaching EBP

Evidence-based practice is identified by both the American Association of Colleges of Nursing and the National League for Nursing Accreditation Commission as an essential component of all levels of nursing education for their member schools—baccalaureate, masters, and DNP preparation. Entry-level nurses should be prepared to differentiate between research and EBP, understand models of EBP, demonstrate retrieval of all types of evidence and evaluate credibility of the source, critique and synthesize the evidence and be able to propose evidence-based solutions, and collaborate in the implementation and dissemination of that evidence into practice (American Association of Colleges of Nursing [AACN], 2008; National League for Nursing Accreditation Commission [NLNAC], 2010a). The master's prepared nurse should be prepared to perform rigorous evaluation of multiple sources of evidence in relation to clinical judgment and perspectives of all health care providers; participate and/or lead teams in practice change implementation; articulate to broad audiences the rationale for EBP changes; and evaluate the impact on quality of EBP changes in a systematic fashion (AACN, 2011, NLNAC, 2010b). The DNP graduate would ideally function at the highest level of EBP—designing and implementing quality improvement activities to improve care; lead substantive EBP changes to practice; collect, analyze, and synthesize evidence; and propose changes for patient populations (AACN, 2006; NLNAC 2010c).

McCurry and Martins (2010) examined the effect of teaching research terminology, research critique, and EBP process using innovative approaches aimed at the "millennial" learner. The innovative strategies were interactive, group focused, or experiential as compared with more traditional teaching methods such as textbook readings, quizzes, library orientation, and didactic content. At the end of the course, students rated the innovative approaches as more effective and instructors found increased classroom participation, more collaborative learning, and greater mastery of the content as compared with traditional approaches.

The effectiveness of small group work has been demonstrated in teaching EBP at the undergraduate level, particularly as it relates to significantly improving the EBP knowledge and skill level of the student (Balakas & Sparks, 2010; Kim, Brown, Fields, & Stichler, 2009; Kruszewski, Brough, & Killeen, 2009; Oh et al., 2010). Results regarding the improvement of attitudes toward EBP and the likelihood of future use of EBP, however, were inconsistent in some of those studies (Oh et al., 2010; Kim et al., 2009).

Barriers to EBP in clinical practice

It has been said that, for practicing RNs, EBP is an "abstraction whose benefits are neither immediately visible nor necessarily compatible with existing practice values, needs, and experiences" (Cronje & Moch, 2010, pp. 24-25). Practicing RNs lack basic EBP knowledge and skills, which will continue to impede the integration of new evidence into practice (Pravikoff, Tanner, & Pierce, 2005).

Practicing nurses are more likely to seek advice from a colleague rather than utilize research or journals (Pravikoff et al., 2005). A significant majority (>80%) have never used a hospital library or sought assistance from a librarian—not surprising, as 77% report they have never learned to use electronic databases. Disappointingly, only 46% of practicing nurses state that they are even familiar with the term *evidence-based practice* (Pravikoff et al., 2005).

Barriers to the use of EBP in the clinical setting cited by practicing nurses include lack of value for research in the clinical setting, lack of understanding of electronic databases, and difficulty gaining access to research (Pravikoff et al., 2005). Additionally, practicing nurses do not feel they have the skills to search for, analyze, or synthesize the evidence. They also cite a lack of organizational resources or support for use of research. It may be as basic as having a computer available on the unit with access to a digital library.

Nurses working in settings other than acute care facilities such as ambulatory and primary care clinics, physician offices, and other delivery areas may have added challenges to assure their practice is based on current evidence. These challenges may include even less evidence available on which to base practice improvement decisions, fewer nurses prepared at an advanced level of EBP, lack of EBP mentors familiar with these settings, and fewer colleagues to form EBP teams. However, the process of EBP is essentially the same regardless of setting. The use of today's technology may be particularly helpful for nurses practicing in these settings as it can facilitate long-distance mentoring and multisite teams from similar settings in evaluating evidence and finding support/advice in implementing EBP.

Examination of these barriers creates an even stronger imperative to set a strong foundation in nursing curricula as new graduates will encounter challenges and barriers as they transition into practice in the "real world." Based on the current evidence about EBP, nursing education in all settings should focus on preparing nurses who see the value and moral imperative to be lifelong consumers of evidence in the quest to provide best care for our patients. The educational environment can be the leader for instilling in learners the value and required skills needed for EBP (Ferguson & Day, 2005).

Teaching strategies

The QSEN project serves to advance competency achievement in nursing to support this new era of health care quality and engages nurse educators to examine the competencies in a new light. Education of learners about EBP is more than teaching the steps of the process and where to find the evidence; it also helps learners explore more deeply—for example, to develop understanding of formal and informal grading of evidence, differentiate between evidence and consensus opinion, to look at the use of evidence and related patient preferences from an ethics perspective, and to develop care plans utilizing not just research evidence but also patient values and clinical judgment. But when is the best time to introduce EBP into the nursing curriculum?

Traditionally, nursing curriculum has been built on a progression of simple to complex concepts—from discrete skills to the increasing complexity of families, organizations, and systems (Barton, Armstrong, Preheim, Gelmon, & Andrus, 2009). It is not unusual for EBP to be introduced later in the nursing program—often as late as the last semester of the senior year in the form of an EBP project.

Barton and colleagues (2009) conducted a web-based modified Delphi study to recommend when the KSAs for the six quality and safety competencies should be introduced and emphasized in a prelicensure program (see Appendix C). The study goal was to reach two-thirds consensus with three survey rounds. Consensus among nurse educator experts was that many of the KSAs for EBP should be introduced primarily in the beginning and intermediate phases of nursing programs, which would allow students time to gain experience in evidence-based applications. Examples of recommended timing for EBP KSAs include the following:

Beginning phase introduction:
- Knowledge of scientific methods/processes
- Description of EBP and sources of evidence
- Skill in developing patient care plans with evidence, patient values, and clinical judgment
- Promotion of the value of EBP to clinical practice

Intermediate phase introduction:
- Knowledge in determining the strength of evidence
- Developing skill in data collection and analysis in reading research and evidence reports
- Skill in finding evidence
- Questioning traditional care practices
- Appreciating the strengths and weaknesses of types of evidence

Advanced phase introduction:
- Differentiate when it's appropriate to use patient requests or clinical judgment to deviate from EBP guidelines
- Skill in preparing the environment to integrate new evidence into practice

It is important to set the stage early for development of knowledge, skills, and attitudes for EBP. Start introduction of the concepts early and expand each year on the competency in order to facilitate building of the foundation (Barton et al., 2009; Rolloff, 2010). Education requires a multipronged approach threaded throughout the curriculum, reinforcing and linking EBP concepts with patient encounters. As students develop critical thinking skills, their critical thinking related to EBP will also develop in relation to the judgment needed to critically evaluate the evidence with a new appreciation of the impact of patient values and the judgment needed to seek advice when considering deviating from guidelines. Providing opportunities for students to learn about organizational structures and institutional culture regarding attitudes toward and support for change will assist new graduates as they transition to practice and apply what they have learned about EBP.

The QSEN Learning Collaborative was a 15-month project funded by the Robert Wood Johnson Foundation to develop the next steps in revising curricula for quality and safety education, trialing innovative teaching strategies, and promoting future educator development (Cronenwett et al., 2009). Innovative teaching strategies continue to be posted on the QSEN website for faculty and clinical educators to share and explore new educational approaches related to evidence-based practice. Below are examples of teaching strategies that can be applied and adapted for the classroom, simulation, and clinical settings.

Didactic strategies

Exposure to EBP models

Using EBP models can guide students through the EBP process. Students can form small groups, each choosing different EBP models to explore. Examples of common EBP models include the Iowa, STAR, Hopkins, and University of Arizona models (Melnyk & Fineout-Overholt, 2004; Newhouse et al., 2005; Rosswurm & Larrabee, 1999; Stetler, 2003; Stevens, 2004; Titler et al., 2001). Assign clinical practice questions to the groups and have them work through the EBP process using their models. Group presentations can be used to discuss the models and results. After all groups have presented, have the entire group compare and contrast differences between the models and evaluate the ease of use of each of the models.

Grading of evidence

Small groups of students can choose both a nursing and a nonnursing grading model. Have the groups compare and contrast differences between the rating models. Using a nursing research study, have the groups explore the feasibility of grading the study using both a nursing and nonnursing grading model. Small group presentations can be used to describe the different grading models and what study designs would best be used with each grading model.

Journal clubs

Assign research articles relevant to current clinical rotations and provide students with a research critique tool. In small groups, have one or two students lead the group through the critique process.

EBP project

An EBP project can be used at both the graduate and undergraduate levels. Have students select an EBP question they have identified from the clinical setting and work through the steps of EBP process. This can be done in small groups with undergraduates and as an individual project with graduate students (Sullivan, 2010a). Course instructors could collaborate by forming groups with members from both undergraduate and graduate students, adding a library student to the group, or having interdisciplinary groups of students. Criteria for evaluating the project could be more stringent for graduate student projects. Objectives would vary based on the formation of the small groups. For instance, having a graduate student facilitate an undergraduate EBP project could prepare them for the practice setting where they will be leading staff in working through a clinical question and implementation of a practice change. Interdisciplinary teams could take similar questions from their discipline perspective and compare the evidence between disciplines, noting how the entire evidence base could be used in an interdisciplinary approach in care of a patient. Involving a library student could allow for development of finding evidence sources on the part of nursing students while giving the library student an opportunity to look at the utility of the literature from a health care perspective.

Simulation or skills lab strategies

Utilize EBP simulation scenarios

Patient scenarios utilized in a simulation lab should be based on evidence with purposeful EBP concepts woven in. Student preparation for the simulation scenario can include reading relevant guidelines, determining the source of the evidence, encouraging students to write down questions of how scenarios and the corresponding evidence may differ from practice in the clinical setting, and review of evidence-based tools for the skill development (e.g., Confusion Assessment Method [CAM] or Confusion Assessment Method for the ICU [CAM-ICU] for delirious patients, handwashing guidelines, CPM for knee replacement surgery, VAP prevention guidelines for suctioning in MV patients, DM guidelines, asthma guidelines in pediatrics) (Jarzemsky, 2010).

Student-led simulation scenarios

Using the example above, students could be assigned to lead the discussion about the EBP components of the simulation scenario.

Clinical strategies

Use of journals for reflection

Encourage students to use journals to reflect on discrepancies between evidence and practices they note in the clinical setting. Nursing students can query preceptors and practicing nurses about the discrepancies they note (Sullivan, 2010b).

Sacred cows contest

Leake (2004) had nursing students ask three questions of practicing nurses when they were in the clinical setting: (1) What is the most traditional nursing practice being done? (2) What is the least logical nursing practice? (3) What is the most time-consuming practice on the unit? Nurses then formed small groups and searched the evidence surrounding the practices they identified. Frequently the evidence found did not support the practice being observed. The assignment could be turned into an EBP project where results are presented to the hospital nursing staff and a practice change implemented if feasible.

Postclinical discussion and debrief

EBP discussions can occur through the routine postclinical discussion and debrief sessions. "Students need opportunities to discuss the credibility of the research-generated evidence from both quantitative and qualitative paradigms and to explore the relative weighting of particular evidence in specific patient situations" (Ferguson & Day, 2005, p. 108). Students could be encouraged to comment on their journal notes if they feel comfortable or the discrepancies they note in their clinical rotations. The instructor can lead students in looking at all the evidence in patient situations and how to deal with the dilemma of preceptors performing interventions that are not evidence-based. Frontline nurses could be encouraged to apply similar opportunities to their daily work, for example, use of journal clubs, opportunities for reflection on differences in practice between staff nurses at forums like nursing practice or research committees, and facilitated discussions about differences between preceptors on what they teach.

Attendance at nursing practice or research committee meetings

Students could be offered the opportunity to attend health care institutions' nursing practice or research committee meetings. They could evaluate the extent of EBP utilized and any models for guiding the work of the committee.

Role playing

Learners can discuss and role play interactions they may have as both students and new graduates in initiating a dialogue with more experienced nurses or physicians about practices that are not evidence based. This develops skill in effective communication, teamwork and collaboration when differing opinions exist, consensus reaching in providing optimal care for patients, role modeling EBP, and approaching a situation in a way as to minimize a defensive reaction.

Academic and clinical partnerships

There are many reasons to foster the partnership between academic and clinical settings, particularly facilitating the ability for students and practicing nurses to promote and cultivate EBP. The academic instructor should be cognizant that preceptors for nursing students may be skilled and experienced practicing nurses but may not be familiar with the concepts of EBP. The academic-clinical partnership can be maximized to ensure openness of the preceptor toward EBP to help both the preceptor and student and provide optimal patient care.

Academic instructors should know the organizational structure of the clinical setting where students have rotations as it relates to advancing EBP student objectives. For instance, does the organization have advanced practice nurses who are accountable for EBP in the clinical setting? Who is accountable for implementing change and for education of the staff if an EBP project is to be fully carried out in the clinical setting? How will a student navigate the system if there are multiple nursing roles accountable for pieces of an EBP implementation in the setting? What are the current organizational priorities that will impact the ability of any particular unit to be involved in an EBP implementation? What is the feasibility of any one unit to absorb multiple EBP projects at one time versus having one student group project for the semester? Who ultimately oversees the content and process of the EBP project to be implemented in the clinical setting—is it the academic instructor or the nursing leadership from the clinical setting? In setting goals and plans, be realistic about the extent of the project that can be feasibly implemented in the time frame of a nursing course. Priorities in a health care organization can change quickly, meaning resources can be quickly diverted to other initiatives.

Ideally, the academic and health care organizational leadership will develop a comprehensive approach to EBP projects completed in the clinical setting. This ensures that course instructors and the organizational leadership have an overview of all projects planned for the semester, including both undergraduate and graduate work. An institution may have multiple levels of students from several academic institutions all needing to complete EBP projects in the same time frame. Student placement managers are acutely aware of the number of students being matched to preceptors by unit throughout the hospital; however, they may not be aware of the course project expectations for those preceptors, students, and nursing leadership and the resulting impact that can have on units, nursing leadership, and the institution. Just as course instructors from the same academic institution may not be aware of other course requirements for students in the clinical setting, nursing leaders at the health care institution may not be aware of projects that are occurring throughout the institution.

This academic and clinical collaboration can include a discussion about organizational priorities during the semester and the learning objectives required for the nursing students. A consistent approach among students and units throughout the organization will help students have the support needed to meet their objectives, and units will not have discrepancies in either benefit from student projects or burden from multiple student projects at the same time.

Conclusion

This is both a challenging and an exciting time to be a health care professional. There are great opportunities to make significant strides in providing excellent evidence-based care—both through nursing practice and as part of an interdisciplinary team that can contribute to improved quality of care. The competencies identified by the IOM and adapted by the QSEN group are the next steps in ensuring patients receive the care they deserve and are expecting. Nursing has a unique opportunity to be at the front of this health care transformation by preparing nurses who are ready to accept the challenge of providing exceptional evidence-based patient care.

References

American Association of Colleges of Nursing. (2006). *The essentials of doctoral education for advanced nursing practice.* Retrieved March 15, 2011, from www.aacn.nche.edu/DNP/pdf/Essentials.pdf

American Association of Colleges of Nursing. (2008). *The essentials of baccalaureate education for professional nursing.* Retrieved March 15, 2011, from www.aacn.org/Education/pdf/BaccEssentials08.pdf

American Association of Colleges of Nursing. (2011). *AACN's essentials of master's education in nursing.* Retrieved March 15, 2011, from www.aacn.nche.edu/Education/pdf/Master'sEssentials11.pdf

Balakas, K., & Sparks, L. (2010). Teaching research and evidence-based practice. *Journal of Nursing Education, 49*(12), 691–695.

Balas, E. A. & Boren, S. A. (2000). Managing clinical knowledge for healthcare improvements. In V. Schattauer (Ed.), *Yearbook of medical informatics* (pp. 65–70). New York: Stuttgart.

Barnsteiner, J. (2010). *Evidence based practice. Enhancing quality and safety in nursing education: Preparing nurse faculty to lead curricular change.* [CDROM] Vol 1, Version 7A. Quality and Safety Education for Nurses/American Association of Colleges of Nursing.

Barnsteiner, J., Palma, W., Preston, A., Reeder, V., & Walton, M. (2010). Fueling a love of knowledge: Promoting evidence-based practice and translational research. *Nursing Administrative Quarterly, 34,* 217–235.

Barton, A. J., Armstrong, G., Preheim, G., Gelmon, S. B., & Andrus, L. C. (2009). A national Delphi to determine developmental progression of quality and safety competencies in nursing education. *Nursing Outlook, 57,* 313–22.

Cronenwett, L., Sherwood, G., Barnsteiner, J., Disch, J., Johnson, J., Mitchell, P., et al. (2007). Quality and safety education for nurses. *Nursing Outlook, 55,* 122–131.

Cronenwett, L., Sherwood, G., & Gelmon, S. B. (2009). Improving quality and safety education: The QSEN learning collaborative. *Nursing Outlook, 57,* 304–312.

Cronenwett, L., Sherwood, G., Pohl, J., Barnsteiner, J., Moore, S., Sullivan, D., T., et al. (2009). Quality and safety education for advanced practice nurses. *Nursing Outlook, 57,* 338–348.

Cronje, R. J., & Moch, S. D. (2010). Part III. Re-envisioning undergraduate nursing students as opinion leaders to diffuse evidence-based practice in clinical settings. *Journal of Professional Nursing, 26*(1), 23–28.

Department of Health and Human Services. (2010a). *Healthcare.gov: Compare quality care.* Retrieved March 15, 2011, from www.hospitalcompare.hhs.gov/staticpages/for-consumers/for-consumers.aspx

Department of Health and Human Services. (2010b). *Healthcare.gov: The national prevention strategy.* Retrieved March 15, 2011, from www.healthcare.gov/center/councils/nphpphc/final_intro.pdf

Ferguson, L., & Day, R. A. (2005). Evidence-based nursing education: Myth or reality? *Journal of Nursing Education, 44*(3), 107–115.

Fineout E., Melnyk, B. M., & Schultz, A. (2005). Transforming health care from the inside out: Advancing evidence-based practice in the 21st century. *Journal of Professional Nursing, 21,* 335–344.

Gibbons, R. J., Smith, S., & Antman, E. (2003). American College of Cardiology/American Heart Association clinical practice guidelines: Part I. Where do they come from? *Circulation, 107,* 2979–2986.

Institute of Medicine. (2001). *Crossing the quality chasm: A new health system for the 21st century.* Washington, DC: National Academies Press.

Institute of Medicine. (2003). *Health professions education: A bridge to quality*. Washington, DC: National Academies Press.

Jarzemsky, P. (2010). Integration of QSEN competencies when designing simulation scenarios. Retrieved March 18, 2011, from http://www.qsen.org/search_strategies.php?id=131

Johnston, L., & Fineout-Overholt, E. (2005). Teaching EBP: "Getting from zero to one." Moving from recognizing and admitting uncertainties to asking searchable, answerable questions. *Worldviews on Evidence-Based Nursing, 2,* 98–102.

Kim, S. C., Brown, C. E., Fields, W., & Stichler, J. F. (2009). Evidence-based practice-focused interactive teaching strategy: A controlled study. *Journal of Advanced Nursing, 65*(6), 1218–1227.

Kruszewski, A., Brough, E., & Killeen, M. B. (2009). Collaborative strategies for teaching evidence-based practice in accelerated second-degree programs. *Journal of Nursing Education, 48*(6), 340–342.

Leake, P. Y. (2004). Teaming with students and a sacred cow contest to make changes in nursing practice. *Journal of Continuing Nursing Education, 35*(6), 271–277.

McCurry, M. K., & Martins, D. C. (2010). Teaching undergraduate nursing research: A comparison of traditional and innovative approaches for success with millennial learners. *Journal of Nursing Education, 49*(5), 276–279.

McKenna, H., Cutcliffe, J., & McKenna, P. (2000). Evidence-based practice: Demolishing some myths. *Nursing Standard, 14*(16), 39–42.

Melnyk, B. M., & Fineout-Overholt, E. (2004). *Evidence-based practice nursing and healthcare: A guide to best practice*. Hagerstown, MD: Lippincott Williams & Wilkins.

Mitchell, S., Fischer, C., Hastings, C., Silverman, L., & Wallen, G. (2010). A thematic analysis of theoretical models for translational science in nursing: Mapping the field. *Nursing Outlook, 58*(6), 287–300.

Moch, S. D., & Cronje, R. J. (2010). Empowering grassroots evidence-based practice: Part II. A curricular model to foster undergraduate student-enabled practice change. *Journal of Professional Nursing, 26*(1), 14–22.

Moch, S. D., Cronje, R. J., & Branson, J. (2010). Undergraduate nursing evidence-based practice: Part I. Envisioning the role of students. *Journal of Professional Nursing, 26*(1), 5–13.

National League for Nursing Accreditation Commission. (2010a). Competencies for graduates of baccalaureate programs. Retrieved May 27, 2011, from www.nln.org/facultydevelopment/competencies/comp_bacc.htm

National League for Nursing Accreditation Commission. (2010b). Competencies for graduates of master's programs. Retrieved May 26, 2011, from www.nln.org/facultydevelopmen/competencies/comp_mast.htm

National League for Nursing Accreditation Commission. (2010c). Competencies for graduates of practice doctorate programs. Retrieved May 26, 2011, from www.nln.org/facultydevelopment/competencies/comp_prac_doc.htm

Newhouse, R., Dearholt, S., Poe, S., Pugh, L. C., & White, K. M. (2005). Evidence-based practice: A practical approach to implementation. *Journal of Nursing Administration, 35*(1), 35–40.

Newhouse, R. P., & Spring, B. (2010). Interdisciplinary evidence-based practice: Moving from silos to synergy. *Nursing Outlook, 58,* 309–317.

Oh, E.G., Kim, S., Kim, S. S., Kim, S., Cho, E., Yoo, J., et al. (2010). Integrating evidence-based practice into RN-to-BSN clinical nursing education. *Journal of Nursing Education, 49*(7), 387–392.

Pravikoff, D. S., Tanner, A. B., & Pierce, S. T. (2005). Readiness of US nurses for evidence-based practice. *American Journal of Nursing, 105*(9), 40–51.

Rolloff, M. (2010). A constructivist model for teaching evidence-based practice. *Journal of Nursing Education Perspectives, 31*(5), 290–293.

Rosswurm, M. A., & Larrabee, J. H. (1999). A model for change to evidence-based practice. *Image: Journal of Nursing Scholarship, 31*(4), 317–322.

Sackett, D. L., Strauss, S. E., Richardson, W. S., Rosenberg, W., & Haynes, R. B. (2000). *Evidence-based medicine: How to practice and teach EBM*. Edinburgh, UK: Churchill Livingstone.

Smith, E. L., Cronenwett, L., & Sherwood, G. (2007). Current assessments of quality and safety education in nursing. *Nursing Outlook, 55*, 132–137.

Stetler, C. B. (2001). Evidence-based nursing: What it is and what it isn't. *Nursing Outlook, 49*(6), 286.

Stetler, C. B. (2003). Role of the organization in translating research into evidence-based practice. *Outcomes Management, 7*(3), 97–105.

Stevens, K. C. (2004). *ACE star model of EBP: Knowledge transformation*. San Antonio, TX: Academic Center for Evidence-Based Practice, University of Texas Health Science Center. Retrieved March 20, 2011, from www.acestar.uthscsa.edu

Straus, S. E., Tetroe, J., & Graham, I. D. (Eds.). (2009). *Knowledge translation in health care: Moving evidence to practice*. Oxford, UK: Wiley-Blackwell.

Sullivan, D. T. (2010a). Evidence-based practice (EBP) project guidelines and grading criteria. Retrieved March 18, 2011, from www.qsen.org/teachingstrategy.php?id=54

Sullivan, D. T. (2010b). Staff RN perspective on evidence supporting practice. Retrieved March 18, 2011, from www.qsen.org/teachingstrategy.php?id=53

Sullivan, D. T., Hirst, D., & Cronenwett, L. (2009). Assessing quality and safety competencies of graduating prelicensure nursing students. *Nursing Outlook, 57*, 323–331.

Tetroe, J., Graham, I., Foy, R., Robinson, Eccles, M. P., Wensing, M., et al. (2008). Health research funding agencies' support and promotion of knowledge translation: An international study. *Milbank Quarterly, 86*(1), 125–155.

Titler, M. G., Kleiber, C., Steelman, V. J., Rakel, B. A., Budreau, G., Everett, L. Q., et al. (2001). The Iowa model of evidence-based practice to promote quality care. *Critical Care Nursing Clinics of North America, 13*(4), 497–509.

Chapter 8

Safety

Jane Barnsteiner, PhD, RN, FAAN

The Institute of Medicine (IOM, 1999) defined patient safety as freedom from accidental injury. It is estimated that upwards of 98,000 people die each year as a result of preventable harm from health care that is supposed to help them. Nurses in executive positions and at the frontlines of care are instrumental in preventing harm to patients and improving patient outcomes. While delivery of health care is extremely complex and there are tremendous system challenges, nurses often have been held accountable for harm to patients, even while they have not had input into system designs and have little understanding of how complex systems leave them vulnerable to making errors. Indeed, the issue of health care safety is so serious, the IOM has produced numerous reports devoted to identifying the issues and recommending how to solve them. Consequently, many organizations have become involved in working to make health care safer. These include the Institute for Healthcare Improvement, The Joint Commission, the American Association of Colleges of Nursing, the National League for Nursing, the American Nurses Association, and the National Patient Safety Foundation, among many others.

The goal of a culture of safety is to "minimize the risk of harm to patients and providers through both system effectiveness and individual performance" (Cronenwett et al., 2007). This acknowledges the influence of complex systems and human factors within the health care delivery system in general and within nursing practice specifically. While a health care culture of safety has been a practice priority in nursing for many years, there has been scant attention to incorporating the specific content related to the science of safety into the education of health care professionals.

There are numerous threats to patient safety and errors that can occur at all interfaces of care delivery. Common situations that are obstacles to a safe system include an extremely complex and inherently risk-prone system that can produce unintended consequences; lack of comprehensive verbal, written, and electronic communication systems; tolerance of individualistic practices and lack of standardization; fear of retribution inhibiting reporting; and organizational lack of ownership for patient safety.

Quality and Safety in Nursing: A Competency Approach to Improving Outcomes, First Edition. Edited by Gwen Sherwood and Jane Barnsteiner.

The work of the IOM has been to move the emphasis to widespread system change to promote safety. The message in IOM's *To Err Is Human* was to prevent, recognize, and mitigate harm from error. Errors are defined as the "failure of a planned action to be completed as intended or the use of a wrong plan to achieve an aim" (IOM, 1999). There are multiple places where errors can take place; the medication prescribing-dispensing-administration cycle, wrong site surgery, equipment designs and failure, and handoffs at change of shift reporting are but a few examples (Mitchell, 2008). Nurses need to be knowledgeable about system vulnerabilities and understand how knowledge, skills, and attitudes promoting utilization of safety science will lead to high-quality care for patients and families (Cronenwett, 2012; Cronenwett et al., 2007; Cronenwett et al., 2009; Finkelman & Kenner, 2009).

Learning about patient safety as a fundamental quality of patient care needs to begin in prelicensure programs and be an integral part of learning in all phases of nursing education and practice (Cronenwett et al., 2007; Cronenwett et al., 2009). This chapter will discuss the mechanism of developing a culture of safety in learning organizations, and how understanding the limits of human factors and appreciating the reasons for comprehensive reporting mechanisms are essential components in the preparation of nurses to be participants in 21st century health care, and how these concepts about safety can be integrated into nursing education in both the clinical and academic settings.

Culture of safety

Elements of a culture of safety in an organization are establishment of safety as an organizational priority, teamwork, patient involvement, openness/transparency, and accountability (Lamb et al., 2003). There are shared core values and goals, nonpunitive responses to adverse events and errors, and promotion of safety through education and training. A balance needs to be achieved between not blaming individuals for errors and not tolerating egregious behavior. This is currently referred to as a "just culture" (Mitchell, 2008; Yates et al., 2005).

Culture is not necessarily uniform within a single organization. Within a health care setting, each discipline may have a different culture as can each patient care area. While differences may benefit the work of the practice group or organization, more frequently it results in communication difficulties, particularly around patient handoffs (Lamb, Studdert, Bohmer, Berwick, & Brennan, 2003; Riensenberg, Leitsch, & Cunningham, 2010, Walsh & Shortell, 2004). In a culture of safety, the focus is on effective teamwork to accomplish the goal of safe, high-quality patient care. Within a culture of safety, when an adverse event occurs, the focus is on *what* went wrong, *not who* is the problem. A culture of blame has been pervasive in health care. The focus has often been to try to determine who has been at fault and, all too often, to mete out discipline. This approach leads to hiding rather than reporting errors and is the antithesis of a culture of safety. More recent efforts have been directed to changing this approach and to encourage people to report problems so they can be addressed (Lamb et al., 2003).

A patient safety culture is nonpunitive and emphasizes accountability, excellence, honesty, integrity, and mutual respect. It incorporates safety principles such as designing jobs and working conditions for safety; standardizing and simplifying equipment, supplies, and processes; and avoiding reliance on memory (Association of Perioperative Registered Nurses, 2006). A safety culture requires strong, committed leadership, and engagement and empowerment of all employees. It entails periodic assessment of the culture by employees about the relationship between the organization culture and the quality and safety within the organization (Wachter & Pronovost, 2009). Numerous tools are available for measuring the health care safety culture within an organization. The most widely used is the Culture of Patient Safety Assessment developed by the Agency for Healthcare Research and Quality (AHRQ; Sorra, Famolaro, & Dyer, 2008; see Table 8.1).

Table 8.1 Safety culture assessment tools

Tool	Website
Agency for Healthcare Research and Quality (AHRQ) Three surveys on patient safety culture: • Nursing Home Survey on Patient Safety Culture • Medical Office Survey on Patient Safety Culture • Hospital Survey on Patient Safety Culture Health care organizations can use these survey assessment tools to: • Assess their patient safety culture • Track changes in patient safety over time • Evaluate the impact of patient safety interventions	http://www.ahrq.gov/qual/patientsafetyculture/
Premier data tool for managing results of AHRQ culture survey	http://www.premierinc.com/quality-safety/tools-services/safety/topics/culture/data-tool.jsp#download
VHA culture survey to assess leadership and organizational culture climate	https://www.vhafoundation.org/portal/server.pt?open=512&objID=1279&PageID=526932&cached=true&mode=2
Westat Patient Safety Culture Improvement Tool (PSCIT)	http://www.longwoods.com/product.php?productid=19604

The IOM outlined the components of quality care as: safe, timely, effective, efficient, equitable, and patient centered. STEEEP is a useful acronym to remember the components (Acronym Finder, 2009). The Quality and Safety Education for Nurses (QSEN) definition of safety is adapted from the IOM and is defined as "minimiz[ing] risk of harm to patients and providers through both system effectiveness and individual performance" (Cronenwett et al., 2007, p. 128).

What students/clinicians need to know about safety

The QSEN project (Cronenwett et al., 2007, 2009) was developed to identify the competencies prelicensure and graduate students need for safe practice. With funding from the Robert Wood Johnson Foundation, a group of experts, with consultation and input from multiple accrediting and professional groups, developed the competencies and disseminated them in publications (Cronenwett, 2012; Cronenwett et al., 2007; Cronenwett et al., 2009;), a website, www.qsen.org, through an annual national forum, and in "train the trainer" workshops to nurse educators across the United States. Didactic, simulation laboratory and clinical fieldwork teaching strategies have been developed to assist educators to in incorporating a culture of safety into the curriculum. This chapter describes the components of the safety competency that needs to be embedded into nursing curricula and strategies for doing so.

The QSEN definition of safety incorporates the need for students to understand that "safe, effective delivery of patient care requires understanding of the complexity of care delivery, the limits of human factors, safety design principles, characteristics of high reliability organizations, and patient safety resources" (Cronenwett et al., 2007). Our traditional focus of education for nursing students and clinicians has been steeped in the care of individual patients and families with understanding of the complexity of care delivery systems being notably absent.

To teach the safety competency requires teaching of all the QSEN competencies (Barnsteiner, 2011). *Patient-centered care* (Walton & Barnsteiner, 2012) ensures the patient and family is at the center of the decision-making process and understands the plan of care that can prevent errors from occurring. *Evidence-based practice* (Tracey & Barnsteiner, 2012) ensures clinicians are using up-to-date science in addition to considering clinical expertise and patient values in designing a plan of care. *Teamwork and collabora*tion (Disch, 2012) ensures the health care team is communicating and working together effectively with shared decision among professionals to achieve safe, high-quality care. *Quality improvement* (Johnson, 2012) provides for trending and analysis of data to be able to benchmark with comparable organizations and identify vulnerabilities in the system needing correction. *Informatics* (Warren, 2012) enables clinicians to use information and technology to communicate, access knowledge, and support decision making to promote safe care. The QSEN project separated quality and safety into two separate competencies, whereas the IOM lists them together, to more comprehensively address the science underlying each of the two and to better describe the knowledge, skills, and attitudes necessary for effective practice (Sherwood, 2011, 2012).

The safety competency

Appendixes A and B list the safety competency knowledge, skills, and attitudes students and clinicians need to know to practice safely. Content includes the elements of a culture of safety, types of health care errors and why they occur, and how to make care safer.

Categories of errors

Students and clinicians need to understand that errors can take place across the health care system. Latent failures, sometimes called the "blunt" end, arise from decisions that affect organizational policies, procedures, and allocation of resources. For example, the decisions made by the purchasing department regarding the types of monitoring equipment to buy without input from frontline clinicians may result in equipment that does not work seamlessly in the daily work at the frontlines of care. Active failures occur at the interface of contact with the patient; for example, a nurse being interrupted during medication administration loses her concentration and pulls the wrong syringe from the medication drawer. This is sometimes referred to as the "sharp" end. Organizational system failures, or indirect failures, are related to management, organizational culture, policies/processes, transfer of knowledge, and external factors, for example, how decisions are made regarding staffing and scheduling. Technical failures are the indirect failure of facilities or resources, such as when a backup generator does not function during an electrical blackout.

A commonly used framework for considering the components related to patient safety is Reason's Adverse Event Trajectory, often referred to as the Swiss cheese model (Reason, 2000). When a system fails, the immediate question should be *why* it failed rather than *who* caused the failure; for example, which safeguards failed. Reason created the Swiss cheese model to explain how faults in the different layers of the system can lead to errors. The Swiss cheese framework describes the numerous triggers that can set up a sequence of events that may cause an error to occur. These include institution triggers such as incomplete or overly complicated procedures and policies, organization triggers such as patient flow pressures, professional triggers such as delegation authority, team triggers such as inadequate communication training, individual triggers such as distractions, and technical triggers such as the use of universal connections. Multiple defenses set up to prevent errors from occurring occasionally line up so that multiple triggers align to allow an accident to occur. Hence, the name Swiss cheese model—the holes are aligned.

Sammer, Lykens, Singh, Mains, and Lackan (2010) identified seven subcultures of patient safety from the research on safety culture; these form a framework that may answer the question, "What is a patient safety culture?" The seven subcultures identified are leadership, teamwork, evidence-based, communication, learning, just, and patient-centered. They align closely with the QSEN competencies.

The Joint Commission established the National Patient Safety Goals to promote specific improvements in patient safety. The requirements highlight problematic areas in health care and describe evidence and expert-based solutions to these problems. The goals that are reviewed and updated annually focus generally on systemwide solutions for hospitals, mental health settings, ambulatory settings, and other health care settings (Joint Commission, 2011).

Making care safer

Students need to understand how nurses may contribute to making care safer. The IOM (2001) described nine categories that provide opportunities to improve patient safety by incorporating these into organizations that have a culture of safety:

1. **User-centered design**. A user-centered design makes it easier for the clinician to do the right action. Approaches include making things visible so the user is able to see actions possible at any time, affordance, constraints, and forcing functions. For example, making something visible would be signs outside a patient door alerting providers the patient is at risk for falls so clinicians passing by the room would look in more frequently to check on the patient. Affordance indicates how something is to be used, such as marking the correct limb before surgery or a sign on a door indicating which way to open it. A constraint makes it hard to do the wrong thing, and a forcing function makes it impossible to do the wrong thing, such as connect equipment to a patient improperly.
2. **Avoid reliance on memory**. Standardizing and simplifying procedures and tasks decreases the demand on memory, planning, and problem solving. The use of protocols and checklists reduces reliance on memory and serves as a reminder for the steps to be followed. Simplifying processes minimizes problem solving. Having the usual dose of a medication as the default in an electronic order entry, or having an easy-to-use checklist in the procedure tray for central line placement outlining correct steps are examples of simplification of processes.
3. **Attend to work safety**. Work hours, workloads, staffing ratios, distractions, and interruptions all affect patient safety. In many health care settings, realizing that interruptions are a major cause of medication administration errors, nurses have chosen to wear something visually apparent such as a vest to indicate they should not be interrupted when they are preparing or administering medications. Standardizing practice with implementation of "red rules," safe zones, and sacred spaces are all

practices that attend to a safe working environment. Having policies and processes in place that require that staff take lunch breaks to recharge promotes patient safety.

4. **Avoid reliance on vigilance**. Checklists, well-designed alarms, rotating staff, and breaks decrease the need for remaining vigilant for long periods. Well-designed alarms that differentiate a potential emergency from a pressing situation decrease the need for continuous vigilance. For example, one alarm may signal a disconnected ventilator needing immediate response, while another may notify of an intravenous pump needing adjustment. Rotating staff assignments and staff taking scheduled breaks and meals also decreases the need for remaining vigilant for long periods.

5. **Training concepts for teams**. The literature is replete with more than 20 years of evidence outlining the importance of teamwork and collaboration. Training programs for effective intra-and interprofessional communication and collaboration include standardizing transitions in care and handoffs, and implementation of crew resource management skill. Many organizations are implementing TeamSTEPPS to provide a framework for interprofessional collaboration and communication and instill a skill set consistent with a safety climate (www.ahrq.gov).

6. **Involve patients in their care**. Patients and families should be in the center of the care process. This includes clinicians obtaining accurate information and including patients and families in decisions about treatments and comprehensive discharge planning and education. Knowing the plan of care, holding rounds in patient rooms, and having patients/families participate promote the concept of patients being at the center and source of control. It allows patients to become knowledgeable about their care and to correct any misinformation. This also means clinicians have a responsibility to assist patients and families to become health literate.

7. **Anticipate the unexpected**. Reorganization and organization-wide changes result in new patterns and processes of care. Introduction of new processes and technologies depends on a chain of involvement of frontline users and the need for pilot testing before widespread implementation to identify vulnerabilities that may affect patient safety. When implementing changes, such as the implementation of an electronic health care record, that call for new ways to deliver care, it would be important to increase organizational vigilance with additional staffing. Additional information system resources during implementation of a new electronic health care record system promotes safe care by anticipating unexpected breakdowns which may happen when putting in a large-scale change.

8. **Design for recovery**. Errors will occur despite the existence of a culture of safety. Designing and planning for recovery will allow reversal or make it hard to carry out irreversible critical functions. Simulation training promotes the practice of processes and rescues using models and virtual reality. Having backup generators in place in the event of an electrical failure, and disaster management programs in place and practiced on a regular basis, help to promote a smooth recovery with minimal harm to patients.

9. **Improve access to accurate, timely information**. Information for decision making needs to be available at the point of care. This includes easy access to drug formularies, evidence-based practice protocols, patient records, laboratory reports, and medication administration records.

Nursing is in a central position to improve the quality and safety of care through patient safety activities as nurses are in the position to coordinate and integrate the multiple aspects of care, monitoring, and identifying hazards and changes in patient conditions before errors and adverse events can occur. Nursing is also in a position to positively affect high-quality, safe care with strong leadership, adequate staffing, and strong interprofessional communication and collaboration.

High-reliability organizations

Safety science posits that safety is dependent on health care systems and organizations and patients should be safe from injury caused by interactions with these systems and organizations of care (Shortell et al., 2005). Organizations that have cultures of safety, foster a learning environment and evidence-based care, promote positive working environments for nurses, and are committed to improving the safety and quality of care are considered to be high-reliability organizations (Carrol & Rudolph, 2006). Characteristics of these organizations include having a safety- and quality-centered culture, direct involvement of top and middle leadership, safety and quality efforts aligned with the strategic plan, an established infrastructure for safety, and continuous improvement and active engagement of staff across the organization (Bagian et al., 2001; Baker, Ray, & Sales, 2006; Shortell et al., 2005). They exhibit characteristics of having all employees fully engaged in the process of detecting high-risk situations, there are resources dedicated to bringing about the changes suggested, everyone is empowered to act in dangerous situations, and there is a work environment that is fair to employees (Page, 2004). The safety and quality of care can be improved by holding systems accountable, redesigning systems and processes to mitigate the effects of human factors, and using strategic improvements.

Work environment

The IOM report *Keeping Patients Safe: Transforming the Work Environment of Nurses* (2004) emphasized the importance of the work environment in which nurses provide care. Recommendations from the report included the need for the following:

1. The chief nurse executive to have a leadership role in the organization. This provides a voice for nursing and safe patient care at the top levels of the organization.
2. Evidence-based staffing models, which decrease stress and workload and positively impact patient outcomes.

3. Evidence-based scheduling, which modulates the effect of fatigue.
4. Safe work environments such as safe patient handling programs, which minimize injury and disability and promote healthy work environments.

The Joint Commission identified the pervasive effect on patient safety related to disruptive behavior among health care clinicians. Disruptive behavior is psychological and physical intimidation and overt and passive activities meant to intimidate or disrupt care. Disruptive behavior/bullying/abuse has a negative effect on quality of care, patient safety, and nurse retention and job satisfaction (Barnsteiner, 2012; Clarke & Donaldson, 2008; Heath, Johanson, & Blake, 2004). The Joint Commission (2009) has identified that disruptive behaviors undermine a culture of safety and has instituted two leadership standards for accreditation that will facilitate civility in the workplace and give staff a mechanism for reporting disruptive behavior:

- EP 4: The hospital/organization has a code of conduct that defines acceptable and disruptive and inappropriate behaviors.
- EP 5: Leaders create and implement a process for managing disruptive and inappropriate behaviors.

In addition to disruptive behavior, components in the design of the physical environment can produce vulnerabilities to patient safety and clinician safety as well. Having "no lift" policies and sufficient patient lifting equipment prevents patient and clinician injuries. Limiting work hours and adequate staffing prevents fatigue. Workspace design that promotes flow of patient care and fewer interruptions decreases the chance of errors.

Work-arounds may present patient safety hazards. Clinicians regularly encounter problems or impediments in delivering care and invent a quick work-around to solve those problems. This first-order change occurs because clinicians are really busy and need to get the problem solved. Examples include using equipment for purposes it was not intended or bypassing the procedure for barcoding medication administration because the process has too many steps. Many organizations do not provide a way to report problems and develop solutions in a timely or effective fashion. This frequently used approach to problem solving leaves systemic problems untreated and potentially is a cause of error.

Human factors

Human factors is the science of the interrelationship between humans, the technology they use, and the environment in which they work (IOM, 1999). Thinking is automatic, rapid, and effortless. Actions often are a result of mental models that are based on recurrent aspects of our lives, such as the way one drives to work or the routine for admitting a postoperative heart transplant patient. Fatigue, distraction, and interruptions affect cognitive abilities and problem solving. Errors result when one is tired, distracted, or interrupted and consequently deviates from safe operating procedures, standards, and policies, which can be routine and necessary (Reason, 2000). Human factors considers the "human condition," or our inability to focus on multiple things at once and perform accurately (Vicente, 2004). Everyone, regardless of the role they play in a health care system, needs to be mindful of the interdependent system factors and their importance in shaping safe care. Recent studies reported that nurses were interrupted on average almost 12 times per hour and 22% of the time while administering medications, as well as frequently while performing safety-critical tasks (Brixey, 2010; Trbovich, Prakash, Stewart, Trip, & Savage, 2010). Understanding the complex and demanding clinical environment helps us be aware of the components and relationships that influence the safety of care. Systems need to be designed to protect against human errors; hence, the focus needs to be on system failures, not human failures, and on meeting the needs of clinicians within the health care system.

Transitions in care and handoffs

Handoff of patient care from one nurse to another is an integral part of nursing practice (Dayton & Henricksen, 2007; Riesenberg et al., 2010; Sexton et al., 2004). The term handover rather than handoff is increasingly being used in practice to indicate the process is not one-sided. Handoff is used in this chapter as it is the more commonly used term. Transitions in care and handoffs create vulnerabilities in health care that require special attention. Central to effective handoffs is effective communication. Ineffective communication and inadequate handoffs have negative consequences for patients. Standardization in the processes of handoffs with face-to-face communication remains key to addressing patient safety concerns (Dayton & Henricksen, 2007; Friesen, White, & Byers, 2008; Saint, Kaufman, Thompson, Rogers, & Chenowith, 2005; Welsh, Flanagan, & Ebright, 2010). The Joint Commission International Center for Patient Safety (2005) defines handoff communication as "the realtime process of passing patient specific information from one caregiver to another or from one team of caregivers to another for the purpose of ensuring continuity and safety of the patient/client/resident's care." Handoffs may be facilitated through the use of standardized change of shift reporting checklists. SBAR (situation, background, assessment, and recommendation) has become a frequently used approach both for interprofessional communication and nurse to nurse communication (Barenfinger, Sauter, & Lang, 2004; Haig, Sutton, & Whittington, 2006; Hanna, Griswold, Leape, & Bates, 2005). At the direct work group/team level, the use of safety huddles has been demonstrated to engage frontline staff in improving patient safety (Gerke, Uffelman, & Chandler, 2010).

Processes for examining safety threats

Root cause analysis (RCA) and failure mode and effects analysis (FMEA) are two methods for examining the factors leading to an adverse event or a close call (Johnson, 2012; Reiling, Knutzen, & Stoecklein, 2003; Rooney & Vanden

Heuvel, 2004). There are numerous resources for RCAs and FMEAs on the AHRQ website (www.patientsafety.gov). The Joint Commission recommends an RCA after all sentinel events to outline the sequence of events that led up to the event, identifying causal factors and root causes. It is followed by defining a course of action to eliminate risks.

FMEA is an evaluation technique used to identify and eliminate known and/ or potential failures, problems, and errors from a system, design, process, and/or service before they actually occur (Hughes & Blegen, 2008). The goal of an FMEA is to prevent errors by attempting to identify all the ways a process could fail, estimate the probability and consequences of each failure, and then take action to prevent the potential failures from occurring. Simulating equipment failures has been shown to be useful to hone provider skills and identify equipment vulnerabilities and to evaluate alternative approaches or procedures (Waldrop, Murray, Boulet, & Kraus, 2009).

Disclosure

Accountability to patients and families is a hallmark of a culture of safety. Disclosure of errors to patients is linked to patient safety efforts and is mandated by many state patient safety requirements. It involves both communicating information as well as addressing the patient's emotions. High-reliability organizations have in place policies, processes, and training directed toward disclosing health care errors and significant near misses to patients and their families. Students and clinicians need to understand the disclosure process for the health care organization and develop disclosure communication skills related to how to deliver difficult news.

External drivers of safety

Voluntary versus mandatory error reporting systems

The IOM (2001) differentiated between mandatory and voluntary reporting of health care errors. Voluntary reports may encourage practitioners to report near misses and errors, thus producing important information that might reduce future errors. However, there is concern that with voluntary reporting, the true error frequency may be many times greater than what is actually reported. Mandatory reporting systems, usually enacted under state law, generally require reporting of sentinel events, adverse events causing patient harm, and unanticipated outcomes such as serious patient injury or death (Schumann, 2012).

The IOM (2001) has called for a nationwide reporting system that would provide funds for state governments to organize systems for reporting errors. The goal is to have a national patient safety center that would receive state reports and aggregate data for intensive analysis. To date, this legislation has not been passed, but there are 22 states that currently have mandatory reporting and that have designed databases to aggregate and report statewide data.

Regulation, legislation, accrediting organizations, linking payment with performance, commitment of professional organizations, and public engagement can impact the safety and quality of nursing care and health care (Schumann, 2012). Numerous states such as Pennsylvania and Texas now have error reporting laws. Accrediting organizations such as the Joint Commission influence patient safety with explicit standards such as the National Patient Safety Goals and handoff communications. The Centers for Medicare and Medicaid Services are linking reporting performance on quality indicators such as pressure ulcer prevalence and central line infections with hospital payment. An initiative of the National Council of State Boards of Nursing, the Practice Breakdown Advisory Panel, was established to study nursing practice breakdown and identify common themes related to events and recommend strategies to correct unsafe practices (National Council of State Boards of Nursing, 2010). It is expected that this work will shift the focus of state boards of nursing from punishment to prevention and correction. The American Nurses Association has widely publicized standards related to prevention of workplace injuries from needle sticks and patient lifting. The American Association of Critical-Care Nurses (2005) promulgated standards for establishing and sustaining healthy work environments. All of these efforts are initiating changes in the work environment for nurses (Antonovsky, Smith, & Silver, 2000; Elnitsky, Nichols, & Palmer, 1997; Evans et al., 2006; Schumann, 2012).

Openness is a critical factor in a culture of safety. It indicates there is acceptance of human elements in error and a means of reporting any error or near miss or identified potential for error. Many errors go unreported by health care workers. A major concern clinicians have is that self-reporting will result in repercussions. Lack of reporting of errors and near misses has consequences for individual clinicians as well as for the organizations in which they work. Unreported errors remove the opportunity of analyzing to improve patient safety, thereby limiting improvements because there is no understanding of what works to prevent the errors. Openness is important so that errors and potential problems are exposed and solved before they endanger others. Within a culture of openness, there is a "just culture" where discipline is limited to reckless or egregious behavior.

Near misses are more common than adverse events and provide valuable information regarding weaknesses in systems that predispose to adverse events (Bagian et al., 2001). Aggregate data from near-miss analyses is used to direct attention to critical safety issues. Discussions of near misses usually do not generate the defensive reaction often associated with discussion of adverse events. Institutional reporting systems system should be nonpunitive and should keep reported information confidential and nondiscoverable. Information should be used for system improvements. The reporting process should be uncomplicated and preferably electronic to lead to rapid analysis. The opportunity for anonymous reporting is thought to lead to greater willingness to report errors. Traditional reporting mechanisms have utilized verbal reports and paper-based incident reports to detect and document clinically significant medical errors, yet the correlation with actual errors has been low (Gallagher, Waterman, Ebers, Frassier, & Levinson, 2003; Weissman et al., 2005).

Reporting errors and near misses through established systems provides opportunities to prevent future similar, and perhaps even more serious, errors. Several factors are necessary to increase error reporting: having leadership committed to patient safety; eliminating a punitive culture and institutionalizing a culture of safety; increasing reporting of near misses; providing timely feedback and follow-up actions and improvements to avert future errors; and having a multidisciplinary approach to reporting (Lawton & Parker, 2002; Nuckols, Bell, Liu, Paddock, & Hillborne, 2007; Thurman, 2001).

Second victim

Health care professionals report feeling worried, guilty, and depressed following serious errors, as well as being concerned for patient safety and fearful of disciplinary actions (Conway, Federico, Stewart, & Campbell, 2010; Rassin, Kanti, & Silner, 2005; Rossheim, 2009; Scott et al., 2010; Wolf, 2005). They also are aware of their direct responsibility for errors. Many nurses accept responsibility and blame themselves for serious-outcome errors. Wu (2000) coined the phrase *second victim* to describe the impact of errors on professionals. The use of the term is controversial. Consumer advocates challenge the use of the term *second victim* on the basis that it takes attention away from the patient who suffered because of an error. However, health care professionals practice the art and science of health care delivery within very complex environments. Rather than allow clinicians to suffer alone after an adverse event, it is imperative that systems be developed to help them understand the event, to stimulate healing, and to improve the health care system (Denham, 2007; Institute for Safe Medication Practices, 2011; White, Waterman, McCotter, Boyle, & Gallagher, 2008).

Integrating a culture of safety into the curriculum

Sherwood (2011) described initiatives taking place worldwide for integrating quality and safety science in nursing education and practice. These include curriculum mapping for spreading the competencies across the curriculum, educational standards for incorporating the competencies into accrediting organizations, curriculum essentials documents, and regional institutes held across the country that use a train-the-trainer development model to help educators transform curricula. Barton, Armstrong, Preheim, Gelmon, and Andrus (2009) used a developmental approach—beginning, intermediate, and advanced stages of the curriculum—in a Delphi study to identify where in the curriculum the 162 QSEN competencies should be introduced and where they should be emphasized (see Appendix C). Early introduction was recommended for the safety competency and indeed should be integrated in all phases of an educational program. The National Council of State Boards of Nursing in their Transition to Practice model recommends the QSEN competencies be incorporated into nurse residency programs for new-to-practice nurses (Spector, Ulrich, & Barnsteiner, 2012). Content related to a safety should be a component of ongoing professional development programs across all health care agencies.

Teaching strategies

How to teach the safety competency

Students and clinicians alike need to understand that safe, effective delivery of patient care requires understanding of the following: the complexity of health care systems, the limits of human factors, safety design principles, characteristics of high-reliability organizations, and patient safety resources. Safety education needs to move from the "background" of implicit learning to the "foreground" of established curriculum. For educators to teach safety they must be knowledgeable and current about the components of a safe culture. Activities that may facilitate up-to-date learning are (1) become members of a clinical agency such as Quality Improvement, Patient Safety, pharmacy, and other quality and safety committees, (2) schools of nursing holding quarterly or twice yearly meetings of clinical agency chief nursing executives and clinical leaders with deans/ directors and key educators, and (3) gaining familiarity with resources to use when teaching, such as on the QSEN website (www.qsen.org). The IHI (Institute for Healthcare Improvement) Open School has courses on quality and safety that are free for faculty and students.

Most nurses, including nurse educators, have not been educated in error prevention or trained as patient safety coaches (Reid & Catchpole, 2011). When a teaching moment presents itself, as with a medication administration near miss by a student, a nurse will typically base educational outcomes on success or failure, automatically designating errors or near misses as failures without analyzing the circumstances surrounding the incident. Curricula should stress the complexity of patient safety, using near misses as well as sentinel events as educational tools to improve delivery of care. A case-based curriculum provides opportunities for role-play in "ideal" models as well as "real" situations. Scenarios should stress truth telling, responsible behavior, error reporting, and follow-up to error reporting. Finally, a comprehensive curriculum should prepare nurses to anticipate the potential for error. Multiple strategies may be employed to teach a culture of safety. These are usually divided into classroom, simulation laboratory, and clinical activities (see Textboxes 8.1–8.3).

Textbox 8.1   Classroom education activities to teach safety competency

- Demonstrate prescribing, dispensing, and medication error vulnerabilities and solutions during pharmacy classes.
- Evaluate the research on work hours and fatigue and have discussion of how these affect quality of care and risk of errors.
- Discuss sentinel event and serious reportable event—"never event"— statistics.
- Discuss The Joint Commission videos such as *Speak Up: Prevent Errors in Your Care*, which may be accessed on YouTube http://www.youtube.com/watch?v=EccuE-_2_2E (retrieved June 28, 2011).
- Use unfolding case studies incorporating multiple QSEN competencies within cases appropriate for the course content. See www.qsen.org website for examples.
- Invite patients and/or their families to tell their stories and what they want from health care providers.
- Incorporate problem-based learning with clinical scenarios in classroom with participants working in teams.
- Develop pocket guides—brief self-contained learning modules on the components of safety—for clinicians and students to use.

Textbox 8.2   Simulation education activities to teach safety competency

- Use a patient model to simulate safety breaches.
- Simulate equipment failures with scenarios to detect and correct equipment problems.
- Set up a clinical room with opportunities to identify and correct multiple hazards and errors.
- Demonstrate how a near-miss or error is documented.
- Practice SBAR for effective handoffs and communication between and among clinicians.
- Use high-fidelity clinical simulations to assess ability to deliver safe care in the clinical setting.
- Read and interpret medication labels, some of which are correct and some of which contain errors. Have participants rewrite labels for clearer understanding.
- Use a complex set of discharge medication orders and set up a schedule of medications; have participants set up a mediset using small candies.

> **Textbox 8.3   Clinical education activities to teach safety competency**
>
> - Observe and evaluate teamwork communication and collaboration while attending patients.
> - Design a checklist for a common procedure, e.g., insertion of foley catheter.
> - Serve as "secret shoppers" and observe staff and other students' technique, such as hand hygiene or interruptions. Track findings and report the data.
> - Discuss near misses and adverse events with staff nurses during clinical experiences.
> - Attend an RCA and/or FMEA.
> - Observe and evaluate teamwork, communication, and collaboration on patient/walk rounds.
> - Develop QI projects in clinical settings and engage an interprofessional team to implement the project. Share project results with students, educators, and agency members.
> - Attend patient safety rounds.
> - Incorporate reflective exercises on patient safety in clinical postconferences.
> - Complete TeamSTEPPS and assess communication and collaboration on interprofessional patient rounds.
> - Develop a safety rounds checklist and have teams make unit rounds to complete the checklist. Have participants share results with staff and initiate a discussion of the findings.
> - Peer review of documentation to assess for any errors in documentation.
> - Set up error/near miss reporting system to trend student errors/near misses.
> - Complete an environmental safety scan of a clinical area and evaluate the lighting, space, and accessibility for patients, families, and staff. Assess traffic and noise, and accessibility of supplies and equipment, including space for medication preparation.
> - Working in teams, a nursing, medical, and pharmacy student examine a complex patient health record and complete a medication reconciliation analysis from admission through discharge.
> - Design approaches to reduce interruptions, such as wearing vests during medication administration and establishing no-interruption zones such as the medication preparation area.

Summary

Making progress on a culture of safety begins with learning how to learn about safety. Change, however, will occur at different stages and speed. Cultural transitions can take 10 years or more. Educators and clinicians need to be proactive and remain persistent in the commitment to help develop the knowledge, skills, and attitudes necessary to reshape the education and practice environment. Reducing health care errors is complex business. Safe, effective delivery of patient care requires understanding of the complexity of health care systems, the limits of human factors, safety design principles, characteristics of high reliability organizations, and patient safety resources. These components are critical to the preparation of safe clinicians and essential for 21st century health care delivery.

References

Acronym Finder (2009). Retrieved on June 29, 2011, from http://www.acronym-finder.com/Safe%2c-Timely%2c Effective%2c-Efficient%2c-Equitable%2c-Patient_Centered-(Care%3b-Baylor-Health-Care-System)-(STEEEP).html.

American Association of Critical-Care Nurses. (2005). AACN standards for establishing and sustaining healthy work environments: A journey to excellence. *American Journal of Critical Care, 14*, 187–197.

Antonovsky, J. A., Smith, A. B., & Silver, M. P. (2000). Medication error reporting: A survey of nursing staff. *Journal of Nursing Care Quality, 15*(1), 42–48.

Association of periOperative Registered Nurses. (2006). *AORN position statement: Creating a patient safety culture.* Retrieved October 20, 2009, from www.aorn.org/PracticeResources/AORNPositionStatements/Position_Creat ingaPatientSafetyCulture,

Bagian, J. P., Lee, C., Gosbee, J., DeRosier, J., Stalhandske, E., Eldridge, N., et al. (2001). Developing and deploying a patient safety program in a large health care delivery system: You can't fix what you don't know about. *Joint Commission Journal on Quality Improvement, 27*(10), 522–532.

Baker, D. P., Day, R., & Sales, E. (2006). Teamwork as an essential component of high-reliability organizations. *Health Services Research, 41*(4), 1576–1598.

Barenfinger, J., Sauter, R. L., & Lang, D. L. (2004). Improving patient safety by repeating (read-back) telephone reports of critical information. *American Journal of Clinical Pathology, 121*, 801–803.

Barnsteiner, J. (2012). Workplace abuse in nursing. In D. Mason, J. Leavitt, & M. Chafee (Eds.), *Politics and policy in nursing and healthcare*, 6th ed. London: Elsevier.

Barnsteiner, J. (2011). Teaching the culture of safety. *Online Journal of Issues in Nursing, 16*(3), Ms. 5.

Barton, A., Armstrong, G., Preheim, G., Gelmon S., & Andrus L. (2009). A national Delphi to determine developmental progression of quality and safety competencies in nursing education. *Nursing Outlook, 57*, 331–332.

Brixey, J., (2010, March/April). Interruptions in workflow for RNs in a level one trauma center. *Patient Safety and Quality Healthcare*, 25-30.

Carrol, J. S., & Rudolph, J. W. (2006). Design of high reliability organizations in health care. *Quality and Safety in Health Care, 15*(Suppl. 1), i4–i9.

Clarke, S., & Donaldson, N. (2008). Nurse staffing and patient care quality and safety. In Hughes, R. G., (Ed.), *Patient safety and quality: An evidence-based handbook for nurses*, (pp. 2-111-2-136). Rockville, MD: Agency for Healthcare Research and Quality, Publication No. 08-0043.

Conway, J., Federico, F., Stewart, K., & Campbell, MJ. (2010). Respectful management of serious clinical adverse events. IHI Innovation Series white paper. Cambridge, MA: Institute for Healthcare Improvement.

Cronenwett, L. (2012). A national initiative: Quality and Safety Education for Nurses (QSEN). In G. Sherwood & J. Barnsteiner (Eds.), *Quality and safety in nursing: A competency approach to improving outcomes*. Hoboken, NJ: Wiley-Blackwell.

Cronenwett, L., Sherwood, G., Barnsteiner, J., Disch J., Johnson, J., Mitchell, P., et al. (2007). Quality and safety education for nurses. *Nursing Outlook, 55*, 122-131.

Cronenwett, L., Sherwood, G., Pohl, J., Barnsteiner, J. Moore, S., Sullivan, D. T., et al. (2009). Quality and safety education for advanced practice nurses. *Nursing Outlook, 57*, 338-348.

Dayton, E., & Henriksen, K. (2007). Communication failure: Basic components, contributing factors, and the call for structure. *Joint Commission Journal on Quality and Patient Safety/Joint Commission Resources, 33*(1), 34-47.

Denham, C. R. (2007). Trust: The 5 rights of the second victim. *Journal of Patient Safety, 3*, 107-119.

Disch, J. (2012). Teamwork and collaboration. In G. Sherwood & J. Barnsteiner (Eds.), *Quality and safety in nursing: A competency approach to improving outcomes*. Hoboken, NJ: Wiley-Blackwell.

Elnitsky, C., Nichols, B., & Palmer K. (1997). Are hospital incidents being reported? *Journal of Nursing Administration, 27*, 40-46.

Evans, S. M., Berry, J. G., Smith, B. J., Esterman, A., Selim, P., O'Shaughnessy, J., & DeWit M. (2006). Attitudes and barriers to incident reporting: A collaborative hospital study. *Quality and Safety in Health Care, 15*, 39-43.

Finkelman, A., & Kenner, C. (2009). *Teaching IOM: Implications of the Institute of Medicine reports for nursing*, 2nd ed. Silver Springs, MD: Nursebooks.org.

Friesen, M. A., White, S. V., & Byers, J. (2008). Handoffs: Implications for nurses. In R. G. Hughes, (Ed.), *Patient safety and quality: An evidence-based handbook for nurses* (pp. 2-285-2-333). Rockville, MD: Agency for Healthcare Research and Quality. Publication No. 08-0043. 34.

Gallagher, T. H., Waterman, A. D., Ebers, A. G., Frassier, V., & Levinson, W., (2003). Patients' and physicians' attitudes regarding disclosure of medical errors. *Journal of the American Medical Association, 289*, 1001-1007.

Gerke, M., Uffelman, C., & Chandler K., (2010, May/June). Safety huddles for a culture of safety. *Patient Safety and Quality Healthcare*, 24-28.

Haig, K. M., Sutton, S., & Whittington, J. (2006). National patient safety goals. SBAR: A shared mental model for improving communication between clinicians. *Joint Commission Journal on Quality and Patient Safety, 32*(3), 167-175.

Hanna, D., Griswold, P., Leape, L. L., & Bates, D. (2005). Communicating critical test results: Safe practice recommendations. *Joint Commission Journal on Quality and Patient Safety, 31*(2), 68-80.

Heath, J., Johanson, W., & Blake, N. (2004). Healthy work environments: A validation of the literature. *Journal of Nursing Administration, 34*(11), 524-530.

Hughes, R. G, & Blegen, M. A. (2008). Medication administration safety. In Hughes, R. G., (Ed.), *Patient safety and quality: An evidence-based handbook for nurses* (pp. 2-397-2-458). Rockville, MD: Agency for Healthcare Research and Quality. Publication No. 08-0043.

Institute of Medicine. (1999). *To err is human: Building a safer health system*. Washington, DC: National Academies Press.

Institute of Medicine. (2001). *Crossing the quality chasm: A new health system for the 21st century*. Washington, DC: National Academies Press.

Institute of Medicine. (2004). *Keeping patients safe: Transforming the work environment of nurses*. Washington, DC: National Academies Press.

Institute for Safe Medication Practices. (2011). Too many abandon the "second victims" of medical errors. *ISMP Safety Alert, 16*(14), 1-3.

Johnson, J. (2012). Quality improvement. In G. Sherwood & J. Barnsteiner (Eds.), *Quality and safety in nursing: A competency approach to improving outcomes.* Hoboken, NJ: Wiley-Blackwell.

Joint Commission. (2009). Leadership committed to safety. Sentinel Event #43, Retrieved from http://www.jointcommission.org/assets/1/18/SEA_43.PDF

Joint Commission. (2011). *2011 National Patient Safety Goals.* Retreived July 10, 2011, from http://www.jointcommission.org/assets/1/6/HAP_NPSG_6-10-11.pdf

Joint Commission International Center for Patient Safety. (2005). *Strategies to improve hand-off communication: Implementing a process to resolve questions.* Retrieved June 29, 2011, from http://www.jcipatientsafety.org/15274/

Lamb, R. M., Studdert, D. M., Bohmer, R. M, Berwick, D. M., & Brennan, T. A. (2003). Hospital disclosure practices: Results of a national survey. *Health Affairs, 22,* 73-83.

Lawton, R., & Parker, D. (2002). Barriers to incident reporting in a health care system. *Quality and Safety in Health Care, 11,* 15-18.

Mitchell, P. (2008). Defining patient safety and quality care. In R. G. Hughes (Ed.), *Patient safety and quality: An evidence-based handbook for nurses* (pp. 1-1-1-6). Rockville, MD: Agency for Healthcare Research and Quality. Publication No. 08-0043.

National Council of State Boards of Nursing. (2010). *Nursing pathways for patient safety.* Mosby St. Louis, MO: Mosby.

Nuckols, T. K., Bell, D. S., Liu, H., Paddock, S., & Hillborne, L. (2007). Rates and types of events reported to established incident reporting systems in two US hospitals. *Quality and Safety in Health Care, 16,* 164-168.

Page, A. (2004). *Keeping patients safe: Transforming the work environment of nurses.* Committee on the Work Environment for Nurses and Patient Safety, Board on Health Care Services. Washington, DC: National Academies Press.

Rassin, M., Kanti, T., & Silner, D. (2005). Chronology of medication errors by nurses: Accumulation of stresses and PTSD symptoms. *Issues in Mental Health Nursing, 26*(8), 873-886.

Reason, J. (2000). Human error: Models and management. *British Medical Journal, 320,* 768-770.

Reid, J., & Catchpole, K. (2011). Patient safety: A core value of nursing—So why is achieving it so difficult? *Journal of Research in Nursing, 16,* 209-223.

Reiling, G. J., Knutzen, B. L., & Stoecklein, M. (2003). FMEA—the cure for medical errors. *Quality Progress, 36*(8), 67-71.

Riensenberg, L. A., Leitsch, J., & Cunningham, J. M. (2010). Nursing handoffs: A systematic review of the literature. *American Journal of Nursing, 110*(4), 24-34.

Rooney, J. J., & Vanden Heuvel, L. N. (2004). Root cause analysis for beginners. *Quality Progress, 37*(7), 45-53.

Rossheim, J. (2011). To err is human—even for medical workers. *Healthcare Monster.* Retrieved June 29, 2011, from http://healthcare.monster.ca/8099_en-CA_pf.asp.

Saint, S., Kaufman, S. R., Thompson, M., Rogers, M., & Chenowith, C. (2005). A reminder reduces urinary catheterizations in hospitalized patients. *Joint Commission Journal on Quality and Patient Safety, 31*(8), 455-462.

Sammer, C., Lykens, K., Singh, K., Mains, D., & Lackan, N. (2010). What is patient safety culture? A review of the literature. *Journal of Nursing Scholarship, 42,* 156-165.

Schumann, M. J. (2012). Policy implications driving national quality and safety initiatives. In G. Sherwood & J. Barnsteiner (Eds.), *Quality and safety in nursing: A competency approach to improving outcomes.* Hoboken, NJ: Wiley-Blackwell.

Scott, S. D., Hirschinger, L. E., Cox, K., McCoig M., Hahn-Cover, K., Epperly, K.M., et al. (2010). Caring for our own: Deploying a systemwide second victim rapid response team. *Joint Commission Journal on Quality and Patient Safety, 36*(5), 233-220.

Sexton, A., Chan, C., Elliott, M., Stuart, J., Jayasuriya, R., & Crookes, P. (2004). Nursing handovers: Do we really need them? *Journal of Nursing Management, 12,* 37–42.

Sherwood, G. (2011). Integrating quality and safety in nursing education and practice. *Journal of Research in Nursing, 16,* 226–239.

Sherwood, G. (2012). Driving forces for quality and safety: Changing mindsets to improve health care. In G. Sherwood & J. Barnsteiner (Eds.), *Quality and safety in nursing: A competency approach to improving outcomes.* Hoboken, NJ: Wiley-Blackwell.

Shortell, S. M., Schmittdiel, J., Wang, M. C., Li, R., Gillies, R., Casalino, L., et al. (2005). An empirical assessment of high-performing medical groups: Results from a national study. *Medical Care Research and Review, 62*(4), 407–434.

Sorra, J., Famolaro, T., & Dyer, N. (2008). Hospital survey on patient safety culture 2008 comparative database report (Prepared by Westat, Rockville, MD, under contract No. 233-02-0087, Task Order 18). Rockville, MD: Agency for Healthcare Research and Quality Publication No. 08-0039.

Spector, N., Ulrich, B., & Barnsteiner, J. (2012). New graduate transition into practice: Improving quality and safety. In G. Sherwood & J. Barnsteiner (Eds.), *Quality and safety in nursing: A competency approach to improving outcomes.* Hoboken, NJ: Wiley-Blackwell.

Thurman, A. E. (2001). Institutional responses to medical mistakes: Ethical and legal perspectives. *Kennedy Institute Ethics Journal, 11*(2), 147–56.

Tracey, M. F., & Barnsteiner, J. (2012). Evidence-based practice. In G. Sherwood & J. Barnsteiner (Eds.), *Quality and safety in nursing: A competency approach to improving outcomes.* Hoboken, NJ: Wiley-Blackwell.

Trbovich, P., Prakash, V., Stewart, J., Trip, K., & Savage, P., (2010). Interruptions during the delivery of high-risk medications. *Journal of Nursing Administration, 40,* 211–218.

Vicente, K. (2004). *The human factor.* New York: Routledge.

Wachter, R. M., & Pronovost, P. J. (2009). Balancing "no blame" with accountability in patient safety. *New England Journal of Medicine, 361*(14), 1401–1406.

Waldrup, W., Murray, D. J., Boulet, J. R., & Kraus J. F. (2009). Management of equipment anesthesia failure: A simulation-based resident skill assessment. *Anesthesia and Analgesia, 109,* 426–433.

Walsh, K., & Shortell, S. (2004). When things go wrong: How healthcare organizations deal with major failures. *Health Affairs, 23,* 103–105.

Walton, M. K., & Barnsteiner, J. (2012). Patient-centered care. In G. Sherwood & J. Barnsteiner (Eds.), *Quality and safety in nursing: A competency approach to improving outcomes.* Hoboken, NJ: Wiley-Blackwell.

Warren, J. (2012). Informatics. In G. Sherwood & J. Barnsteiner (Eds.), *Quality and safety in nursing: A competency approach to improving outcomes.* Hoboken, NJ: Wiley-Blackwell.

Weissman, J. S., Annas, C. L., Epstein, A. M., Schneider, E., Clarridge, B., Kirle, L., et al. (2005). Error reporting and disclosure systems: Views from hospital leaders. *Journal of the American Medical Association, 293,* 1359–1366.

Welsh, C., Flanagan, M., & Ebright, P. (2010). Barriers and facilitators to nursing handoffs: Recommendations for redesign, *Nursing Outlook, 58,* 148–154.

White, A. A., Waterman, A., McCotter, P., Boyle, D., & Gallagher, T. H. (2008). Supporting health care workers after medical error: Considerations for healthcare leaders. *Journal of Clinical Outcomes Management, 15,* 240–247.

Wolf, Z. R. (2005). Stress management in response to practice errors: Critical events in professional practice. *PA-PSRS Patient Safety Advisory, 2*(4), 1–4.

Wu, A. W. (2000). Medical error: The second victim. The doctor who makes mistakes needs help too. *British Medical Journal, 320*(7237), 726–727.

Yates, G. R, Bernd, D. L., Sayles, S. M., Stockmeier, C. A., Burke, G., & Merti, G. E. (2005). Building and sustaining a systemwide culture of safety. *Joint Commission Journal on Quality and Patient Safety, 31,* 684-689.

Resources

Agency for Healthcare Research and Quality (AHRQ). www.ahrq.gov

AHRQ SBAR (situation-background-assessment-recommendation). http://www.innovations.ahrq.gov/disclaimer.aspx?redirect=http%3a%2f%2fwww.ihi.org%2flHI%2fTopics%2fPatientSafety%2fSafetyGeneral%2fTools%2fSBARTechniqueforCommunicationASituationalBriefingModel.htm

American Hospital Association. http://www.aha.org/

American Nurses Association. http://nursingworld.org/

American Society of Health System Pharmacists. http://www.ashp.org/

AORN Information for Surgical Patients. http://www.aorn.org/aboutaorn/whoweare/informationforsurgicalpatients/

Center for Disease Control. www.cdc.gov

Center for Medicare and Medicaid Services. http://www.cms.hhs.gov/center/quality.asp

Consumers Advancing Patient Safety. www.patientsafety.org

Emergency Care Research Institute. www.mdsr.ecri.org

Food and Drug Administration. www.fda.gov

Institute for Healthcare Improvement. http://www.ihi.org/ihi

Institute for Healthcare Improvement Open School for Health Professions. www.ihi.org/OpenSchool

Institute for Safe Medication Practices. www.ismp.org

Institute of Medicine. http://www.iom.edu/

The Joint Commission (formerly known at JCAHO). http://www.jointcommission.org/

The Joint Commission International Center for Patient Safety. http://www.jcipatientsafety.org/

The LeapFrog Group. http://www.leapfroggroup.org/about_us

Massachusetts Coalition for the Prevention of Medical Errors. http://www.macoalition.org/

Medical Error and Patient Safety Learning. www.medicalerrorreduction.com

Medwatch. http://www.fda.gov/medwatch/index.html

National Coordinating Council for Medication Error Reporting and Prevention. http://www.nccmerp.org/

National Center for Patient Safety. http://www.patientsafety.gov/

National Family Caregivers Association. http://www.thefamilycaregiver.org

National Patient Safety Foundation. http://www.npsf.org/

National Quality Forum. http://www.qualityforum.org/

Partnership for Patient Safety. www.p4ps.org

P.U.L.S.E. (Persons United Limiting Substandards and Errors in Healthcare). www.pulseamerica.org

Quality and Safety Education for Nurses. www.qsen.org

VA National Center for Patient Safety—Patient Safety Resources. www.va.gov/NCPS/resources.html

Voice4Patients.com. http://www.voice4patients.com/

World Health Organization—International Alliance for Patient Safety. http://www.who.int/en/

Chapter 9

Informatics

Judith J. Warren, PhD, RN, BC, FAAN, FACMI

In attempting to arrive at the truth, I have applied everywhere for information, but in scarcely an instance have I been able to obtain hospital records fit for any purposes of comparison. If they could be obtained they would enable us to decide many other questions besides the ones alluded to. They would show the subscribers how their money was being spent, what amount of good was really being done with it, or whether the money was not doing mischief rather than good. Florence Nightingale (1863, p. 176)

Florence Nightingale, an informatics nurse at heart, demonstrated what could be done with data and information to improve patient care. In her quote above, she alludes to the uses of organized patient records that would reveal the contributions of nursing to cost effective, safe, quality patient care. As information and computer technologies have evolved, they have been identified as strategies to ensure safe patient care (Institute of Medicine [IOM], 2001). The patient safety series of books commissioned by IOM have consistently identified informatics as a major infrastructure component of patient safety: presenting patient information as a structure that supports clinical decision making, as are providing alerts, reminders, and clinical decision support; serving as a communications tool for the health care team; and supporting quality improvement and clinical research. As information and computer sciences have matured, the vision of health information technology and electronic health records is being achieved. Now the challenge is to educate our educators, students, and clinicians on how to take advantage of these new clinical tools in patient care.

Nursing informatics is emerging into the forefront of patient care issues as a result of three major innovations: the maturing of health information technology, national legislation requiring the transformation of health care through the use of health information technology, and nursing education initiatives responding to the technology and legislative trends. Health

Quality and Safety in Nursing: A Competency Approach to Improving Outcomes, First Edition. Edited by Gwen Sherwood and Jane Barnsteiner.
© 2012 John Wiley & Sons, Inc. Published 2012 by John Wiley & Sons, Inc.

information technology (HIT) has evolved and produced electronic health records (EHRs) that are able to store and organize the information captured during clinical work flows and return that information in views designed to support clinical design making. As work has progressed on sharing patient information within an organization, health information exchange between organizations has become important. This ensures that a patient's information follows them wherever they need care. For health information exchange to work in a safe, secure manner, the importance of harmonizing health information through evidence-based protocols, quality measures, health informatics standards, and standardized health and nursing terminologies has emerged as major efforts in the delivery of patient care. Social networking is another powerful information technology being used in patient care. Health care providers are using Facebook, LinkedIn, Twitter, RSS feeds, Listservs, virtual worlds, and dynamic web pages to interact with patients, providing services, information, and education (Mayo Clinic, 2011). Being competent in the use of these technologies is becoming essential for the nursing and the health care team.

Health care reform has been the initiator of transformations in the use of HIT in recent years, creating an intense focus on the implementation and use of information in patient care through use of EHRs and health information exchange. The Health Insurance Portability and Accountability Act (HIPAA) of 1996 was the first major legislation to influence the use of standards and terminology in patient records, as well as insuring the privacy and confidentiality of those records (HIPAA, 1996). These regulations have come to be known as administrative simplification. The American Recovery and Reinvestment Act of 2009 included provisions for the infusion of resources and funding for HIT in health care. The section of the act that focused on HIT has become known as the Health Information Technology for Economic and Clinical Health (HITECH) Act (HITECH, 2010). HITECH provided funds for education and research in informatics and financial incentives for the "Meaningful Use" of electronic health records (Office of the National Coordinator for Health IT, 2011). Providers must demonstrate meaningful use of EHRs between 2011 and 2015 to qualify for the financial incentives. Features of this demonstration include a patient problem list and quality measures, among other requirements. In 2010, the Patient Protection and Affordable Care Act was passed with additional requirements for the use of HIT in patient care, mainly in the form of administrative simplification aimed at reducing health care costs (Affordable Care Act, 2010). These three landmark pieces of legislation, and their resultant regulations, have created a demand for health care professionals who are competent in meaningfully using HIT, including EHRs.

The final innovation is education's response to the maturing of technology and the legalization demand for meaningful use of that technology (Warren & Connors, 2007). IOM, as part of their patient safety series of reports, issued a call to health professions educators to transform professional education to include patient-centered care, teamwork and collaboration, evidence-based practice, quality improvement, and informatics (Greiner & Knebel, 2003). They saw these five areas of competency as essential to providing safe patient care. The Quality and Safety Education for Nurses (QSEN) project was a major nursing response to this call (Cronenwett et al., 2007; Cronenwett et al., 2009). As a result of the QSEN work, both the American Association of the Colleges of Nursing and the National League for Nursing have integrated the work in their accreditation criteria for schools of nursing. Until these criteria were published, nursing informatics was viewed as a nursing specialty taught in graduate programs, and only a few of those existed.

Development of the QSEN informatics competencies

The first step in developing competencies is to define the domain for the work. The American Nurses Association defines the specialty of nursing informatics as the facilitation of the integration of data, information, knowledge, and wisdom to support patients, nurses, and other providers in decision making. This is accomplished through the use of information structures and information technology. Nursing informatics is the study and implementation of structures and algorithms to improve communication, understanding, and management of nursing information. Informatics nurses develop symbolic representations of nursing information that can be processed in information systems, regardless of the type of technology used. Structures and algorithms are essential and distinguish nursing informatics from other nursing specialties where the information context is the distinguishing feature. The core phenomena of nursing informatics are (1) all data, information, and knowledge involved in nursing; and (2) the symbolic representation of nursing phenomena (American Nurses Association, 2008). The challenge now is to determine the informatics competencies needed in general and in advanced nursing practice and how to educate our workforce.

Informatics competencies

Early work on defining informatics competencies was conducted by Staggers, Gassert, and Curran (2001, 2002) as they studied competencies for four levels of practice: staff nurses, administrative nurses, informatics nurses, and informatics researchers. This Delphi study was composed of a panel drawn from informatics experts and informatics educators. Subsequent work on informatics competencies is based on this foundational study. Curran expanded the competencies by identifying those for nurse practitioners (Curran, 2003). As this work was being completed in the United States, Australia (Smedley, 2005) and Canada (Booth, 2006) were developing informatics competencies using the work of Staggers and colleagues. Most of the competencies identified were basic computer competencies, literacy competencies, and information management (informatics) competencies.

The TIGER (Technology Information Guiding Educational Reform) Summit was convened to create a nursing profession-wide consortium to promote informatics and technology competencies (Ball et al., 2011). Again the work of

Staggers was used to begin the work of identifying informatics competencies. The QSEN informatics competencies were then added to the analysis (Cronenwett et al., 2007; Cronenwett et al., 2009). Computer competencies, though not part of QSEN, were added to the TIGER work. The work of Hobbs (2002) was consulted for adding these competencies. Other competency work being conducted in education and staff development was used to refine the list of informatics competencies (Barton, 2005; Desjardins, Cook, Jenkins, & Bakken, 2005; McNeil et al., 2003; McNeil et al., 2005; Sackett, Jones, & Erdley, 2005; Simpson, 2005). Finally, information literacy was included in the competencies. The information literacy competencies are based on the work of the National Forum on Information Literacy (n.d.).

The development of the QSEN informatics competencies also was based on the Staggers work. However, the decision was made not to include computer literacy and basic computer skills. The IOM report (Greiner & Knebel, 2003) concerning informatics was clear that computer skills were not included; the focus was on the information management and representation portion of the informatics domain. Information literacy was included as that is essential not only for informatics competencies but also the evidence-based practice competencies. The competencies were then leveled for prelicensure students and advanced nursing practice students (Cronenwett et al., 2007; Cronenwett et al., 2009). The final competencies are listed in Appendixes A and B. The informatics competency threads through all six QSEN competencies. Managing patient history, data, and preferences in the EHR enables patient-centered care (Walton & Barnsteiner, 2012). The tools and strategies utilized in developing evidence-based standards of care are based on informatics application (Tracey & Barnsteiner, 2012). Quality improvement can only happen through technology-based tools and decision support software (Johnson, 2012). Safety alerts, error reporting systems and management, and system improvements use informatics application (Barnsteiner, 2012). Interprofessional teams communicate and manage collaborative relationships via technology (Disch, 2012). Informatics is integrated to some degree throughout quality and safety.

Educational strategies for teaching informatics

Educating nurse educators

A significant percentage of nurse educators lack education or experience in informatics, as this area of expertise has only recently evolved. As nursing students require more informatics knowledge, skills, and attitudes, it is imperative that nurse educators master the QSEN advanced nursing practice informatics competencies so that they may create curricula and learning strategies to help students become competent in this area. Academic administrators must encourage and support nursing educators to get involved in lifelong learning activities concerning informatics (Bakken et al., 2004; Booth, 2006). Bakken and colleagues (2004) recommend three strategies to achieve nurse educator competence: seminars and small workshops related to informatics, consultation with informatics nurses on developing assignments to insure informatics content, and having informatics nurses as guest lecturers or as part of the course team. A fourth strategy is to partner with a clinical agency that has an EHR and have educators spend time at the agency learning how the EHR is designed, built, implemented, and used on a daily basis. Talk with them about the impact of federal legislation and reimbursement policies on the demand for electronic information. Other strategies would be to work with QSEN consultants (http://www.qsen.org/consultants.php) and to attend QSEN conferences.

Creating curricula

There are two tools that may help educators integrate informatics knowledge, skills, and attitudes into their courses: curriculum/course maps and course sequencing guides. A curriculum map lays out the content and its relationships so that educators can ensure that essential content and requirements are taught. As educators plot the content in a curriculum map and propose learning activities, they should investigate the way students are taught to manage patient data, not only the documentation of care but the retrieval of information about the patient for care and quality purposes. It is the representation and manipulation of data and information that is informatics, regardless of technology used. The content reveals the discipline of nursing. Second, a national Delphi study was conducted to provide guidance on sequencing QSEN competencies in the undergraduate curriculum (Barton, Armstrong, Preheim, Gelmon, & Andrus, 2009). The results of this survey will assist in knowing where and when in the curriculum to introduce and reinforce informatics content and competencies.

A second approach to curriculum and course design is mind mapping. Mind mapping provides an opportunity to look at related concepts that can be combined to teach a variety of competencies. See Figures 9.1 and 9.2 for examples of mind maps using the QSEN prelicensure and advanced nursing practice informatics competencies as source material. When the material is presented as a map with relationships, new ideas of working with the competencies or placing them in courses may emerge.

Educating students

There are many strategies for teaching informatics competencies. The most obvious are lectures with readings, slides, or handouts highlighting the most critical competencies. Attitudes may also be taught in this manner, with the educator serving as role model and mentor—most professional attitudes are learned through this approach. Online courses present learning material through the use of modules that contain overviews, objectives, readings, resources (videos, software, web pages, podcasts, virtual worlds, and games), and assignments (quizzes, discussion boards, projects, papers, concept maps, mind maps, website evaluations, etc.) to teach all three types of competencies. The QSEN web page has numerous activities with directions and resources for

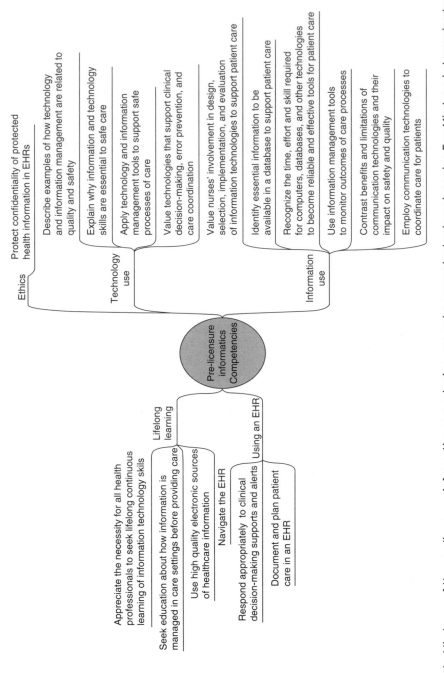

Figure 9.1 Mind map of the pre-licensure informatics competenices group by conceptual categories using FreeMind, a mind mapping tool, available at http://freemind.sourceforge.net/wiki/index.php/Download

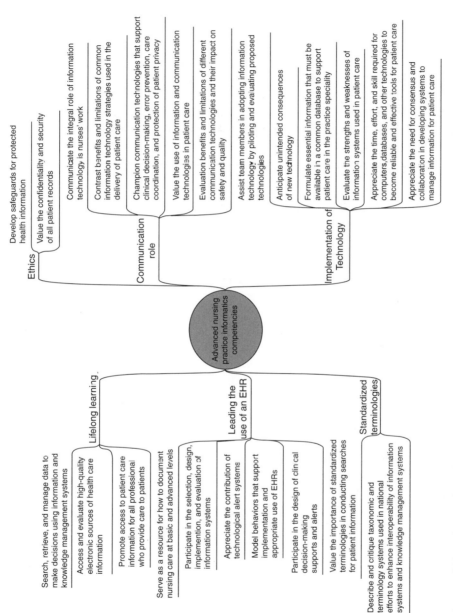

Figure 9.2 Mind map of the advanced nursing practice informatics competenices group by conceptual categories, using FreeMind.

educators to adapt and use to develop assignments for lectures and modules (http://www.qsen.org/view_strategies.php).

Assignments fostering information literacy are essential for students who must live and work in the information age. Flood, Gasiewicz, and Delpier (2010) have developed a sequence of five assignments to increase a student's ability to recognize the need for knowledge. In the first assignment the students are taught to search and evaluate the literature. The second assignment is the development of a teaching brochure based on a literature review. In the third assignment, the student identifies an organizational policy or procedure, conducts a literature review, compares the policy to the evidence, and then makes recommendations. The fourth assignment is a care plan for a complex patient based on a literature review and evidence evaluation. The final assignment has the student selecting a clinical setting and identifying how informatics and health information are used to make decisions. Planning activities with library literature searches meets one of the informatics competencies. Including information literacy is essential as it is part of the QSEN and TIGER competencies, yet many do not consider this as part of informatics (Dixon & Newlon, 2010).

Another literature evaluation activity is to evaluate a website that provides health information. Eight questions guide a good critique: What can the URL tell you? Who wrote the page and are they a qualified authority? Is it dated, current, timely? Is the information cited authentic? Does the page have overall integrity and reliability as a source? Are there biases in the presentation of information? Could the page or site be ironic, like a satire or a spoof? If you have questions or reservations, can you ask them? The QSEN website has other web page evaluation criteria and activities. This activity helps the student learn how to select a good website to recommend to a patient and family and how to tell a patient and family whether the information they are getting from the web is accurate and safe to use.

Engaging students in evaluating their own competency achievement is a powerful strategy to promote engagement in learning and rich feedback. Table 9.1 depicts an assessment form for the student to complete. While the assessment tool can be used in a variety of ways, the tool that best helps students focus is the completion of the self-assessment at the beginning of a course. Then the student can develop a personal action plan to achieve or enhance their competency attainment. During the semester, they should work on the plan. At the end of the course, students should complete the self-assessment again and evaluate their strategies for attaining competency.

The next strategy is to review current assignments. If the assignment is about patient information management or care planning, is it done on paper? If it is on paper, consider replacing that assignment with managing the patient data electronically using software such as a spreadsheet, a database, or an EHR. Review the patient simulations, both low and high fidelity, and include electronic documentation of the patient information in an EHR optimized for academic uses (the software selection is growing to meet a variety of needs) to increase the fidelity and to add informatics skills. Also, include retrieval of

Table 9.1 Quality and safety education for nurses (QSEN) informatics competencies for prelicensure nursing students worksheet

Name:

QSEN defines informatics as the use of information and technology to communicate, manage knowledge, mitigate error, and support decision making.

In the grid below, please rate the degree of your achievement of this competency. Place an X in the appropriate box.

QSEN Competency	Very competent	Moderately competent	Somewhat competent	Not competent
Explain why information and technology skills are essential for safe patient care				
Seek education about how information is managed in care settings before providing care				
Apply technology and information management tools to support safe processes of care				
Appreciate the necessity for all health professionals to seek lifelong, continuous learning of information technology skills				
Identify essential information that must be available in a common database to support patient care				
Contrast benefits and limitations of different communications technologies and their impact on safety and quality				
Navigate the electronic health record				
Document and plan patient care in an electronic health record				
Employ communication technologies to coordinate care				

(Continued)

Table 9.1 *(Continued)*

QSEN Competency	Very competent	Moderately competent	Somewhat competent	Not competent
Value technologies that support clinical decision making, error prevention, and care coordination				
Protect confidentiality of protected health information in electronic health records				
Describe examples of how technology and information management are related to the quality and safety of patient care				
Recognize the time, effort, and skill required for computers, databases, and other technologies to become reliable and effective tools for patient care				
Respond appropriately to clinical decision-making supports and alerts				
Use information management tools to monitor outcomes of care processes				
Use high-quality electronic sources of health care information				
Value nurses' involvement in design, selection, implementation, and evaluation of information technologies to support patient care				

In the space below, develop a Personal Action Plan for enhancing or achieving the above nursing informatics competencies.

Adapted from "Quality and Safety Education for Nurses," by L. Cronenwett, G. Sherwood, J. Barnsteiner, J. Disch, J. Johnson, P. Mitchell, D. T. Sullivan, and J. Warren, 2007, *Nursing Outlook*, 55(3), pp. 122–131.

patient information for purposes of gathering information for clinical decision making, quality improvement analysis, administrative reporting, and clinical research.

Every curriculum contains education concerning ethics. HIPAA and the Affordable Care Act have very strong requirements for safeguarding the confidentiality, privacy, and security of patient records, both paper and electronic. Most hospitals require HIPAA training before students are allowed to care for their patients. Be sure to identify this education as achieving both informatics knowledge and attitude competencies. If the information and practice about managing usernames and passwords is added to the lesson, then a skill competency also is achieved.

Nursing care plans are another teaching strategy. From an informatics perspective, this is the overarching representation structure of nursing knowledge. We teach students about assessment data, nursing problem lists, goals, interventions, and outcomes. Most EHRs have designed and structured nursing information in accordance with this representation. The structure may be displayed similarly to a paper format of a care plan or it may put each of the care plan structures in a different location. Either way, students need to be taught about the components in order to learn how to navigate an EHR to enter and find the patient information they need. An added benefit of teaching the components of a nursing care plan in an EHR is that it provides images to the student of what is being discussed. By adding this teaching strategy, visual learners are supported and nursing process skills are improved (Kennedy, Pallikkathavil, & Warren, 2009). As we move to EHRs, the use of standardized languages becomes imperative. It is only through coded structured data that we can aggregate, summarize, and analyze nursing's contribution to patient care outcomes (Lundberg et al., 2008). The American Nurses Association has recognized both nursing-specific and health care-specific terminologies and classifications to represent nursing in a structured way; see their website: http://nursingworld.org/npii/terminologies.htm. This website provides links to learn about each terminology and classification and is a good resource for educators. Introducing standardized language representing nursing knowledge is critical. Most often this knowledge is taught during the nursing process learning activities.

Finally, add experiences with EHRs, both real and simulated. Initially, hospitals were reluctant to grant EHR privileges to students. As health care reform has evolved, more hospitals are implementing EHRs and are automating all patient information. They have more resources to manage EHRs and to train users. As this expertise grows, hospitals are beginning to grant EHR privileges to all students. This is another opportunity to partner with clinical agencies to provide opportunities for student to attain informatics skills in working with EHRs. Clinical agencies are beginning to realize they will be educating nurses either before or after graduation. It is better for students to learn a clinical work flow that includes EHRs than to learn one that includes paper only and then have to learn a new work flow involving EHRs. Review the competencies and add clinical activities that foster the mastery of the competencies.

In early 2001, the need for an EHR optimized for academic purposes was identified (Connors, Weaver, Warren, & Miller, 2002). In a pilot project, a production EHR was adapted for use in the classroom and clinical laboratory. An insight was that the design of forms and order sets could facilitate learning by using learning theories concerning the gestalt (field/ground), advance organizers, constructivism, reinforcement, and active engagement. By interacting with the academic EHR, students learn about the data, information, and knowledge of nursing while attaining informatics skill competencies (Connors, Warren, & Weaver, 2007; Warren, Fletcher, Connors, Ground, & Weaver, 2004; Warren, Meyer, Thompson, & Roche, 2010). Assignments in the EHR were completing case studies by entering assessment data and planning care, scavenger hunts to learn navigation, graded care plans based on patients from the clinical settings (taking precautions to be HIPAA compliant), and reviewing information on forms and orders as preparation for class. Evidence-based nursing protocols were integrated into the EHR so that students could experience, analyze, and appreciate how these protocols are deconstructed and then implemented into an EHR (Weaver, Warren, & Delaney, 2005). As a result of the success of this pilot, more than 40 schools have adopted this particular learning strategy. Furthermore, simulated EHRs have joined the market to fill the need of having students engage with EHRs.

Combining the EHR with simulations, both low and high fidelity, creates an optimal learning environment. Students can engage in simple and complex scenarios while performing workflows required in clinical practice. The EHR requires point of care documentation. Clinicians depend on the information in the EHR to be accurate and current. Clinicians, once they thoroughly integrate the EHR in their work flows, base their decision on the information available. The information age has taught us that we can go to one electronic source and have all information brought to us—the EHR vendors sell their products based on this fact. Learning to give care and document at the point of care is a necessary skill and must be learned—simulations provide the place to begin this learning. A typical simulation would have the students accessing the EHR to find information about the patient in their simulation. During the simulation they would document the care given, looking up labs, orders, and other tasks done in the clinical setting. Debriefing would explore how the student accessed information and responded in the case. In a low-fidelity simulation, such as a skills check off, documenting the skill in the EHR would be the last step in the check off, as this is the preferred clinical work flow (Warren et al., 2010).

Implications for nursing practice

Nurses are expected to provide safe care in an increasingly technical environment. This technology has changed the role of the nurse and significantly altered the interactions between the nurse and patient. Nurses who have not mastered basic informatics competencies will be at a disadvantage as health care moves to achieve 100% EHR adoption by 2014, a presidential goal. To meet this challenge, The TIGER Summit was convened (http://www.tigersummit.com/Competencies_New_B949.html). The membership of the summit was drawn from professional nursing organizations from the areas of practice, education, administration, and research. The goals of the summit were to develop a strategic plan in which all organizations could work collaboratively to achieve the challenge. A team composed of volunteers was established with the summit to develop informatics competencies for the practicing nurse. The competency model consists of basic computer competencies, information literacy, and information management (including use of an EHR; TIGER Summit, n.d.). The work of QSEN was shared with this team. This competency work is foundational to the work of the other teams for staff development, educator development, and leadership development. The work of the TIGER Summit also identified development needs for educators that may be used to help them gain informatics competencies (Hebda & Calderone, 2010).

The HITECH act has insured that informatics competencies are a high priority for all health care organizations. The legislation provides funds for HIT training, regional EHR support for small practices and hospitals, research on the use of HIT, and state health information exchange initiatives. A second part of the legislation ties Medicare and Medicaid reimbursement at a preferential rate to those providers who can demonstrate "meaningful use." The criteria for this demonstration are the use of patient problem lists, allergy lists, immunization records, discharge summaries, computerized provider order entry, and quality measures. Furthermore, there is a requirement for reimbursement information to be submitted electronically to Medicare and Medicaid. This requirement has created a major stimulus for purchasing and implementing EHRs that are certified for this purpose. Health care organizations are challenged with not only implementing EHRs but also training their workforce to be meaningful users. There is a need for new graduates who are entering the workforce to have informatics competencies.

Kaiser-Permanente provides an exemplar of the challenges in nursing practice when implementing EHRs. The nursing department wanted an information system that promoted evidence-based practice, supported a professional practice framework, and enabled point of care documentation (Chow & Fong, 2010). Nurses in leadership and staff positions were involved in the selection, design, and implementation of the EHR—a major informatics competency. The design included a requirement to compare information across their practice sites in order to promote quality patient care and to identify normal variances in practice. Terminology had to be standardized and brand names eliminated from care documentation. They also created standard data definitions for describing common patient observations, for example, pain, falls, and pressure ulcers. Evidence-based scales were selected to insure data quality and standardization. Assessment forms from multiple sites were harmonized so that core documentation would occur at all Kaiser-Permanente sites. What is described is a new environment for the practice of nursing that is heavily influenced by technology and informatics. Both practice and academia need to retool and partner with each other to insure the success of nursing practice in this environment.

In 2008, the Robert Wood Johnson Foundation and the IOM collaborated on a project to assess and transform the nursing profession: *The Future of Nursing: Leading Change, Advancing Health* (IOM, 2011). Two of the recommendations include informatics initiatives. Recommendation 2 was to "Expand opportunities for nurses to lead and diffuse collaborative improvement efforts." Private and public funders are charged with providing funds to advance research on models of care and innovative solutions, including information technology that will contribute to improved health and health care. Health care organizations must engage nurses to work with developers in the design, development, purchase, implementation, and evaluation of EHRs. Recommendation 6 was to "Ensure that nurses engage in lifelong learning." The recommendation encouraged educators to partner with health care organizations to develop and prioritize competencies so curricula can be updated regularly to insure that graduates at all levels are prepared to meet the current and future health needs of the population.

Conclusion

Transforming health care requires the integration and mastery of the QSEN competencies to achieve safe, quality, cost-effective care. While this chapter focused on informatics, all the competencies must work together to produce this outcome. Collaboration and partnerships between academia and practice are critical to ensure a competent nursing workforce that must use health information technology and EHRs in daily practice.

References

Affordable Care Act. (2010). Retrieved from http://frwebgate.access.gpo.gov/cgi-bin/getdoc.cgi?dbname=111_cong_bills&docid=f:h3590enr.txt.pdf

American Nurses Association. (2008). *Scope and standards of nursing informatics practice*. Washington, DC: American Nurses Publishing.

American Recovery and Reinvestment Act. (2009). Retrieved from http://frwebgate.access.gpo.gov/cgi-bin/getdoc.cgi?dbname=111_cong_bills&docid=f:h1enr.pdf

Bakken, S., Cook, S. S., Curtis, L., Desjardins, K. Hyun, S., Jenkins, M., et al. (2004). Promoting patient safety through informatics-based nursing education. *International Journal of Medical Informatics, 73*, 581–589.

Ball, M. J., DuLong, D., Newbold, S.K., Sensmeier, J. E., Skiba, D. J., Troseth, M.R., et al. (2011). *Nursing informatics: Where technology and caring meet*. New York: Springer.

Barnsteiner, J. (2012). Safety. In G. Sherwood & J. Barnsteiner (Eds.), *Quality and safety in nursing: A competency approach to improving outcomes*. Hoboken, NJ: Wiley-Blackwell.

Barton, A. J. (2005). Cultivating informatics competencies in a Community of Practice. *Nursing Administration Quarterly, 29*(4), 323–328.

Barton, A. J., Armstrong, G., Preheim, G., Gelmon, S. B., & Andrus, L. C. (2009). A national Delphi to determine developmental progression of quality and safety competencies in nursing education. *Nursing Outlook, 57*(6), 313–322.

Booth, R. G. (2006). Educating the future eHealth professional nurse. *International Jouranl of Nursing Education Scholarship, 3*(1), Article 13. Retrieved from http://www.bepress.com/ijnes/vol3/iss1/art13

Chow, M. P., & Fong, V. (2010). Nursing leadership and impact. In L. L. Liang & D. M. Berwick (Eds.), *Connected for health: Using electronic health records to transform care delivery* (pp. 69–81). San Francisco: Jossey-Bass.

Connors, H. R., Weaver, C., Warren, J. J., & Miller, K. (2002). An academic-business partnership for advancing clinical informatics. *Nursing Education Perspectives, 23*(5), 228–233.

Connors, H., Warren, J. J., & Weaver, C. (2007). HIT plants SEEDS in healthcare education. *Nursing Administration Quarterly, 31*(2), 129–133.

Curran, C. R. (2003). Informatics competencies for nurse practitioners. *AACN Clinical Issues: Advanced Practice in Acute and Critical Care, 14*(3), 320–330.

Cronenwett, L., Sherwood, G., Barnsteiner, J., Disch, J., Johnson, J., Mitchell, P., et al. (2007). Quality and safety education for nurses, *Nursing Outlook, 55*(3), 122–131.

Cronenwett, L., Sherwood, G., Pohl, J., Barnsteiner, J., Moore, S., Sullivan, D. T., et al. (2009). Quality and safety education for advance nursing practice. *Nursing Outlook, 57*(6), 338–348.

Desjardins, K. S., Cook, S. S., Jenkins, M., & Bakken, S. (2005). Effect of an informatics evidence-based practice curriculum on nursing informatics competence. *International Journal of Medical Informatics, 74*, 1012–1020.

Disch, J. (2012). Teamwork and collaboration. In G. Sherwood & J. Barnsteiner (Eds.), *Quality and safety in nursing: A competency approach to improving outcomes.* Hoboken, NJ: Wiley-Blackwell.

Dixon, B., & Newlon, C. M. (2010). How do future nursing educators perceive informatics? Advancing the nursing informatics agenda through dialogue. *Journal of Professional Nursing, 26*(2), 82–89.

Flood, L. S., Gasiewicz, N., & Delpeir, T. (2010). Integrating information literacy across a BSN curriculum. *Journal of Nursing Education, 49*(2), 101–104.

FreeMind. Retrieved from http://freemind.sourceforge.net/wiki/index.php/Download

Greiner, A. C., & Knebel, E. (Eds.), Institute of Medicine Committee on the Health Professions Education Summitt. 2003. *Health professions education: A bridge to quality.* Washington, DC: National Academies Press.

Health Information Technology for Economic and Clinical Health (HITECH) Act. (2010). Retrieved from http://www.hipaasurvivalguide.com/hitech-act-text.php

Health Insurance Portability and Accountability Act. (1996). Retrieved from https://www.cms.gov/hipaageninfo

Hebda, T., & Calderone, T. L. (2010). What nurse educators need to know about the TIGER initiative. *Nurse Educator, 35*(2), 56–60.

Hobbs, S. D. (2002). Measuring nurses' computer competency: An analysis of published instruments. *CIN: Computer, Informatics, Nursing, 20*(2), 63–73.

Institute of Medicine. 2001. *Crossing the quality chasm: A new health system for the 21st century.* Washington, DC: National Academies Press.

Institute of Medicine. 2011. *The future of nursing: leading change, advancing health.* Washington, DC: National Academies Press.

Johnson, J. (2012). Quality improvement. In G. Sherwood & J. Barnsteiner (Eds.), *Quality and safety in nursing: A competency approach to improving outcomes.* Hoboken, NJ: Wiley-Blackwell.

Kennedy, D., Pallikkathavil, L., & Warren, J. J. (2009). Using a modified electronic health record to develop nursing process skills. *Journal of Nursing Education, 2,* 96–100.

Lundberg, C., Warren, J., Brokel, J., Bulechek, G., Butcher, H., Dochterman, J. M., et al. (June, 2008). Selecting a standardized terminology for the electronic health record that reveals the impact of nursing on patient care. *Online Journal of Nursing Informatics, 12*(2). Retrieved from http://www.ojni.org/12_2/lundberg.pdf

Mayo Clinic Center for Social Media. http://socialmedia.mayoclinic.org

McNeil, B. J., Elfrink, V. L., Bickford, C. J., Pierce, S. T., Beyea, S. C., Averill, C., & Klappenbach, C. (2003). Nursing information technology knowledge, skills, and preparation of student nurses, nursing faculty, and clinicians: A U.S. survey. *Journal of Nursing Education, 42*(8), 341–349.

McNeil, B. J., Elfrink, V. L., Pierce, S. T., Beyea, S. C., Bickford, C. J., & Averill, C. (2005). Nursing informatics knowledge and competencies: A national survey of nursing education programs in the United States. *International Journal of Medical Informatics, 74,* 1021–1030.

National Forum on Information Literacy. (n.d.). *Information literacy competency standards for higher education.* Retrieved from www.infolit.org

Nightingale, F. (1863). *Notes on hospitals.* London: Longman, Green, Longman, Roberts and Green, p. 176.

Office of the National Coordinator for Health IT. (2011). Retrieved from http://healthit.hhs.gov/portal/server.pt/community/healthit_hhs_gov__meaningful_use_announcement/2996

Sackett, K., Jones, J., & Erdley, W. S. (2005). Incorporating healthcare informatics into the strategic planning process in nursing education. *Nursing Leadership Forum, 9*(9), 98–104.

Simpson, R. L. (2005). Practice to evidence to practice: Closing the loop with IT. *Nursing Management, 36*(9), 12–17.

Smedley, A. (2005). The importance of informatics competencies in nursing: An Australian perspective. *CIN: Computers, Informatics, Nursing, 23*(2), 106–110.

Staggers, N., Gassert, C. A., & Curran, C. (2001). Informatics competencies for nurses at four levels of practice. *Journal of Nursing Education, 40*(7), 303–316.

Staggers, N., Gassert, C. A., & Curran, C. (2002). A Delphi study to determine informatics competencies for nurses at four levels of practice. *Nursing Research, 51*(6), 383–390.

TIGER Summit, Informatics Competencies. (n.d.). Retrieved from http://www.tiger-summit.com/Competencies_New_B949.html

Tracey, M. F., & Barnsteiner, J. (2012). Evidence-based practice. In G. Sherwood & J. Barnsteiner (Eds.), *Quality and safety in nursing: A competency approach to improving outcomes.* Hoboken, NJ: Wiley-Blackwell.

Walton, M. K., & Barnsteiner, J. (2012). Patient-centered care. In G. Sherwood & J. Barnsteiner (Eds.), *Quality and safety in nursing: A competency approach to improving outcomes.* Hoboken, NJ: Wiley-Blackwell.

Warren, J. J., & Connors, H.R. (2007). Health information technology can and will transform nursing education. *Nursing Outlook, 55*(1), 58–60.

Warren, J. J., Fletcher, K. A., Connors, H. R., Ground, A., & Weaver, C. (2004). The SEEDS Project: From health care information system to innovative educational strategy. In P. Whitten & D. Cook (Eds.), *Understanding health communication technologies* (pp. 225–231). San Francisco, CA: Jossey-Bass.

Warren, J. J., Meyer, M. N., Thompson, T., & Roche, A., (2010). Transforming nursing education: Integrating informatics and simulations. In Weaver, Delaney, Weber, & Carr (Eds.), *Nursing and informatics for the 21st century: An international look at practice, trends and the future* (pp. 145–161). Chicago: HIMSS Press.

Weaver, C. A., Warren, J. J., & Delaney, C. (2005). Bedside, classroom and bench: Collaborative strategies to generate evidence-based knowledge for nursing practice. *International Journal of Medical Informatics, 74,* 989–999.

Section 3

Strategies to Build a Culture of Quality and Safety

Chapter 10

The Imperative to Transform Education to Transform Practice

Gwen Sherwood, PhD, RN, FAAN

Unprecedented attention to health care quality and safety has led to regulatory requirements to stimulate improvements in the health care industry. Regulations alone, however, cannot improve our systems; to improve quality and safety, all health professionals must have the knowledge, skills, and attitudes to assess the scientific evidence to determine what constitutes good care, identify gaps between good care and actual care in their setting, and know the actions necessary to lead change. To address these expectations, the Institute of Medicine (2003) recognized education as the bridge to quality if health professionals are to be able to lead and work in redesigned systems. To transform the system requires transformation of health professions education to achieve the six competencies critical to health care improvement: patient-centered care, teamwork and collaboration, quality improvement, evidence-based practice, safety, and informatics. Although familiar terms, there are new applications to create system change. These competencies have been endorsed by major health care professional organizations and credentialing agencies for inclusion in curricula (Bataldan, Leach, & Ogrinc, 2009).

Shifts in nurses' role responsibilities place greater emphasis on quality and safety. Nurses contribute critical information about patients to the health care team. They are the largest group of health professionals and spend the most time with patients. In acute care, nurses are responsible for constant surveillance and in all settings help to coordinate complex care across multiple providers.

Impetus for a focus on quality and safety derives from multiple perspectives: moral, ethical, and economical. Health professionals have a fundamental value of helping people live more wholesome lives and base care decisions on ethical frameworks. The opportunity to do one's work well contributes to

Quality and Safety in Nursing: A Competency Approach to Improving Outcomes, First Edition. Edited by Gwen Sherwood and Jane Barnsteiner.
© 2012 John Wiley & Sons, Inc. Published 2012 by John Wiley & Sons, Inc.

satisfaction and meaning in work, which helps build a positive work environment. Nurses who work in systems focused on quality and safety report higher satisfaction; satisfaction has an impact on retention of workers; turnover costs organizations both intellectual capital and the high expense of orienting new employees, adding further to the high costs of health care errors and poor outcomes (Spector, Ulrich, & Barnsteiner, 2012). Nurses demonstrate the motivation to contribute to safe, high-quality work but need tools and resources to be able to integrate quality and safety into their daily work. This chapter describes the changing roles and responsibilities for nurses in quality and safety and the imperative to transform nursing education in all settings to assure that nurses achieve the competencies needed to help redesign and to work in systems focused on quality and safety.

A new mindset for health care

New views of quality and safety science are changing mindsets in the health care industry, in delivery settings as well as academic institutions. While quality and safety are intertwined concepts in the attempt to deliver exemplary patient care, quality refers to the gap between desired and ideal outcomes (Johnson, 2012), and safety is the focus on eliminating unintended consequences of care delivery (Barnsteiner, 2012). Nurses have not always been trained or educated for the new roles they must play in ensuring patient care quality and safety. The Institute of Medicine (IOM) report *The Future of Nursing* (2010) is the latest call for nurses to be prepared to lead quality improvements across health care settings and maintain patient safety; however, curriculum updates in nursing education are necessary for nurses to have the knowledge, skills, and attitudes for helping lead health care redesign and improvement efforts. Nurses' proximity to patients and care coordination across the continuum of care requires unique partnerships with other health professionals to facilitate quality improvement and safety initiatives, whether in hospitals, schools, homes, clinics, or long-term care settings.

In the classic double helix, changes in one area demand changes in another; health care changes demand changes in health professions education, and transformed curricula likewise advance role responsibilities. It varies across settings whether education or care delivery institutions lead the change. As new role responsibilities emerge, profound changes are required in both pre- and postlicensure nursing education. A competency-based approach to include a systems orientation emphasizes evidence-based practice, teamwork and collaboration, quality improvement, safety, and informatics within patient-centered care models that situate within complex delivery systems. The complexities of care require competency in a variety of technological tools and complex information management systems, as well as analysis and synthesis to improve quality and effectiveness of care. Nurses are expected to coordinate care and collaborate with a myriad of health professionals such as physicians, social workers, physical therapists, and pharmacists, most of whom have graduate degrees, across varied settings.

Emerging roles in quality and safety: what nurses need to know

In the wake of the staggering reports from the IOM, regulatory agencies are requiring health care organizations meet new standards and implement new initiatives to improve outcomes (IOM, 2000; Schumann, 2012; Sherwood, 2012). Implementing these new standards helped launch quality improvement initiatives and new applications of safety with new roles and responsibilities for nurses (Johnson, 2012; Barnsteiner, 2012). Because nurses are often the first line for communication with patients and their families, both as the constant provider with inpatients and the first link for communication in outpatient settings, they have an essential role on health care teams for coordinating, integrating, and facilitating care delivery. Nurses practicing within complex health care environments manage a variety of issues, including the disease processes of their patients with related care demands, the clinicians and others who are part of the health care team, informatics and technologies needed in care, the policies and procedures that guide practice, and the resources required to manage the complexities of care (Hughes, 2008). Nurses participate in and may lead quality improvement teams, which require coordinating input from the multiple disciplines involved in improving a particular aspect of care. These new levels of leadership require knowledge, skills, and attitudes in negotiation, problem solving, and communication (Disch, 2012).

Two studies cite the increasing role and influence by nurses in quality initiatives. Chief nurse executives report it is the area of their greatest focus (Arnold et al., 2006), and the Center for Studying Health System Change identifies the ways nurses participate in quality initiatives (Draper, Felland, Liebhaber, & Melichar, 2008). Nurses gather data used to help develop and implement protocols required to meet regulatory standards and economic incentives. Nurses use data derived from patients, providers, and systems to monitor the outcomes of care and design and apply improvement methods to test changes (Johnson, 2012). Nurses may lead improvement activities on patient care units as well as those launched by organizational leaders; it is often a challenge to balance both while meeting the demands of patient care. Roles vary according to the hospital's organizational culture and investment in a quality culture. Organizations that have supportive leadership, embrace a philosophy of quality as everyone's responsibility, promote individual accountability, identify physician and nurse champions, and seek effective feedback have more staff engagement in quality and safety (Bodrock & Mion, 2008).

Nurses participate in building a culture of patient safety by applying new approaches to error prevention and management (Sammer, Lykens, Singh, Mains, & Lackan, 2010). Organizations build a safety culture only as individual, unit, and organizational commitment to quality and safety values, attitudes, perceptions, competencies, and behavior patterns is lived out. Safety checks ensure that certain actions and precautions are taken by clinicians to protect patients during care delivery. Nurses participate in recognizing and reporting errors and near misses, root cause analysis (RCA) and failure mode and effects analysis (FMEA), and work with risk management and other team members in disclosing adverse events with patients and their families (Barnsteiner, 2012).

Nurses must have the knowledge, skills, and attitudes as well as the resources to do the right thing the right way the first time with the tools and resources to document care outcomes. Nurses have a responsibility to speak out, speak up, and call the question when they observe actions that jeopardize patient safety or care that falls short of evidence-based care standards. Nurses work with interdisciplinary teams to help create new care protocols, design care pathways to set standards of care, use safety reporting systems to identify safety risks, examine benchmark data for areas of improvement, and help design system changes derived from analysis of data (Sherwood & Jones, 2010). The American Nurses Association's National Center for Nursing Quality project for nurse-sensitive outcomes is a repository of nursing care quality projects, provides quality and safety educational resources and tools, and examines the quality of the work environment for nurses (Johnson, 2012; Schumann, 2012).

For nurses to move from passively observing system dysfunction to changing the system, the first step in building a quality improvement and safety culture is staff acknowledgement of breakdowns in communication, work flow hampered by work-arounds that have become the norm, and care processes that are ineffective. The unit manager helps lead staff to recognize process breakdowns and implement strategies to eliminate, improve, or redesign for improvement. The manager monitors outcomes of care delivery on their patient care unit and compares with benchmarks and other quality and safety indicators. To underscore the importance of quality and safety, nurse manager performance may be based on meeting targets for quality-related metrics, including patient satisfaction.

Impact of quality and safety culture on the work environment

Patients and their families, nurses, and the health care system pay a high price when nurses are unable to implement best practices in their everyday nursing activities and continue to observe unanswered compromises to safety. The growing focus on providing high-quality care not only benefits patients but also stimulates satisfaction and joy in nurses' work by honoring their basic values for contributing to good (Hall, Moore, & Barnsteiner, 2008). Nurses experience ethical conflict when their values are not in synch with the system in which they work, contributing to dissatisfaction. Nurses with the skills and empowerment to deliver the kind of care they know meets best practice express higher satisfaction that helps build a more positive work environment (Hall, Doran, & Pink, 2008) and contributes to higher patient satisfaction (Lindberg & Kimberlain, 2008). In fact, many system issues that influence nurses' job satisfaction can be addressed through quality improvement, such as patient flow problems, safe management of high census periods, communication problems around complex patients, and improving medication safety (Hall, Moore, & Barnsteiner, 2008).

Changing the way nurses practice can be challenging, but there are incentives and motivations to invest in best practice and provide opportunities to contribute to systematic changes in the health care system. *Keeping Patients Safe: Transforming the Work Environment of Nurses* (Page, 2004) examined the link between nurses, their work environment, and patient safety and quality of care with recommendations for organizations to honor the responsibility to provide a satisfying and rewarding work environment, assure adequate nurse staffing, and provide continued learning opportunities for both new and experienced nurses. Trust is built between nurses and organizational leaders when nurses are given a voice in patient care delivery through effective nursing leadership and participation in executive decision making and through support for interdisciplinary collaboration (Page, 2004). These recommendations are consistent with the Magnet designation recognizing excellence in nursing leadership and service (Lundmark, 2008; Triolo, 2012).

While we can articulate the roles and responsibilities for nurses in quality and safety, there are other challenges. Although nurses are a constant presence with patients, serve as advocates, apply clinical knowledge and reasoning, and bring skills in change agency, individual vigilance alone is not an adequate safety defense. Nurses and other professionals must have additional training and skills to identify clinical questions, describe processes for changing current practice, and evaluate the outcomes of improvement strategies. Clinical educators must address implications for staff development to help the generations of practicing professionals whose education did not include quality improvement and safety science. We need continued efforts to guide responses to the myriad of human factors that influence quality and safety work. Organizations have been lax in addressing vulnerabilities that are the result of human factors. Workload fluctuations, interruptions, multitasking, complacency, fatigue, task fixation, failure to follow up or follow protocol, and poorly managed handoffs can stifle improvement efforts. All professionals need to improve interpersonal interactions to alleviate safety risks associated with ineffective communication, excessive professional courtesy, power gradients, fear of speaking up, and hidden agendas.

Transforming nursing education

To achieve the ambitious goals for quality and safety, how do we begin to rethink nursing educational approaches that go beyond caring for the individual patient? How best to introduce learners to health care systems and the way in which individual patients live in and are cared for within those systems? Nursing is unique among health professions with multiple educational pathways for entry level practice licensure. Regardless of educational entry, all nurses have accountability to deliver evidence-based, safe, quality, patient-centered care across all settings. The gap between prelicensure education and expanded practice expectations has contributed to longer and more costly orientation programs for nurses to achieve the competencies required for this level of practice (Sherwood & Drenkard, 2007) and to the high turnover rate of new graduates during the first year of employment (Spector, Ulrich, & Barnsteiner, 2012). Innovative partnerships between schools of nursing and clinical agencies can begin to close the disparity between nursing curricula and practice responsibilities with graduates more prepared for practice, reduce the burden on orientation and staff development, and provide smoother transition to practice.

QSEN: integrating new views of quality and safety in nursing education

The national Quality and Safety Education for Nurses project (Cronenwett et al., 2007; Cronenwett, 2012; Sherwood, 2011) responded to the challenge for integrating the IOM (2003) competencies by adopting a bold approach to redefine a good nurse as one who embraces quality and safety as a part of his or her daily work. A national expert panel defined the six competencies (patient-centered care, teamwork and collaboration, evidence-based practice, quality improvement, safety, and informatics) and used an iterative process to identify 162 knowledge, skills, and attitude (KSA) objectives for the six competencies (Cronenwett et al., 2007; Appendix A). While the definitions remain the same across all nursing practice, the QSEN team defined graduate-level competencies to aid the progression of novice to expert (Cronenwett et al., 2009; Appendix B).

The QSEN team implemented a 15-pilot school learning collaborative to model integration of the six QSEN competencies in prelicensure nursing education across educational entry programs (Cronenwett, Sherwood, & Gelmon, 2009), much like a PDSA (plan, do, study, act) cycle as a small test of change (Johnson, 2012). Schools mapped ways to integrate the competencies, led faculty development for understanding the competencies, and worked with a clinical partner to implement demonstration projects for transforming their curricula. The QSEN website (www.QSEN.org/pilot) reports curricular strategies developed by schools with their practice partners to model integration of the competencies (Cronenwett, Sherwood, & Gelmon, 2009). Barton, Armstrong, Preheim, Gelmon, and Andrus (2009) report a Delphi study for placement of the 162 KSAs defining the six quality and safety competencies for beginning, intermediate, and advanced learners (Appendix C). Cronenwett et al. (2009) and Pohl et al. (2009) discuss graduate placement.

Developing educational models

Content-based nursing curricula that are already overcommitted can be reframed with an organizing framework based on quality and safety (Chenot & Daniel, 2010). Curriculum development is based on consideration of emerging health needs, values, and beliefs that shape educational philosophy, and factors within the environmental context. Quality and safety have emerged as critical societal needs based on values and beliefs; health care professionals are motivated for excellence when they have the tools and resources to do so; and the current environment is poised for transition. New curriculum models based on competency development (Chenot & Daniel, 2010) require rethinking pedagogy to develop new strategies to engage learners in beginning to think like a nurse in contemporary practice (Ironsides & Cerbi, 2012). Citing rapid and profound change in science, technology, and nursing practice, Benner, Sutphen, Leonard, and Day (2010) call for radical transformation in nursing education to redesign the prevailing educational frameworks of the past 40 years. Questions that challenge us to move outside our comfort zone:

- How do we challenge embedded assumptions about how we prepare nurses?
- What are ways to organize clinical learning experiences beyond one clinical faculty and a small group of students who are guests on a unit where each student cares for an individual patient?
- What are the safety risks of a clinical faculty supervising 6–10 students, each caring for at least one patient, and risks when students change clinical sites with every course?

The six quality and safety competencies can be integrated across a curriculum, threading through existing courses, clinical experiences, simulations, learning assignments, and case studies, thus reducing content burden on curriculum. The same is true for educational units in practice settings. The QSEN pilot learning collaborative (Cronenwett, Sherwood, & Gelmon, 2009; Armstrong, Sherwood, & Tagliareni, 2008) found that questions embedded in case studies, redesigned clinical learning experiences, debriefings in postclinical conferences, mentoring through participation in quality improvement initiatives, and application of the competencies in simulated learning experiences are ways to work with existing curricula. Learning experiences should be focused on more than the individual patient to position the patient within the system of care. Developing mindful inquiry leads to a questioning attitude that is the first step in a quality and safety practice orientation (Day & Smith, 2007).

Competency-based education challenges traditional organization of nursing fundamentals that teaches discrete skills to one nurse, one patient at a time (Preheim, Armstrong, & Barton, 2009). Schools of nursing skills labs have been organized around individual skill competence such as sterile technique, IV insertion, and provision of bed baths and other hygiene needs. To provide complex care in the current environments, we must rethink the traditional psychomotor skills lab. Highly orchestrated clinical learning labs can be organized around physiologic systems, such as the cardiac-compromised patient; skills may be thus emphasized in bundled sets via high-fidelity simulation to more closely resemble an actual nursing situation, in some cases creating a virtual hospital (Durham & Alden, 2012). Learners can engage longer with simulated patients to better understand how a patient situates within a larger system, and can participate with interprofessional team members to better grasp the various scopes of practice.

Innovations to transform learning

Educators can engage learners through innovative pedagogical approaches to integrate quality improvement and safety into existing curricula. Ironsides and Cerbie (2012) discuss application of narrative pedagogies to develop unfolding case studies that help learners explore multiple concepts from a patient centered perspective. Both high- and low-fidelity simulation exercises (Durham & Alden, 2012) help learners develop KSAs for teamwork and collaboration, medication administration safety and other safety alerts, patient-centered care, communication both with the patient and family and with other team members, and electronic health records. Clinical partners can help design learning opportunities for developing or updating evidence-based care standards, environmental safety assessments, and teamwork.

Nurses need skills to apply quality improvement techniques to improve and standardize care processes based on current evidence (Hughes, 2008; Tracey & Barnsteiner, 2012), all of which requires competency in informatics (Warren, 2012). Nurses, students, or educators may learn about quality improvement through participation in an improvement initiative with an interprofessional team or through high-fidelity patient simulation exercises (Durham & Sherwood, 2008). Learning activities, particularly for experienced nurses or graduate students, can be based on analysis of clinical pathways or developing clinical algorithms to standardize nursing care (Jones, Mayer, & Mandelkehr, 2009). The QI Knowledge Application Tool (Varkey, Reller, Smith, Ponto, & Osborn, 2006) determined that medical and nursing participants in an interdisciplinary quality improvement initiative significantly improved their capacity to make changes using quality improvement methods. Helping learners form inquiry-based practice can help develop clinical reasoning important for making decisions in current practice.

Nurses and students may apply reflective learning to uncover gaps in their own care delivery or within the system and develop improvement strategies. Using reflection to analyze case studies, narrative pedagogies, practice events, and other learning experiences consciously examines consistency of actions with beliefs and attitudes (Ironsides & Cerbie, 2012) to improve one's work. More than just recording daily events, reflection is a systematic way of thinking about one's actions and responses to change future actions and responses (Freshwater, Taylor, & Sherwood, 2008). Reflection is asking questions; the quality and safety goals are based on a spirit of inquiry, the art of asking questions both to determine the evidence for why actions are implemented but also asking if there is a better way to do one's work. Thinking about one's work opens the possibility of change through a spirit of inquiry to identify potential gaps in the system where errors may occur, where values and actions clash, or where change is needed. A spirit of inquiry is part of becoming an analytical practitioner able to ask questions, the first stage of any improvement or change in safety awareness, and apply clinical reasoning.

Reflection can help develop emotional intelligence, leadership capacity, mindfulness, and engagement in work activities and thus lead to improvement (Horton-Deustch & Sherwood, 2008). Reflecting in or on action helps develop greater awareness of behavior, skills, and attitudes, and helps accept accountability for actions. The goal of reflection is to learn from experience by considering one's knowledge, beliefs, and values within the context of one's actions. Reflection helps one make sense of events, which leads to feeling more effective and satisfied, both personally and within one's environment. Benner (1984) asked nurses to write exemplars of meaningful patient encounters and through reflection examine the meaning of these events to the patient, family, and themselves, thus developing patient-centered care based on understanding the illness experience, and progressing from novice to expert.

Reflection can be used for group dialogue, particularly among novice and seasoned nurses. Learners in pre- and postlicensure can use the outline in Textbox 10.1 to write about a particular event that stands out in their mind or has unresolved consequences. Reflecting-on-Action can be used as a part of the briefing process in planning care, as well as to guide conversation in the handoff between providers or in leading interdisciplinary patient-centered care rounds to set daily goals for the patient. Reflecting-on-action can be applied at the end of the day to consider events to learn for the future or as a debriefing after a particular event, asking learners to write one-minute papers on their experiences. Reflecting-in-action can be used

---

Textbox 10.1   Reflective guide in making sense of practice

Describe what happened, objectively giving details of the event.

Examine feelings that arose in the moment and in the aftermath.

Consider the event from multiple perspectives, evaluating positive and negative aspects of the event and how others may have viewed it.

Analyze the description to make sense of the event by considering knowledge and attitudes that influenced what happened.

Consider alternatives; ask what else could you have done? What gaps in knowledge affected what happened?

Determine the appropriate response by setting an action plan for future situations.

Adapted from "The Scholarship of Reflective Practice," by D. Freshwater, S. Horton-Deutsch, G. Sherwood, and B. Taylor, 2005, Sigma Theta Tau International Task Force on the Scholarship of Reflective Practice. Available for download at http://www.nursingsociety.org/aboutus/PositionPapers/Pages/position_resource_papers.aspx

for team huddles to address complex problems, clarify miscommunication, integrate the patient or family in care, or "get everyone on the same page." Team huddles can discuss a near miss and what to do to avoid the situation in the future.

Critical reflection based on appreciative inquiry can be applied to evaluate or assess achievement of learning objectives, guide learners in self-assessment, or contribute to a professional portfolio for career development. Changes in attitudes or movement toward professional maturity may not be revealed in standardized tests, multiple choice questions, or traditional performance evaluations, but they may be visible in reflections. Educators may develop rubrics to respond to reflective learning activities, simulations, or case studies. An appreciative inquiry guide leads the learner to reflect on times of success using the following reflective questions:

- What were standout events (this semester/this work period) when I felt successful?
- Describe the events.
- What about the events made me feel worthwhile?
- What roles and responses did others have?
- How was this different from other events?
- What are lessons learned to guide my actions in the future?

Changing our mental models: educator development for competency-based education

Participants in the QSEN Pilot School Learning Collaborative found educator development in both clinical and academic settings necessary to advance quality and safety (Armstrong et al., 2009; Brown, Feller & Benedict, 2010; Cronenwett, Sherwood & Gelmon, 2009; Finkelman & Kenner, 2009). Faculty development has continued with QSEN regional workshops through the American Association of Colleges of Nursing and the annual QSEN National Forums (Cronenwett, 2012).

Finkelman and Kenner (2009) challenged educators to move out of their comfort zone and focus teaching on relevancy of concepts and competencies consistent with contemporary practice. Educators must understand the background and rationale driving quality and safety (Sherwood, 2012), the impact of clinical performance measures, and the various ethical, moral, economic, and regulatory perspectives (Schumann, 2012; Thornlow & McGuinn, 2010). Accreditation standards for most health professions now require experiences in interdisciplinary learning, quality improvement, and safety science (Batalden et al., 2009). Quality improvement processes require participation across the disciplines, yet health professions students have few interprofessional learning experiences such as that described by Achieving Competence Today (http://www.ihi.org/IHI/Programs/IHIOpenSchool/TeachingResourceACT.htm?tabId=0), a course for learners from different disciplines to develop a quality improvement project (Ladden, Bednash, Stevens, & Moore, 2006).

Whether in clinical or academic settings, it can be a challenge to know how to begin to integrate the competencies into educational programs. Two studies provide prelicensure student assessment data that can help guide educators. Sullivan, Hirst, and Cronenwett (2009) report student self-assessment of the quality and safety competencies following their schools' participation in the QSEN Pilot Learning Collaborative. Chenot and Daniel (2010) assessed student awareness of the competencies. Barton and colleagues (2009) report a Delphi to assist educators in determining beginner, intermediate, and advanced placement of the KSAs for the QSEN competencies (Appendix C).

Textbox 10.2 suggests questions for educator discussions to explore change. For any change, early adopters will almost certainly face challenges. To champion change, first be clear about the vision, goal, and rationale to accomplish. Seek understanding of factors behind any resistance to change. Identify the most effective communication to reach the intended audience and the resources available. Quality and safety applications can be a regular item in faculty meetings, curriculum committee meetings, agency newsletters, and websites. Capitalize on the social influence of those who have passion for achieving the desired goals. Stakeholders can use appreciative inquiry to examine and build on past successes in curricular change. Developing the QSEN competencies can be the theme of an educator retreat. Active learning can engage educators in a personal PDSA project such as planning how to manage sleep deprivation or increase an exercise regime, thus mastering quality improvement based on evidence-based standards through a small quick-change process that can be used as a model to inspire curricular change.

Textbox 10.2   Key questions to guide educator discussions in academic and clinical settings

What are the driving forces for improving quality and safety health care?
What are influences on the changing role of nurses?
What do nurses need to know to work in and lead redesigned systems?
Where are gaps in our educational programs to help nurses achieve the knowledge, skills, and attitudes required to improve quality and safety?
How do we begin to work toward common goals across education and practice settings?
What educational approaches will engage nurses in achieving quality and safety competencies?
What pedagogical approaches engage learners in developing a system perspective?
What are ways to integrate student learning experiences into clinical settings and with other disciplines?
What are assessment strategies to determine achievement of knowledge, skills, and attitudes?

Partnerships to create change

Bridging education and practice is a group process; quality and safety transformation of our health care system cannot occur in isolation. Academic and clinical partners can begin by engaging in new conversations to discuss the strengths of each in order to design the best partnership model (Sherwood, 2006). Representation on each other's committees, councils, or advisory boards can integrate faculty and clinical leaders. Clinical partners can help with periodic updates or share educator retreats to provide the perspective of the health care system, and educators can share advancements in education, thereby keeping each appraised of developments and leveraging the power of collaboration. Textbox 10.3 provides broad questions for discussion that can lead to specific topics. For example, paticipants could discuss changes required by the latest Joint Commission National Patient Safety Goals or the National Quality Forum Serious Reportable Events (often known as never events) and how these are being integrated into practice in the clinical setting, or discuss preventable errors (e.g., wrong site surgery) and Red Rules that apply standards without exception in a particular process (e.g., reconciling the sponge count during surgery; Barnsteiner, 2012).

Textbox 10.3   Questions to guide organizational change

Beginning with self-assessment: Change comes individual by individual

What is my mindset about quality and safety? How do I define my own approach and commitment to improving outcomes?

What are changes in knowledge, skills and attitudes I have made in regards to quality and safety?

What am I willing to invest to create change?

Assessing nurses' roles:

What are changes in nurses' roles and responsibilities for improving quality and safety in our setting?

Are quality and safety integrated into our organization's mission and vision?

What partnerships could help us achieve the knowledge, skills, and attitude objectives that define the six quality and safety competencies?

Transforming the organization:

How do we engage people in changing mindsets, programs, and/or organizations?

What are the challenges?

What are examples of success?

What lessons can we learn from these success stories?

How do we demonstrate that we recognize that people's lives depend on the work we do?

Discussing student feedback, particularly when based on appreciative inquiry, about their experiences at clinical sites can guide improvements in learning from both clinical and academic perspectives. Academic and clinical partners can work together to plan internships or externships, discuss how students and faculty can contribute to care in clinical sites, and consider ways for students and faculty to participate in improvement projects. Working with the clinical agency, educators can identify patients and families involved as consumer advocates in clinical organizations, now required in some states. These patients and families may be invited to share their experiences with learners to help develop care based on patient preferences, values, and beliefs. Educators in both settings must complete certain assessments to meet regulatory requirements; they can compare lists of required skills to be sure students and new graduates or other learners are meeting expectations, discuss how competencies are measured and evaluated to avoid repetitious work and share measurement tools, and plan orderly transition to practice to ease new graduate adaptation. Dedicated education units are relatively new partnerships between clinical and academic institutions that concentrate on innovative learning to help faculty and students move from guest on the unit to an integrated learning system.

There is little evidence to guide the balance of time spent in didactic and clinical learning; the question is less about how much time is spent in clinical but the quality of the time while there. Schools have traditionally integrated clinical learning into or concurrent with didactic courses to allow students to apply classroom and skill learning into the clinical setting. Students may spend 1 to 2 days per week in clinical for roughly 8 to 12 weeks per semester. Internationally, schools are more likely to have concentrated blocks of didactic and skills learning followed by blocks of clinical experiences to apply what has been learned. Does this allow students to have more continuity in clinical to be able to see the results of their care, observe patient changes over time, and gain confidence in their skills? If students remained in one agency for their clinical learning over their course of study, would they be able to focus more intently on learning the system and gaining confidence, thus saving time spent in constant orientation and reducing safety risks involved in adjusting to a new setting?

Learning from other models

Competency-based education models are evolving. The Oregon Consortium for Nursing Education (OCNE, 2010) developed a competency-based model that embeds the IOM competencies discussed in this chapter and has influenced development of other models. The Massachusetts Department of Education's (2010) "Nurse of the Future: Nursing Core Competencies" document, which includes the six quality and safety competencies in the model, is based on the OCNE model and includes 10 competencies. The 6 QSEN quality and safety competencies are effecting changes in nursing education policy with adoption into the curriculum essentials documents for undergraduate

(American Association of Colleges of Nursing [AACN], 2009), master's (AACN, 2011), and Doctor of Nursing Practice (AACN, 2008) programs from the AACN, as well as the competency work for all levels of nursing education from the National League for Nursing (2010).

A collaboration between the Robert Wood Johnson Foundation (RWJF) and the Institute for Health Care Improvement, Transforming Care at the Bedside (or TCAB), was initiated in 2003 to recognize "nursing's critical but commonly overlooked role" in care delivery (Lavizzo-Mourey & Berwick, 2009, p. 3). The QSEN quality and safety competencies were incorporated into curriculum objectives to improve hospital performance (Hasmiller & Bolton, 2009). A step-by-step guide for implementing innovations from TCAB is provided in the TCAB toolkit, made available through the Robert Wood Johnson Foundation (2008).

The Agency for Healthcare Research and Quality (AHRQ) recognized the critical role of nurses in quality and safety by joining with the Robert Wood Johnson Foundation to publish a handbook for nurses on patient safety and quality that could be used in education and practice, titled *Patient Safety and Quality: An Evidence-Based Handbook for Nurses* (see Hughes, 2008). AHRQ also provides a free multimedia curriculum to improve teamwork performance, TeamSTEPPS (2009), which has been adopted by many schools and health care agencies, and has guidelines for developing high-reliability organizations that mitigate quality and safety issues (www.AHRQ.gov).

Summary

To achieve the goals set forth by the IOM requires significant changes in health professions education and educator development. This chapter has addressed the imperative to transform nursing curricula by integrating the six quality and safety competencies identified and defined by the QSEN project. The goal is to change nursing role identify formation so that a good nurse is described as one who practices from a spirit of inquiry, engages in mindful practice attentive to safety science, explores best practices based on current evidence, constantly seeks improvements in practice, participates in and leads interprofessional teams, effectively applies informatics, and includes patients and families as full partners in care. New KSAs to support these goals are identified to guide learners in pre- and postlicensure education programs to function effectively in contemporary practice in which quality and safety are integrated as part of nurses' daily work. Health professions education programs must stay abreast with the changes taking place in health care to assure clinicians have the requisite KSAs. New approaches to partnerships between practice and academic settings, among the various health care disciplines, and from agency to agency are essential to integrate current practice with curricula and develop interprofessional learning experiences. To improve patient care outcomes, it is imperative to have well-prepared professionals who understand the complexity of the health care system and pressures to implement change. As educators continue embedding quality and safety competencies into educational programs both in the clinical area and in academic programs, we can hasten the uptake of effective quality improvement and patient safety practices, which will ultimately result in higher quality, safe care to patients.

References

Achieving Competence Today. http://www.ihi.org/IHI/Programs/IHIOpenSchool/TeachingResourceACT.htm?tabId=0

American Association of Colleges of Nursing. (2008). *The essentials of doctor of nursing practice*. Washington, DC: Author.

American Association of Colleges of Nursing. (2009). *The essentials of baccalaureate education for professional nursing practice*. Washington, DC: Author.

American Association of Colleges of Nursing. (2011). *The essentials of master's education for professional nursing practice*. Washington, DC: Author.

Armstrong, G., Sherwood, G., & Tagliareni, E. (2009). Quality and Safety Education in Nursing (QSEN): Integrating recommendations from IOM into clinical nursing education. In T. Valiga & N. Ard (Eds.), *Clinical nursing education: Critical reflections* (pp. 207-226). New York: National League for Nursing Press.

Arnold, L., Campbell, A., Dubree, M., Fuchs, M., Davis, N., Hertzler, B., et al. (2006). Priorities and challenges of health system chief nursing executives: Insights for nursing educators. *Journal of Professional Nursing, 22*(4), 213-220.

Barnsteiner, J. (2012). Safety. In G. Sherwood & J. Barnsteiner (Eds.), *Quality and safety in nursing: A competency approach to improving outcomes*. Hoboken, NJ: Wiley-Blackwell.

Barton, A., Armstrong, G., Preheim, G., Gelmon, S., & Andrus, L. (2009). A national Delphi to determine developmental progression of quality and safety competencies in nursing education. *Nursing Outlook, 57*(6), 313-322.

Batalden, P. B., Leach, D., & Ogrinc, G. (2009). Knowing is not enough: Executives and educators must act to address challenges and reshape healthcare. *Healthcare Executive, 24*(2), 68-70.

Benner, P. (1984). *From novice to expert: Excellence and power in clinical nursing practice*. Menlo Park, CA: Addison Wesley.

Benner, P., Sutphen, M., Leonard, V., & Day, L. (2010). *Educating nurses: A call for radical transformation*. San Francisco: Jossey-Bass.

Bodrock, J. A., & Mion, L. C. (2008). Pay for performance in hospitals: Implications for nurses and nursing care. *Quality Management in Health Care, 17*(2), 102-111.

Brown, R., Feller, L., & Benedict, L. (2010). Reframing nursing education: the Quality and Safety Education for Nurses initiative. *Teaching and Learning in Nursing, 5*, 115-118. doi:101016/j.teln.2010.02.005

Chenot, T., & Daniel, L. (2010). Frameworks for patient safety in the nursing curriculum. *Journal of Nursing Education, 49*(10), 559-568. doi:10.3928/01484834-20100730-02

Cronenwett, L. (2012). A national initiative: Quality and Safety Education for Nurses (QSEN). In G. Sherwood & J. Barnsteiner (Eds.), *Quality and safety in nursing: A competency approach to improving outcomes*. Hoboken, NJ: Wiley-Blackwell.

Cronenwett, L., Sherwood, G., Barnsteiner, J., Disch, J., Johnson, J., Mitchell, P., et al. (2007). Quality and safety education for nurses. *Nursing Outlook, 55*(3), 122-131.

Cronenwett, L., Sherwood, G., & Gelmon, S. (2009). Improving quality and safety education: The QSEN learning collaborative. *Nursing Outlook, 57*(6), 304-312.

Cronenwett, L., Sherwood, G., Pohl, J., Barnsteiner, J., Moore, S., Sullivan, D. T., et al. (2009). Quality and safety education for advanced practice nursing practice. *Nursing Outlook, 57*(6), 338-348.

Day, L., & Smith, E. L. (2007). Integrating quality and safety content into clinical teaching in the acute care setting. *Nursing Outlook, 55*(3), 138-143.

Disch, J. (2012). Teamwork and collaboration. In G. Sherwood & J. Barnsteiner (Eds.), *Quality and safety in nursing: A competency approach to improving outcomes.* Hoboken, NJ: Wiley-Blackwell.

Draper, D. A., Felland, L. E., Liebhaber, A., & Melichar, L. (2008, March). The role of nurses in hospital quality improvement. Center for Studying Health System Change Research Brief No. 3. Retrieved from http://hschange.org/CONTENT/972/972.pdf

Durham, C., & Sherwood, G. (2008). Education to bridge the quality gap: A case study approach. *Journal of Urologic Nursing* [Special issue], *28*(6), 431-438.

Finkelman, A., & Kenner, C. (2009). *Teaching IOM: Implications of the Institute of Medicine reports for nursing,* 2nd ed. Silver Spring, MD: American Nurses Association.

Freshwater, D., Horton-Deutsch, S., Sherwood, G., & Taylor, B. (2005). *The scholarship of reflective practice* [Resource paper]. Available at Sigma Theta Tau International website: http://www.nursingsociety.org/aboutus/PositionPapers/Pages/position_resource_papers.aspx

Freshwater, D., Taylor, B., & Sherwood, G. (Eds.). (2008). *International textbook of reflective practice in nursing.* Oxford: Blackwell Publishing & Sigma Theta Tau Press.

Hall, L. M., Doran, D., & Pink, L. (2008). Outcomes of interventions to improve hospital nursing work environments. *Journal of Nursing Administration, 38*(1), 40-46.

Hall, L. W., Moore, S. M., & Barnsteiner, J. H. (2008). Quality and nursing: moving from a concept to a core competency. *Urologic Nursing: Official Journal of the American Urological Association Allied, 28*(6), 417-425.

Hassmiller, S. B., & Bolton, L. B. (2009). The development of TCAB. *American Journal of Nursing, 109*(11), 4.

Horton-Deutsch, S., & Sherwood, G. (2008). Reflection: An educational strategy to develop emotionally competent nurse leaders. *Journal of Nursing Management, 8,* 946-954.

Hughes, R. G. (2008). *Patent safety and quality: An evidence-based handbook for nurses* (AHRQ Publication No. 08-0043). Rockville, MD: Agency for Healthcare Research and Quality. http://www.ahrq.gov/qual/nurseshdbk

Hughes, R. G. (2008). Tools and strategies for quality improvement and patient safety. In R. G. Hughes (Ed.), *Patient safety and quality: An evidence-based handbook for nurses,* Vol. 3 (pp. 3-1-3-40). Rockville, MD: Agency for Healthcare Research and Quality.

Institute of Medicine. (2000). *To err is human: Building a safer health system.* Washington, DC: National Academies Press.

Institute of Medicine. (2003). *Health professions education: A bridge to quality.* Washington, DC: National Academies Press.

Institute of Medicine (2010). *The future of nursing: Leading change, advancing health.* Washington, DC: National Academies Press.

Ironsides, P., & Cerbie, E. (2012). Narrative teaching strategies to foster quality and safety. In G. Sherwood & J. Barnsteiner (Eds.), *Quality and safety in nursing: A competency approach to improving outcomes.* Hoboken, NJ: Wiley-Blackwell.

Johnson, J. (2012). Quality improvement. In G. Sherwood & J. Barnsteiner (Eds.), *Quality and safety in nursing: A competency approach to improving outcomes*. Hoboken, NJ: Wiley-Blackwell.

Jones, C. B., Mayer, C., & Mandelkehr, L. K. (2009). Innovations at the intersection of academia and practice: Educating graduate nursing students about quality improvement and patient safety. *Quality Management in Health Care, 18*(3), 158–164.

Ladden, M. D., Bednash, G., Stevens, D. P., & Moore, G. T. (2006). Educating inter-professional learners for quality, safety and systems improvement. *Journal of Interprofessional Care, 20*, 497–505.

Lavizzo-Mourey, R., & Berwick, D. M. (2009). Nurses transforming care. *American Journal of Nursing, 109*(11), 3.

Lindberg, L., & Kimberlain, J. (2008). Quality update. Engage employees to improve staff and patient satisfaction. *Hospital & Health Networks, 82*(1), 28–29.

Lundmark, V. (2008). Magnet environments for professional nursing practice. In R. G. Hughes (Ed.), *Patient safety and quality: An evidence-based handbook for nurses*, Vol. 3 (pp. 3-69-3-90). Rockville, MD: Agency for Healthcare Research and Quality. Retrieved June 17, 2010, from http://www.ahrq.gov/qual/nurseshdbk

Massachusetts Department of Education. (2010). *Nurse of the future: Nursing core competencies*. Retrieved July 15, 2011, from http://www.mass.edu/currentinit/documents/NursingCoreCompetencies.pdf

National League for Nursing (2010). *Outcomes and competencies for graduates of practical/vocational, diploma, associate degree, baccalaureate, masters, doctoral and research doctorate programs in nursing*. New York: National League for Nursing.

Oregon Consortium for Nursing Education. (2010). *Curriculum model*. Retrieved July 15, 2011, from http://ocne.org/curriculum.html

Page, A. (2004). *Keeping patients safe: Transforming the work environment of nurses*. Committee on the Work Environment for Nurses and Patient Safety, Board on Health Care Services. Washington, DC: National Academies Press.

Pohl, J., Savrin, C., Fiandt, K., Beauchesne, M., Drayton-Brooks, S., Scheibmeir, M., & Brackley, M. (2009). Quality and safety in graduate nursing education: Cross-mapping QSEN graduate competencies with NONPF's NP core and practice doctorate competencies. *Nursing Outlook, 57*(6), 349–354.

Preheim, G. J., Armstrong, G. E., & Barton, A. J. (2009). The new fundamentals in nursing: Introducing beginning quality and safety education for nurses' competencies. *Journal of Nursing Education, 48*(12), 694–697.

Robert Wood Johnson Foundation. (2008). *Transforming care at the bedside toolkit*. Retrieved June 30, 2010, from http://www.rwjf.org/pr/product.jsp?id=30051

Sammer, C. E, Lykens, K., Singh, K. P., Mains, D. A., & Lackan, N. A. (2010). What is patient safety culture? A review of the literature. *Journal of Nursing Scholarship, 42*(2), 156-165.

Schumann, M. J. (2012). Policy implications driving national quality and safety initiatives. In G. Sherwood & J. Barnsteiner (Eds.), *Quality and safety in nursing: A competency approach to improving outcomes*. Hoboken, NJ: Wiley-Blackwell.

Sherwood, G. (2006). Appreciative leadership: Building customer driven partnerships. *JONA, 36*(12), 551–557.

Sherwood, G. (2011). Integrating quality and safety science in nursing education and practice. *Journal of Research in Nursing, 16*(3), 226–240. doi:10:1177/1744987111400960.

Sherwood, G. (2012). Driving forces for quality and safety: Changing mindsets to improve health care. In G. Sherwood & J. Barnsteiner (Eds.), *Quality and safety in nursing: A competency approach to improving outcomes*. Hoboken, NJ: Wiley-Blackwell.

Sherwood, G., & Drenkard, K. (2007). Quality and safety curricula in nursing education: Matching practice realities. *Nursing Outlook, 55*(3), 151–155.

Sherwood, G., & Jones, C. (2011). Quality improvement in nursing. In W. Sollecito & J. Johnson (Eds.), *CQI in healthcare* (4th ed., pp. 485–511). San Francisco: Jossey-Bass.

Spector, N., Ulrich, B., & Barnsteiner, J. (2012). New graduate transition into practice: Improving quality and safety. In G. Sherwood & J. Barnsteiner (Eds.), *Quality and safety in nursing: A competency approach to improving outcomes*. Hoboken, NJ: Wiley-Blackwell.

Sullivan, D. T., Hirst, D., & Cronenwett, L. (2009). Assessing quality and safety competencies of graduating prelicensure nursing students. *Nursing Outlook, 57*(6), 323–331.

TeamSTEPPS. (2009). http://teamstepps.ahrq.gov/ Accessed June 30, 2011.

Thornlow, D., & McGuinn, K. (2010). A necessary sea change for nurse faculty development: Spotlight on quality and safety. *Journal of Professional Nursing, 26*(2), 71–81.

Tracey, M. F., & Barnsteiner, J. (2012). Evidence-based practice. In G. Sherwood & J. Barnsteiner (Eds.), *Quality and safety in nursing: A competency approach to improving outcomes*. Hoboken, NJ: Wiley-Blackwell.

Triolo, P. (2012). Creating cultures of excellence: Transforming organizations. In G. Sherwood & J. Barnsteiner (Eds.), *Quality and safety in nursing: A competency approach to improving outcomes*. Hoboken, NJ: Wiley-Blackwell.

Varkey, P., Reller, M. K., Smith, A., Ponto, J., & Osborn, M. (2006). An experiential interdisciplinary quality improvement education initiative. *American Journal of Medical Quality, 21*(5), 317–322.

Warren, J. (2012). Informatics. In G. Sherwood & J. Barnsteiner (Eds.), *Quality and safety in nursing: A competency approach to improving outcomes*. Hoboken, NJ: Wiley-Blackwell.

Resources

Agency for Healthcare Research and Quality. http://www.ahrq.gov

American Association of Colleges of Nursing. www.aacn.nche.edu

American Association of Critical Care Nurses. Clinical Practice Resources. http://www.aacn.org/DM/MainPages/PracticeHome.aspx?lastmenu=divheader_clinical_practice

American Organization of Nurse Executives. http://www.aone.org/

Center for Studying Health System Change. http://hschange.org/

Institute for Healthcare Improvement. www.ihi.org

Institute for Healthcare Improvement Open School for Health Professions. www.ihi.org/OpenSchool

International Council of Nurses. http://www.icn.ch/

Massachusetts Nurse of the Future Core Curriculum.

http://www.mass.edu/currentinit/currentinitNursingNurseFutureComp.asp

The National Center for Nursing Quality Indicators. American Nurses Association.

https://www.nursingquality.org/

National League for Nursing. http://www.nln.org

National Patient Safety Foundation. http://www.npsf.org/
Nursing Alliance for Quality Care. http://www.gwumc.edu/healthsci/departments/nursing/naqc/
Quality and Safety Education for Nurses. www.QSEN.org
Oregon Consortium of Nurse Educators. http://ocne.org/index.html
Robert Wood Johnson Foundation. http://www.rwjf.org/
TeamSTEPPS. http://teamstepps.ahrq.gov&sol

Chapter 11

Narrative Teaching Strategies to Foster Quality and Safety

Pamela M. Ironside,
PhD, RN, FAAN, ANEF
Elizabeth Cerbie, MSN, RN

The goal of the Quality and Safety Education for Nurses (QSEN) initiative is to transform nurses' professional identity such that every nurse has a commitment to improve the quality and safety of health care wherever and whenever it is delivered (Cronenwett et al., 2007). To that end, educators across the country are working diligently to embed the QSEN competencies as well as knowledge, skill, and attitude statements into their courses and curricula. To be successful, however, these efforts must go far beyond merely providing learners with more content knowledge about particular aspects of quality and safety or more skills they can proficiently and habitually perform. Rather, achieving a transformation in nurses' professional identity will require a change in how educators think about nursing practice and how we prepare learners to engage in that practice.

Teaching nursing practice

The predominant approach to teaching nursing in both academic and practice settings is conventional pedagogy, which focuses heavily on cognitive gain and skill acquisition as the basis of all learning encounters. Two common assumptions of this approach are that (a) content knowledge is best presented beginning with simple aspects and progressing to those that are more complex, and (b) when learners have acquired the prespecified content knowledge, they can then apply it in assigned practice settings in a linear, direct, and corresponding manner to provide evidence of their learning (Ironside, 2001). This approach to teaching is pervasive in the discipline, and educators rarely question the utility or limits of using just one pedagogy to prepare learners to

Quality and Safety in Nursing: A Competency Approach to Improving Outcomes, First Edition. Edited by Gwen Sherwood and Jane Barnsteiner.
© 2012 John Wiley & Sons, Inc. Published 2012 by John Wiley & Sons, Inc.

provide safe, quality care. Because of this overreliance on conventional pedagogy, teachers often mistake the mere adoption of innovative strategies as the means by which the QSEN goal can be met.

It is clearly important for students to obtain knowledge of the field and proficiency in practice skills before they enter the workforce. Yet, knowledge and skills alone are insufficient to prepare students for practice. Indeed, research is increasingly explicating the complexity of nurses' work (Ebright, Patterson, Chalko, & Render, 2003; Ebright, Urden, Patterson, & Chalko, 2004) and the complex web of interconnected, interdependent, and diverse elements (Lindberg, Nash, & Lindberg, 2008) that make up the systems within which care is delivered. Navigating the complexity of care delivery systems requires that students learn diverse skills, such as managing ambiguity and uncertainty, dealing with interruptions and distractions, making qualitative distinctions between different manifestations of health disruptions or different patients' and families' responses to health and illness, and understanding differing perspectives of practice encounters. Teaching these aspects of nursing practice will require new pedagogies.

Narrative pedagogy

Narrative pedagogy, a research-based, phenomenological pedagogy, was first identified during a longitudinal study of the experiences of teachers, students, and clinicians in nursing education (Diekelmann, 1995, 2001; Diekelmann & Diekelmann, 2009). Consistent with its philosophical underpinnings in hermeneutic phenomenology, educators enacting narrative pedagogy shift their attention from merely delivering or demonstrating specific content and skills to co-creating experiences in which they work *with* students to explore their experiences in nursing education and to challenge their preconceived notions and habitual ways of thinking. As teachers and students think together about the situations they encounter, they challenge their assumptions and reflect on, question, and reinterpret their shared experiences. In so doing, they discover new possibilities for learning and practice that are local, at hand, and context-specific.

Importantly, narrative pedagogy is an inclusive pedagogy in that it also embraces research in higher education, including attention to issues such as power (critical pedagogy), voice (feminist pedagogy), and the meta-narratives that shape nursing education and practice (postmodern pedagogy; Cho, 2008; Giroux, 2004; Ironside, 2001; Pegues, 2007; Stephenson, 2010; Webber, 2006). These diverse pedagogies (conventional, critical, feminist, phenomenological, and postmodern) are not mutually exclusive but rather extend and enhance one another. Bringing multiple pedagogies to bear on learning and teaching in nursing, teachers enacting narrative pedagogy create learning experiences that invite students and clinicians to think differently (in new ways and from different perspectives) and to be open to new understandings and possibilities for improving education and practice.

When narrative pedagogy is enacted, teachers, students, and clinicians share their experiences communally, most frequently by writing accounts and reading them aloud (Dahlberg, Ekebergh, & Ironside, 2003) or posting them in discussion forums. Writing the account of an experience involves rethinking the experience and making it intelligible to others by filling in details, concerns, and contextual factors that give the account its meaning and set up the possibility of better understanding the experience. For instance, a graduate student began her account as follows:

> It was colder than I ever remember a January night to be. With the fullest, brightest moon, the deepest wind chill, and our Emergency Department no less busy for the weather. The wind was fierce and unforgiving, and the moon in the clearest night of the year lit the way to our doors. It was a cruel night for lost souls. There were more than the usual feverish, fretful children; tired, despondent single mothers; impatient, irritated youth; the homeless and rejected needy. There were too few of our own nurses, a tired and overworked pair of physicians, and no one had thought to bring "treats." I was in charge of it all.[1]

Because understanding is always already situated, contextual, and directed toward possibilities (Heidegger, 1927/1962), descriptions such as this draw the listener/reader into the experience as they hear this charge nurse describe her worries and concerns in the context of a bitterly cold night, a busy emergency department, short staffing, and "no treats." The listener/reader is drawn into the experience, not as a distanced observer, but as an engaged participant. The listener is right there in the account (Gadamer, 2001) and, together with the teller, must attend to the context, challenges, and opportunities influencing the possibilities for care (Webber, 2006). Sharing narrative accounts also reveals preconceived notions, oversights, and misunderstandings brought into the experience, as this prelicensure student shared as he began the story of his experience caring for a patient with end-stage renal disease:

> I got report from the night nurse who said my patient, who had end-stage renal disease, was refusing dialysis. I couldn't believe he would do this! He had been on dialysis for awhile and things were going well. Obviously I would need to do some teaching about his disease and reinforce the consequences of refusing treatment. But when I met the patient and his wife, he said he hadn't refused dialysis. I was surprised by this because I was sure the night nurse had said he had refused. So then I started wondering if he was confused or if he was lying or what. I mean, maybe he just didn't want his wife to know he wanted to refuse. Why would I hear this in report if it wasn't true?

[1] Story presented by S. Voss as part of a collective paper presentation: *Creating a narrative pedagogy in teaching and learning nursing theory: The voices of teachers and students*, by P. M. Ironside, M. Fuhrman, D. Hogan, K. Kavanaugh, M. Ryan, & S. Voss. (1998). Chicago: Chicago Institute for Nursing Education.

> ## Textbox 11.1
>
> Please reflect on your experiences today in clinical. What stands out for you in this experience? As you think about this time, write the story of your experience. Your story may be of breakdown when nothing went right *or* of making a difference, when everything "fell into place." Include as much detail as possible and tell your story in first person, rather than stepping back and analyzing or describing "objectively." Consider what was running through your head at the time, what you were seeing and hearing. Any little fact of the story you can recall belongs with your experience. After you have given the details of your story, please describe why this story is important to you and what it means to you.
>
> **Interpretive Questioning**
>
> - How was your attention shifting as the experience unfolded? What were you watching for? distracted by? worried about? surprised by?
> - What is the *relationship* between X & Y? By whose account?
> - Whose voice is missing /silent? Whose interests were being served?
> - You had certain expectations and goals when you came into this experience. Can you say more about if/how these changed as the situation evolved?
> - Have you encountered a situation like this before? How was this situation like (or different from) that one?
> - What were you hearing from colleagues, faculty, other team members, and the patient/family during this time? How did you understand this and what did it mean to you?

Teaching students how to make qualitative distinctions between different patients' responses to health and illness requires the exploration of the assumptions that inform their thinking about particular situations. Narrative accounts of experiences and collaboratively engaging in cycles of interpretation provide opportunities for teachers and students to appreciate multiple perspectives and to think through preconceived notions.

To elicit narrative accounts of experiences, some teachers ask students to write an account of their most memorable experience in a particular clinical setting or to write an account in response to prompts such as, "Today I wondered about. … ," "I was worried when …," "I didn't know what to do or say when. …," or "I was surprised to find …" (Andrews, 1998; Dahlberg, Ekebergh, & Ironside, 2003). Other teachers have invited beginning students to share an experience that stands out for them in which they cared for, or were cared for by, another person (Ironside, 2003b). Similarly, when orienting new nurses, staff educators have asked new nurses to bring narrative accounts of a time during the orientation when they were unsure about what was going on clinically with a patient or about a memorable moment they encountered during the orientation. In each case, the teacher/educator encourages students to describe their experience as it happened, highlighting what was "going through their head" at the time or what they were thinking "while they were in the thick of it," rather than stepping back and giving a general overview or listing of what they did or said during the experience (Textbox 11.1). As experiences are shared, teachers and students engage in cycles of interpretation, exploring the meaning and significance of the experience, the assumptions underlying the ways the experience is understood, and the new insights about and possibilities for improving nursing education and practice revealed by this communal and collaborative thinking.

Cycles of interpretation

Teachers enacting narrative pedagogy engage students and clinicians in cycles of interpretation of their shared experiences by listening and coresponding, raising questions that provoke thinking. Together they explore the meaningfulness of the story, holding the understanding each brings to the account open and problematic. Seeking new ways to understand, they together attend to multiple perspectives (scientific, critical, feminist, postmodern, phenomenological, as well as perspectives of other team members, the patient, and the family). They also challenge assumptions, critique prevailing perspectives and the limits of current knowledge, and explore the meaning and significance of their interpretations for the emerging practice of the students and new nurses. Importantly, these efforts are not directed specifically toward identifying which perspective or action among those explored is best, most efficient, or most correct. Rather, consistent with the philosophical underpinnings of narrative pedagogy, all understanding is considered tentative as the complexity, uncertainty, and ambiguity of the encounter, as well as the fallibility of current knowledge and understandings, are preserved by cycles of interpretation. Through these cycles of interpretation, students learn to ask unsettling questions rather than rush to judgment about how to intervene in a particular situation.

Again, enacting narrative pedagogy and engaging in cycles of interpretation begin by hearing shared accounts of practice experiences. Consider this experience. Shelly has been a nurse for two years on a pediatric medical unit at City United Hospital, a large urban, acute care hospital. She shared the following:

Shelly's story

It's 3:30 p.m. on a busy pediatric medical unit. Afternoons are always busy because we are sending patients off the floor for tests, many of the medical teams are in seeing their patients, all of the consults are in progress, and we begin to get admissions and process discharges. I am assigned four busy patients and have just discharged my easiest patient (asthma exacerbation) to home. Then the charge nurse tells me there is a patient in the emergency department (ED) who needs to be admitted on our unit and I'm up for the admission. Geez, I think to myself, can't I just have 30 minutes to catch up? I haven't charted all day and I need to spend time with my family in room 27; they have so many questions about their child's new diabetes diagnosis and they need some support. But I just smile at my charge nurse, and tell her OK. Inside I say a little prayer, hoping they won't bring the patient for a good long while. I check in on my patient in room 31 who doesn't have any family with him, but a child life specialist is in playing with him right now (thank goodness!). I decide the charting can wait—it's waited this long—and I head into room 27. The child's grandparents have now arrived and are taking turns playing with the adorable 5-year-old. The mom looks at me and I can see the raw emotion in her eyes. She is exhausted, confused, and terrified of what this new diagnosis means for her child and their family. Just as I pull up a chair to sit next to them, I get called overhead that I have a phone call. Of course I do. (SIGH!) I take the call in the hall and it is Theresa from the ED. She is calling report on my new patient and wants to know if she can bring him up in 10 minutes. I explain that I am with a patient and family right now and need to check on the room before she brings him to the floor, so it will be awhile before we are ready. She gets very impatient and says that she is bringing the patient up in 10 minutes, that should be enough time for the room to be ready, and hangs up the phone. OK, then. I flag the charge nurse down, verify that the room will be ready and go back into room 27. I am able to spend at least a little time with this family, answer some of their questions, assure them that the diabetes educators and dietician will be here shortly to spend some time with them. Then I tell them I have to go but will be back and get ready to take this admission. But Theresa is already rolling onto the floor with Brandon, a 15-year-old boy with cystic fibrosis. I know Brandon; he has been on our unit a lot. He looks pretty good, considering, so I breathe a sigh of relief. Theresa quickly gives me all of the charting that she brought with her, gives quick report, and as she asks me if I have any questions, she starts backing away from Brandon and me; it is pretty clear to me that she isn't interested in my questions. I know Brandon well, but with the unit so busy I'm really worried that I'll overlook or forget something. I try to get Brandon settled in his room, but he can't seem to get comfortable and asks for something to eat. This is going to be a long shift! Times like these are so frustrating! I don't know how I am supposed to keep up. Besides, what's the big rush to get Brandon to the unit and why was Theresa so pushy! Can't she see how busy we are! I mean, I'm new here, give me a break!

By sharing experiences, the teller reveals to the listeners how he/she understands (interprets) the experience. But using narrative pedagogy is not just sharing experiences or responding to the teller's understanding; it is communally and collaboratively questioning the experience. It is a call to thinking deeply about everything present and absent in the experience (Diekelmann & Diekelmann, 2009). In adopting this interpretive stance, teachers, students, and clinicians come to explore in a new way the traditions they inherit, what currently occurs in practice, and what is possible.

After taking a few moments for listeners to consider the shared experience, teachers using narrative pedagogy frequently begin with an open question, such as, What stands out for you in this story? Open questions are a call to thinking and reveal what students notice, what catches their attention or piques their interest in the experience. By its very nature, this question is substantively different and sets up a different kind of conversation than asking questions from within conventional pedagogy, such as, If you were in Shelly's position, what's the first thing you would do? Importantly, the conversation that ensues as teacher and students engage in cycles of interpretation brings multiple perspectives and experiences, current literature, and further questioning to bear on better understanding this experience and on exploring the meaning and significance it has for nursing practice. For instance, as students comment on the tension between Shelly's desire to spend time with a distraught family and a new admission, the teacher may ask: What does it mean to nurses to face competing demands such as an exhausted, confused, and terrified family on one hand and a new admission with a recurrent exacerbation of his cystic fibrosis on the other? How do nurses decide how to spend their limited time? When the needs of a patient and the system conflict, how do nurses decide what approach to take?

Importantly, these shared narratives are dynamic tellings/showings of the possibilities for nursing practice as well as the ambiguity, uncertainty, limits, and disruptions inherent in day-to-day practice. They are simultaneously about the individual nurse (teller), others involved in the encounter, the context or system in which the encounter occurred, and the traditions of nursing being learned by the student (for better or worse). Even when written about a particular experience (e.g., clinical experiences of times students made a difference to a patient or family; Ironside, Diekelmann, & Hirschmann, 2005a, b), there is always an excess of meaning for teachers, students, and clinicians to explore as matters of concern circulate, stand out, or fade into the background (Diekelmann & Diekelmann, 2009).

Teachers may also engage students in cycles of interpretation across the narratives shared by students and clinicians. In some cases, these narratives tell of experiences around a common theme (e.g., a time when you cared for, or were cared for by, another person), whereas in others they may include tellings of a shared experience (e.g., the experiences of several people involved in a particular situation). For example, Theresa, also a nurse at City United Hospital, is a highly experienced nurse in the emergency department.

Theresa's story

My shift was supposed to start at 0700 this morning, but my phone rang at 0400 asking me if I'd come in a little early. One of the night shift nurses had a family emergency and had to leave. They often call me when they need help. I've been in this ED for 15 years, love what I do, and I'm pretty good at it. Plus, I am recently divorced and need the extra shifts for the money to pay the medical bills for my son. He is 7 years old and was born with a congenital heart malformation. He is doing well, but the medical bills are extensive and he'll always require some care. Luckily, my family is extremely supportive and they help whenever they can. Because I live with my sister and her family, they can watch my son so I can work the extra shifts.

When I arrive this morning, the ED is busy as usual. I take my assignment—three children, two who need some teaching before being discharged home and one who is being admitted. I am also to take over as charge nurse for the day shift. I jump right in so the night nurses can finish their shift and head home. We've been short staffed for days, but after 15 years, I guess you learn how to make anything work. This is less than ideal, but we would manage. As our morning goes on, we are working hard, but everything seems to be moving right along. I keep a close eye on everyone, just to be sure that no one gets overwhelmed. All the rooms are filled with patients and there are a few in the hall; the waiting room is packed. The hospital is full, so it is taking forever to get beds. As ED nurses, we are prepared to quickly diagnose, treat, and transfer, not to give care over a long period of time, so having such a backup of patients waiting to transfer can be really stressful for some long-term ED nurses.

I finish my discharges so I can focus on my other patient. His name is Brandon and he has cystic fibrosis. He seems to be doing fine but is being admitted for a "tune-up." We are just waiting for a bed to open up. I have just started talking with Brandon when the call comes in that we are getting a 7-year-old gunshot wound. What? Did they say a 7-year-old? I let the trauma team know and get ready to assist. When the ambulance arrives, team members jump and we all start working quickly.

The victim is a beautiful 7-year-old boy who was outside playing in front of his house. He lived in a bad part of town, probably one of the worst, but it was a beautiful summer morning, probably the first one of the year. Unfortunately, as Isaac was playing outside, a stray bullet from a drive-by gang shooting hit him. In the ED we see too many senseless deaths! This is a hard one on our whole team! We work for almost an hour trying to stabilize him so he can get to surgery, but we lose our battle, and we lose him. The family is being called; only the mom is with him in the ED. She is, of course, devastated! She keeps saying, "I knew I shouldn't have let him play outside. Why did I let him play outside?" As I'm consoling her, I look up from where we are and see Brandon sitting up on his cart, looking across the hall at all of this, his big blue eyes just staring. So now I'm thinking, when is that bed going to be ready? What could be taking so long? He does not need to be down here seeing and hearing all this commotion! I motion to the unit secretary to check on the room for Brandon so we can get him out of here and comfortable in his own room, and give him a wave to let him know we're OK and I'll be over soon. I move the mom down the hall to a grief room. The secretary lets me know the bed is open and that I can give report to Shelly. About then the dad arrives and is just realizing what has happened to his son. I take him to his wife and get them settled into a private visitor's room. But by now I'm really worried that no one is checking in with Brandon. As soon as I can, I call to give report so I can get him into a more comfortable place and away from all this commotion and sadness. When I get the nurse, Shelly, on the phone, she says she knows Brandon (Great, I think, that should speed things up!), but I can tell she doesn't want to take this admission right now; she keeps trying to put me off. I mean, come on! Brandon has already been down here for 4 hours, and this is obviously not a good place for him right now! As I'm trying to get off the phone as quickly as I can, more family members arrive and they are sobbing and yelling in the hall near Brandon's room. I tell Shelly that I'll be bringing him up in 10 minutes and quickly hang up to go support the newest family member who has arrived and learned of their loss.

I go back in to check on mom and dad, and ask them if they want to see Isaac, their little boy, one last time. I can see the fear in their eyes, but I tell them I will be right there with them. They are relieved and say they want to say their goodbyes. I tell them to take some time right now with the chaplain, and I'll get the room ready for them. I don't want them to see Isaac this way, so I need a few minutes to prepare him and the room. I'm moving as fast as I can when another experienced nurse walks in, so I ask him to get Isaac ready for his parents while I take Brandon upstairs. He agrees, and shares that Betsy, one of our newer nurses, is extremely upset by this loss so he has sent her to take a short break. I thank him and say we'll have to do some debriefing after this one—seeing a 7-year-old victim is hard on everyone! I reassure him I will check on Betsy when I get back. I quickly grab Brandon and his stuff, and we head upstairs. He's really quiet, but when I ask he says he is fine. "It's been a tough morning for you, hasn't it?" I ask. Brandon stays quiet. We roll onto the unit and find Shelly. Since she knows Brandon I give her a quick report, ask if she has any questions. I tell Brandon goodbye and quickly head back down to the ED. I now have one of the hardest parts of my job—helping parents say goodbye to their baby! This makes me think of my own 7-year-old for a moment. I can't imagine what his parents are going through. I take the few seconds in the elevator to gather my thoughts. I take a deep breath. Here I go.

The strength of narrative pedagogy lies in seeking to understand an experience and the possibilities for engaging with it as a nurse. In contrast to conventional pedagogy's focus on the application of knowledge or theories (learned elsewhere and applied in a specific situation), with narrative pedagogy, teachers invite students and clinicians to think about the situations they encounter in new ways and from multiple perspectives, using their knowledge and experience as the background for questioning the meaning and significance of the experience. The background, theories, or specific clinical data may be brought to bear in interpreting an account (e.g., understanding Shelly's and Theresa's experiences draws on knowledge of newly diagnosed diabetes and cystic fibrosis in children, family dynamics, grief, and handoffs and communication among team members and across departments), but the focus is on seeking to understand the experience before considering what knowledge to apply, or when and how it might be applied (Doane & Brown, 2011).

Further, hearing the narratives shared and the conversations that ensue as teacher, students, and clinicians collaboratively and communally engage in cycles of interpretation reveals how teachers, students, and clinicians understand the situations they encounter and ascertain what knowledge to use when and how. They also consider the limitations of their knowledge and experience (e.g., what do I know and what do I need to know?), current disciplinary knowledge and evidence to guide practice (e.g., what could be wrong with using best practices in this case?), and inherited, idealized views of nursing practice that do not account for the context in which care is given (e.g., what does it mean to nurses to be unable to provide "good" nursing care because of competing demands for their time?). The shift in using narrative pedagogy is to bring the complexity and the multifaceted, interrelated problems facing nurses on a day-to-day basis into the conversation rather than try to simplify or mitigate the complexity of nursing practice in order to teach isolated skills such as communication, organization, or priority setting. Indeed, phenomenologically, it is only through understanding an experience that decisions about what knowledge/skills to apply as well as when and how to apply them in a particular situation are possible.

Experiences are never straightforward or linear, and it is often the case that cycles of interpretation include "unsettling" an experience by persistently asking questions from multiple perspectives (scientific, critical, feminist, postmodern, and phenomenological). This is in stark contrast to the conventional approach of moving linearly from question to answer without considering questions such as the position of the nurse in the experience and how the particular problem being solved became identified as a problem in the first place. With narrative pedagogy, a shared experience is not simply a description of a discrete event; it brings with it past and current experiences and the available possibilities given the situation. Thus, cycles of interpretation are never acontextual or abstract but are rooted through and through in the pressures and contingencies, the norms and policies, the cultures and traditions, and the values and ethics of the environments in which the experience occurred. As teachers, students, and clinicians communally and collaboratively engage in cycles of interpretation, they bring their background knowledge and experience (i.e., past), their perspective (i.e., present), and their anticipated sense of possibilities (i.e., future) into the conversation. Like the hermeneutic circle, understanding is circular, never ending, and always already situated in the experiences teachers, students, and clinicians bring into conversation.

As teachers participate in cycles of interpretation, they approach each conversation as a learner—seeking to learn more about nursing practice and how students learn nursing in the complex and evolving health care system. They also gain insight into the students' thinking. At times, students' thinking shows great depth and insight, and teachers are amazed at the ways students are thinking about their practice (Dahlberg et al., 2003, Ironside, 2003a, 2006). At other times, students' preconceived notions, oversights, prejudices, and misunderstandings are revealed. For example, after hearing Shelly's story, students frequently want to critique Theresa's practice and to contrast it to an idealized notion of good practice, positing the "right" thing for Shelly to do or say (Doane & Brown, 2011). Yet, when Theresa's narrative is heard, those interpretations quickly become problematic and students must consider new perspectives and ways of thinking about practice. Teachers using narrative pedagogy pose questions to keep students' emerging understandings in play and, together with the students, to learn more about nursing practice. For instance, they might ask: What are the issues of power, control, and authority embedded in Shelly's and Theresa's accounts? Whose voice is missing from these tellings? What assumptions are we making about what constitutes good practice? How are these assumptions influencing our current understanding? What does this experience mean to you as a new nurse (student nurse)? Relying solely on pedagogies directed toward achieving predetermined outcomes or changes in behavior covers over what is to be learned by questioning how we come to understand experiences, the assumptions we make, and the importance of nurses learning together and keeping their practice open and problematic.

Narrative pedagogy and Quality and Safety Education for Nurses

The Quality and Safety Education for Nurses (QSEN) goal of transforming nurses' professional identity such that every nurse has a commitment to improving the quality and safety of health care wherever and whenever it is delivered presents both a challenge and an opportunity for nursing educators (Cronenwett, 2012). The QSEN competencies and the explication of the knowledge, skills, and attitudes required to achieve those competencies sound deceptively straightforward (Appendixes A and B). At first glance, it appears that teaching skills such as *act with integrity, consistency, and respect for differing views,* or *provide patient-centered care with sensitivity and respect for the diversity of human experience* (Cronenwett et al., 2007) requires only that teachers transmit these skills to students such that students recognize and can assimilate and articulate these aspects of practice. Teachers can then evaluate students' acquisition of these skills in subsequent classroom, clinical, or simulation experiences. The prevalence of this approach can be seen in faculties' efforts to map the 6 competencies and the 162 knowledge, skill, and attitude statements (KSAs) across the curriculum so that faculty members, administrators, and regulators are aware of where each of the competencies and KSAs are taught and learned. Yet, research has shown that relying on this approach is problematic because nursing curricula are already overloaded with content and skills to the point where there is little time for thinking (Ironside, 2004). Loosening our grasp on conventional pedagogy as the only, or even the best, approach to teaching nursing creates opportunities for teachers, students, and clinicians to co-create different kinds of experiences in which prevailing views, extant knowledge, assumptions, and the meaning and significance of practice experiences can be communally and collaboratively explored.

Using narrative pedagogy or other research-based pedagogies requires that teachers reconsider how they spend their time with students. Working with students and clinicians to co-create experiences that focus on thinking and extending our understanding of nursing practice, with all the complexities that entails, becomes as important as content knowledge or the demonstration of particular skills. For example, relying solely on conventional pedagogy, a teacher might talk with students about the importance of nurses *acting with integrity, consistency, and respect for differing views* and may create case studies about patients with differing views to see if students are able to identify the best way to proceed in each particular situation. Using narrative pedagogy, teachers invite students to think about the complexity of *respecting different views* and may raise questions such as: Do patients/families experience nursing care as respectful? As a nurse, how would you know if a patient you were caring for felt respected or not? How do nurses exude respectfulness when encountering patients who are predators or who are racist, violent, inappropriate, noncompliant, or aggressive? Could there be times that despite our best efforts to be respectful, patients experience the opposite?

Such questions are unanswerable. That is, the complexity of these questions keeps our experiences, knowledge, and assumptions in play as teachers, students, and clinicians engage in conversation, exploring differing perspectives and thinking together about these aspects of practice. Importantly, because these questions are situated in (and arise from) narrative accounts of experiences, they also show how interrelated the KSAs are in nursing practice. For instance, as teachers, students, and clinicians explore the question of how nurses can exude respectfulness when encountering patients who are predators or who are racist, violent, inappropriate, noncompliant, or violent, they are simultaneously engaging students in thinking about numerous KSAs (e.g., *act with integrity, consistency, and respect for differing views; provide patient-centered care with sensitivity and respect for the diversity of human experience; seek learning opportunities with patients who represent all aspects of human diversity; recognize personally held attitudes about working with patients from different ethnic, cultural, and social backgrounds; willingly support patient-centered care for individuals and groups whose values differ from own*, and so forth; Cronenwett et al., 2007). When providing care, the QSEN KSA statements are not isolated or discreet aspects of practice to be learned separately and later synthesized into a competency. They are embedded in practice situations in both positive and negative ways. Thus, much is to be gained from expanding our pedagogical repertoire by using pedagogies grounded in teachers', students', and clinicians' experiences so that conversations about the competencies and KSA statements occur in ways consistent with and reflective of the complexity of current practice.

Narrative pedagogy is not a strategy teachers employ in the service of teaching quality and safety, but it is a way of persistently thinking about nursing education and practice *with* students and clinicians and of communally and collaboratively exploring new possibilities for improving the quality and safety of care provided. Co-creating experiences that focus on thinking together and understanding experiences in new ways and from multiple perspectives extends conventional pedagogy by developing students' interpretive skills (skills related to thinking in new ways and from multiple perspectives). This means that teachers enacting narrative pedagogy can't plan in advance where the conversation around a narrative experience will go or the understandings that will be uncovered. As participants in the conversation, teachers enacting narrative pedagogy focus on questioning current understanding (e.g., whose interests are being served? What does it mean to patients to have these encounters with nurses?), rather than providing or describing one particular view over others. This questioning cultivates deeper consideration of students', teachers', and clinicians' experiences and holds the possibility of new perspectives and ways to improve nursing education and practice.

Teachers enacting narrative pedagogy reclaim for their teaching practice an emphasis on the importance of always questioning the best practices of nursing care, the strengths and weaknesses of current evidence, and the ways in which nurses listen and respond to those in their care. But more than just critiquing current nursing care (although an important practice), teachers enacting narrative pedagogy foster thinking broadly about the tentativeness of answers in clinical practice and the importance of persistently questioning, holding everything currently assumed to be true open and problematic. This is consistent with the literature that shows how navigating the uncertainty and fallibility embedded in current (and future) practice has become as important for nurses as content knowledge and skill mastery and that interpreting (learning to read) situations is as important as intervening (Cook, Ironside, & Ogrinc, 2011; Ironside, 2003b).

Summary

The importance of preparing students and new nurses to provide safe, quality care cannot be overestimated. The QSEN delineation of specific competencies and of knowledge, skills, and attitude statements identifies important aspects of practice all nurses entering the workforce should possess (Cronenwett et al., 2007). As nursing faculties strive to embed QSEN competencies into their curricula, it is crucial that the complexity of these competencies and KSAs be appreciated and incorporated into teaching and learning encounters in nursing. Using diverse pedagogies, such as narrative pedagogy, affords teachers the opportunity to create substantively different experiences with students and clinicians, experiences focused on thinking together in new ways and from multiple perspectives about the complexities of practice and the possibilities for improvement.

References

Andrews, C. A. (1998). Engendering community: Writing a journal to clinical students. *Journal of Nursing Education, 37*, 358-360.

Cho, S. (2008). Politics of critical pedagogy and new social movements. *Educational Philosophy and Theory, 42*, 310-325.

Cook, M., Ironside, P. M., & Ogrinc, G. (2011). Mainstreaming quality and safety: A reformulation of quality and safety education for health professions students. *Quality and Safety in Health Care, 20*(Suppl 1), 179-182.

Cronenwett, L. (2012). A national initiative: Quality and Safety Education for Nurses (QSEN). In G. Sherwood & J. Barnsteiner (Eds.), *Quality and safety in nursing: A competency approach to improving outcomes*. Hoboken, NJ: Wiley-Blackwell.

Cronenwett, L., Sherwood, G., Barnsteiner, J., Disch, J., Johnson, J., Mitchell, P., et al. (2007). Quality and safety education for nurses. *Nursing Outlook, 55*, 122-131.

Dahlberg, K., Ekebergh, M., & Ironside, P. M. (2003). Converging conversations from phenomenological pedagogies: Toward a science of health professions education. In N. Diekelmann & P. Ironside (Eds.), *Teaching practitioners of care: New pedagogies for the health professions* (Vol. 2, pp. 22-58). Madison: University of Wisconsin Press.

Diekelmann, N. L. (1995). Reawakening thinking: Is traditional pedagogy nearing completion? *Journal of Nursing Education, 34*, 195-196.

Diekelmann, N. L. (2001). Narrative pedagogy: Heideggerian hermeneutical analyses of lived experiences of students, teachers, and clinicians. *Advances in Nursing Science, 23*(3), 53-71.

Diekelmann, N., & Diekelmann, J. (2009). Schooling learning teaching: Toward narrative pedagogy. Bloomington, IN: iUniverse Press.

Doane, G. H., & Brown, H. (2011). Recontextualizing learning in nursing education: Taking an ontological turn. *Journal of Nursing Education, 50*, 21-26.

Ebright, P. R., Patterson, E. S., Chalko, B. A., & Render, M. L. (2003). Understanding the complexity of registered nurse work in acute care settings. *JONA, 33*, 630-638.

Ebright, P. R., Urden, L., Patterson, E., & Chalko, B. (2004). Themes surrounding novice nurse near-miss and adverse-event situations. *JONA, 34*, 531-538.

Gadamer, H.-G. (2001). *Gadamer in conversation: Reflections and commentary*. (R.E. Palmer, Ed. and Trans.). New Haven, CT: Yale University Press.

Giroux, H. A. (2004). Critical pedagogy and the postmodern/modern divide: Towards a pedagogy of democratization. *Teacher Education Quarterly, 31*, 31-47.

Heidegger, M. (1962). *Being and time* (J. Macquarrie & E. Robinson, Trans.). San Francisco: HarperCollins. (Original work published 1927).

Ironside, P. M. (2001). Creating a research base for nursing education: An interpretive review of conventional, critical, feminist, postmodern, and phenomenologic pedagogies. *Advances in Nursing Science, 23*(3), 72-87.

Ironside, P. M. (2003a). New pedagogies for teaching thinking: The lived experiences of students and teachers enacting narrative pedagogy. *Journal of Nursing Education, 42*, 509-516.

Ironside, P. M. (2003b). Trying something new: Implementing and evaluating narrative pedagogy using a multi-method approach. *Nursing Education Perspectives, 24*(3), 122-128.

Ironside, P. M. (2004). "Covering content" and teaching thinking: Deconstructing the additive curriculum. *Journal of Nursing Education, 43,* 5-12.

Ironside, P. M. (2006). Using narrative pedagogy: Learning and practicing interpretive thinking. *Journal of Advanced Nursing, 55,* 478-486.

Ironside, P. M., Diekelmann, N. L., & Hirschmann, M. (2005a). Learning the practices of knowing and connecting: The voices of students. *Journal of Nursing Education, 44,* 153-155.

Ironside, P. M., Diekelmann, N. L., & Hirschmann, M. (2005b). Student voices: On listening to experiences in practice education. *Journal of Nursing Education, 44,* 49-52.

Ironside, P. M., Fuhrman, M., Hogan, D., Kavanaugh, K., Ryan, M., & Voss, S. (1998). *Creating a narrative pedagogy in teaching and learning nursing theory: The voices of teachers and students.* Chicago: Chicago Institute for Nursing Education.

Lindberg, C., Nash, S., & Lindberg, C. (2008). On the edge: Nursing in the age of complexity. Bordentown, NJ: PlexusPress.

Pegues, H. (2007). Of paradigm wars: Constructivism, objectivism, and postmodern stratagem. *The Educational Forum, 71,* 316-330.

Stephenson, S. S. (2010). "Faces" and complexities of continuing higher education units: A postmodern approach. *Journal of Continuing Higher Education, 58,* 62-72.

Webber, M. (2006). Transgressive pedagogies: Exploring the difficult realities of enacting feminist pedagogies in undergraduate classrooms in a Canadian university. *Studies in Higher Education, 31,* 453-467.

Chapter 12

Integrating Quality and Safety Competencies in Simulation

Carol F. Durham, EdD, RN, ANEF
Kathryn R. Alden, EdD, MSN, RN, IBCLC

In nursing education, the term *simulation* typically evokes images of a life-size high-fidelity manikin that breathes, has pulses, and can even speak. In recent years, simulation-based education using human patient simulators has soared in popularity as an instructional strategy in nursing and health professions education. Numerous publications cite the benefits of simulation learning activities while others describe how simulation is used in specific courses and settings. However, there is comparatively less information specific to the effective use of simulation to teach quality and safety in nursing practice (Durham & Alden, 2008, 2010; Henneman & Cunningham, 2005; Henneman, Cunningham, Roche, & Curnin, 2007; Henneman et al., 2010; Larew, Lessans, Spunt, Foster, & Covington, 2006). Furthermore, there is minimal information regarding how to incorporate Quality and Safety Education for Nurses (QSEN) competencies (patient-centered care, teamwork and collaboration, evidence-based practice, quality improvement, safety, and informatics) into simulation learning activities, whether for student, transition to practice, or clinician education (Ironside, Jeffries, & Martin, 2009; Jarzemsky, McCarthy, & Ellis, 2010).

The value of human patient simulation in promoting safe practice is reflected in the Institute of Medicine (IOM) report *To Err is Human: Building a Safer Health Care System*. The IOM recommends simulation as a strategy that can be used to prevent errors in the clinical setting: "Health care organizations and teaching institutions should participate in the development and use of simulation for training novice practitioners, problem solving, and crisis management, especially when new and potentially hazardous procedures and equipment are introduced" (Kohn, Corrigan, & Donaldson, 2000, p. 179).

Quality and Safety in Nursing: A Competency Approach to Improving Outcomes, First Edition. Edited by Gwen Sherwood and Jane Barnsteiner.
© 2012 John Wiley & Sons, Inc. Published 2012 by John Wiley & Sons, Inc.

A decade later, Benner, Sutphen, Leonard, and Day (2010) called for a radical transformation in educating nurses. The authors identified simulation-based education as effective pedagogy.

This chapter focuses on the use of simulation-based education as an instructional strategy and includes information on how to integrate specific QSEN competencies into simulation-based learning activities. Educators have realized only the tip of the iceberg in terms of the potential use of simulation-based education in teaching students about quality and safety in nursing practice.

Simulation and safety are concepts often aligned with one another as educators consider instructional strategies for various courses and situations. It is important for the educator to select or design simulation-based activities to fit learning objectives, needs of the learners, and the setting. In some cases, a variety of simulated-based education approaches can be used in a single patient care scenario. As a prelude to information about using high fidelity simulation to teach QSEN competencies, it is helpful to understand the various types of simulation-based activities used in nursing education.

Types of simulation

The term *simulation* refers to a device or an activity that is used in an attempt to create a realistic representation of the real world (Gaba, 2004). Devices and activities can range from the simplicity of an orange used to teach students injection techniques to the complexity of a high-fidelity computerized manikin that can be used for critical care scenarios.

Simulation activities attempt to replicate real-life situations that occur in various patient care settings. These simulations can vary from simple to complex and are intended to engage learners in realistic learning activities that promote development and utilization of cognitive and psychomotor skills.

Fidelity refers to the degree to which a device or activity represents actual reality. Fidelity is based on physical characteristics and the ability of the technology and scenario to parallel the complexity of a real-life experience. *Low-fidelity simulators* (task, part-task, or skill trainers) are generally used to introduce and practice psychomotor skills, but they lack the realism that promotes immersion into a patient care scenario. An example of a low-fidelity simulator is a part-task trainer that represents a portion of the body such as an arm for teaching venipuncture technique. *Intermediate or medium fidelity* simulators include full body manikins that allow learners to perform a variety of assessments, skills, and interventions, but they limit the interactivity, technical response, and feedback provided by a high-fidelity simulator. *High-fidelity* simulators represent the highest level of realism. The epitomy of high fidelity is standardized patients who are live actors trained to role play as simulated patients. The most technologically advanced human patient simulators are full body manikins that imitate the human response in real time, are physiologically based, and are capable of respiration, breath sounds, heart sounds, pupillary reaction, and urinary output. Simulator manufacturers offer a variety of models representing various ages and genders. Simulators are also designed for specific purposes, such as birthing simulators.

Benefits of high-fidelity simulation

High-fidelity simulation is a learner-centered approach to nursing education. The focus is not on the educator as the "sage on the stage" but on the learner. It is an immersive, hands-on, experiential learning activity in which learners can assume an active role in a patient care scenario. Using simulation, educators can provide students with risk-free, controlled learning opportunities that bridge the gap from theory and laboratory knowledge to actual patient care situations. During simulation, students must use their own knowledge to collect and analyze patient data, and must utilize clinical reasoning skills to decide on appropriate interventions. They can practice assessment and psychomotor skills. Students can evaluate the effectiveness of their actions based on observed responses by the simulator. Students are assisted to visualize the physiologic responses of the "patient" to medications and other interventions. Because simulation does not endanger the lives of real patients, students are permitted to make mistakes, correct those mistakes, and learn from them while in a supportive environment. In most cases, the nonthreatening nature of simulation learning activities promotes inquiry as students actively apply knowledge and skills. Simulation requires learners to utilize cognitive, technical, and behavioral skills as they interact with the manikin and other actors in the scenario, such as family members or health team members. High-fidelity simulation promotes self-efficacy and increases the self-confidence of learners in their ability to perform technical skills, to care for actual patients, and to handle unexpected situations in the clinical setting (Leigh, 2008). This enhances their ability to provide safe, quality care to patients.

High-fidelity simulation learning activities allow for consistency in clinical learning experiences and provide opportunities to care for patients in critical care, emergent, or life-threatening scenarios. Prelicensure students who encounter critical care scenarios, rapid response situations, or cardiopulmonary arrests in the clinical setting are most often asked to step aside while the staff members intervene with the patient. Yet it is important that they understand how to provide appropriate care to patients in these situations. Human patient simulation is an excellent strategy for teaching students how to provide safe, effective, quality care to patients with acute needs.

Simulation is one means of bridging the gap between education and practice for new graduates, thus easing the transition to practice (Kaddoura, 2010). Used as synthesis experiences in their last semester of the nursing curriculum and as part of new nurse orientation programs, simulation can facilitate adaptation from the role of student to professional nurse. In settings where multiple simulators are available, students can care for multiple patients, versus the one or two that they typically were assigned on the actual nursing units during their prelicensure program (Ironside et al., 2009).

Versatility of simulation

One of the most appealing aspects of simulation-based education is its versatility. Its adaptability and flexibility allow for a broad range of uses in undergraduate and graduate nursing education, continuing education, staff development, and interprofessional education.

Prelicensure nursing education programs

Pre-licensure nursing education programs utilize simulation in a variety of courses. Using Benner's (1984) theory of novice to expert as a framework, one can trace the utility of human patient simulation in educating nurses for safe practice. High-fidelity patient simulators can be used by novice learners in foundational nursing courses to practice physical assessment and fundamental nursing skills. As they perform psychomotor skills, students can also practice therapeutic communication skills as the simulator or facilitator responds to the student. Before novice students begin their first clinical practicum, scenarios with the human patient simulator can help prepare them for what they will encounter with real patients, thus reducing their anxiety and stress (Bremner, Aduddell, Bennett, & VanGeest, 2006). As their anxiety is reduced, they are less likely to make mistakes that can affect patient safety.

As students advance in the nursing curriculum, it is ideal for them to have ongoing opportunities to participate in human patient simulation scenarios that are relevant to each course. For example, students in the maternity course can participate in scenarios using a birthing simulator to focus on high-risk intrapartum care, which they may not experience in the hospital but need to know (e.g., prolapsed cord or shoulder dystocia). Integrating content from more than one course into simulation learning activities enhances the learning experiences for students. For example, pediatric and mental health educators can work together to create scenarios that address care of an acutely ill child and the associated psychological responses and needs of the parents.

For the student who is approaching graduation, simulation scenarios can be designed as synthesis learning experiences. During capstone nursing courses, students can participate in complex patient care scenarios that require application of knowledge and performance of a variety of psychomotor skills to provide safe, quality patient care. Leadership and management skills can be incorporated into scenarios.

While many simulation scenarios are situated in hospital settings, educators can expand their use of simulation scenarios to include patient care environments such as long-term care, outpatient psychiatric care, or community health.

Graduate nursing education

High-fidelity simulation can be used to teach advanced practice skills and concepts to nurse practitioner, clinical nurse specialist, nurse anesthetist, and DNP students. Simulation scenarios provide opportunities for these advanced practice nursing students to apply knowledge while utilizing diagnostic reasoning and assessment skills (Henrichs, Rule, Grady, & Ellis, 2002; Hravnak, Tuite, & Baldisseri, 2005; Scherer, Bruce, Graves, & Erdley, 2003; Shepherd, Kelly, Skene, & White, 2007).

There is great potential for the use of high-fidelity simulation in preparing future nurse educators who will supervise students in the clinical setting. Simulation-based activities provide excellent opportunities for graduate students or new educators to facilitate learning with prelicensure students as though they are in the clinical setting.

Continuing education and staff development

As an alternative or adjunct to the traditional lecture format for continuing education activities, simulation-based learning provides a more experiential learning opportunity for nurses seeking to improve their practice (Nehring & Lashley, 2004).

With concerns about transition to practice for new graduates of nursing education programs, health care agencies can utilize simulation to facilitate the shift from the student role to the role of professional nurse as the new nurses participate in realistic scenarios that involve policies, procedures, protocols, and equipment that are specific to that particular institution (Ackerman, Kenny, & Walker, 2007; Beyea, von Reyn, & Slattery, 2007; Nagle, McHale, Alexander, & French, 2009). Simulation can be used to improve critical thinking, clinical decision-making, and confidence of new graduates (Kaddoura, 2010). Competency evaluation of new and existing personnel in health care agencies can be accomplished using simulation (Paparella, Mariani, Layton, & Carpenter, 2004).

Interprofessional simulation

Simulation learning activities present an excellent opportunity to teach students about interprofessional or interdisciplinary care and to help them understand the roles of other health care professionals. Through involvement of a variety of health care providers and ancillary personnel, nurses gain an awareness and appreciation of the team approach to providing safe and effective patient care.

Collaboration between professional schools within a college university is prerequisite to offering interprofessional simulation learning activities (Willhaus, 2010). Within health care institutions, interprofessional team training to promote patient safety can be accomplished using simulation-based education (Miller, Riley, Davis, & Hansen, 2008; Smith & Cole, 2009; Strouse,

2010). The term *in situ simulation* refers to simulation activities that take place on actual patient care units; participants are real health team members.

QSEN competencies and simulation

The competencies identified by the QSEN project (patient-centered care, teamwork and collaboration, evidence-based practice, quality improvement, safety, and informatics; Cronenwett et al., 2007) are inherent to most high-fidelity simulation-based learning activities, whether or not educators purposefully include them. The prelicensure (Appendix A) or graduate-level competencies (Appendix B), as appropriate, can often be integrated into current courses, skills labs, and simulation scenarios without significant revisions (Cronenwett et al., 2007; Cronenwett et al., 2009). Through careful examination of what is currently being done and re-envisioning the focus on QSEN competencies, educators can make meaningful additions to patient quality and safety. Helpful tools on the QSEN website (www.QSEN.org) include a checklist that educators can use to examine existing scenarios for QSEN competencies; it can also be used to develop new scenarios (Alfes, 2010). In addition, Jarzemsky (2009) provides a template for development of scenarios that incorporate the competencies.

The following section will examine the incorporation of QSEN competencies in various simulation-based learning activities. While this section is organized according to the QSEN competencies, it is important to note that the pedagogy of simulation allows for the integration of multiple QSEN competencies simultaneously. Table 12.1 provides examples of integration of the QSEN competencies into prelicensure and graduate education.

Patient-centered care

Definition: Recognize the patient or designee as the source of control and full partner in providing compassionate and coordinated care based on respect for patient's preferences, values, and needs. (Cronenwett et al., 2007, p. 123).

Nurses are quick to affirm that their care is patient-centered, but the knowledge, skills, and attitudes (KSAs) in the QSEN competencies broaden expectations (Walton & Barnsteiner, 2012). Patient-centered care goes beyond considering the patient's preferences for timing of care, management of pain, and providing comfort to truly integrating the patient as part of the care team (see Chapter 3). Care management moves from those delivering the care to the patient receiving the care (Berwick, 2009). One of the 26 recommendations proposed by Benner and colleagues (2010) to transform nursing education is "Develop pedagogies that keep students focused on the patient's experience," (p. 220). The educator should teach pathology and psychosocial components of the illness in the context of the patient's experience.

The Joint Commission implemented Patient-Centered Communication standards in 2010 (Arocha & Moore, 2011). Patient-centered care goes beyond

Table 12.1 Examples of select knowledge, skills and attitudes and simulation learning activities for prelicensure and graduate students

QSEN Competency	Prelicensure Knowledge, Skills, Attitudes (KSAs) (Cronenwett et al., 2007)	Simulation Learning Activity	Graduate Knowledge, Skills, Attitudes (Cronenwett et al., 2009)	Simulation Learning Activity
Patient-centered care	K: Integrate understanding of multiple dimensions of patient-centered care: physical comfort and emotional support. S: Elicit patient values, preferences, and expressed needs as part of clinical interview, implementation of care plan, and evaluation of care. A: Value seeing health care situations through patients' eyes.	*Presimulation:* Ostomy exercise–students apply and wear ostomy appliance and reflect on experience *Simulation:* Care for post-op patient with newly created ostomy, focus on comfort, emotional needs, teaching *Postsimulation:* Debriefing: discuss how pre-sim activity impacted nursing care; describe how having an ostomy affects all aspects of a patient's life.	K: Analyze multiple dimensions of patient-centered care. S: Elicit patient values, preferences, and expressed needs as part of clinical interview, diagnosis, implementation of care plan, and evaluation of care. A: Value the patient's expertise with own health and symptoms.	*Presimulation:* Learners reflect on care they or their family have received and examine where there were gaps in best practices for patient-centered care. *Simulation:* Imbedded patient-centered care opportunities around values, preference, and expressed needs with patient and family *Postsimulation:* Ask advanced practice nurse to identify the patient's values, expressed needs they solicited during the interview, diagnosis, implementation of care, and evaluation of care. Solicit feedback on how they felt they were listened to, how they were integrated as a member of the team, and whether their values and expressed needs were considered in the plan of care.

(Continued)

Table 12.1 *(Continued)*

QSEN Competency	Prelicensure Knowledge, Skills, Attitudes (KSAs) (Cronenwett et al., 2007)	Simulation Learning Activity	Graduate Knowledge, Skills, Attitudes (Cronenwett et al., 2009)	Simulation Learning Activity
Teamwork and collaboration	K: Describe scopes of practice and roles of health care team members. S: Function competently within own scope of practice as a member of the health care team. A: Value the perspectives and expertise of all health care team members.	*Presimulation:* Students view a TeamSTEPPS video on teamwork and collaboration, answer targeted questions. Roles of team are assigned; primary nurse leads team huddle before simulation. *Simulation:* Communicator uses SBAR (situation, background, assessment, recommendation) when contacting MD about change in patient's condition *Postsimulation:* Debriefing: discuss effectiveness of team, how each member felt during scenario, interaction between members, use of SBAR	K: Describe examples of the impact of team functioning on safety and quality of care. S: Follow communication practices that minimize risks associated with handoffs between providers, and across transitions in care. A: Value the solutions obtained through systematic, interprofessional collaborative efforts.	*Presimulation:* Learners receive training using the TeamSTEPPS curriculum. Analyze opportunity and success vignettes to highlight communication techniques. *Simulation:* Imbed communication opportunities for learners to provide handoffs involving interprofessional team members across a transition in care point for the patient. *Postsimulation:* Debrief interprofessional team members together to allow enhanced understanding of roles and effective communication techniques.
Evidence-based practice	K: Explain the role of evidence in determining best clinical practice. S: Participate in structuring the work environment to facilitate integration of new evidence into standards of practice.	*Presimulation:* Assign specific policy or protocol used in clinical agency; have students search current nursing/medical literature to locate evidence to support policy and to	K: Analyze how the strength of available evidence influences the provision of care (assessment, diagnosis, treatment, and evaluation).	*Presimulation:* Inform learner of the content areas for the simulation and ask them to come prepared with standards and protocols for the treatment of the patient.

A: Value the need for continuous improvement in clinical practice based on new knowledge.	identify inaccuracies. Example: protocol for patient with excessive bleeding postbirth. *Simulation:* In a postpartum hemorrhage (PPH) scenario, follow agency protocol, implement standing orders. *Postsimulation:* Debriefing: discuss effectiveness of actions in stopping hemorrhage; discuss latest medications being used for PPH; revise protocol based on research evidence	S: Develop guidelines for clinical decision making regarding departure from established protocol/standards of care. A: Acknowledge own limitations in knowledge and clinical expertise before determining when to deviate from evidence-based best practices.	*Simulation:* Create controversy within the simulated case which causes the practitioner to consider departure from established protocols and standards of care. *Postsimulation:* Extend debriefing time to allow the practitioner to explain their decision making based on the evidence they brought with them and what they, along with the patient, decided was the most appropriate plan of care. Allow time to reflect on how they felt, what concerns they have, and when this type of divergence would not be appropriate.
Quality improvement	K: Recognize that nursing and other health professions students are parts of systems of care and care processes that affect outcomes for patients and families. S: Participate in a root cause analysis of a sentinel event. A: Appreciate that continuous quality improvement is an essential part of the daily work of all health professionals.	*Presimulation:* Read current journal article on root cause analysis. *Simulation:* In a capstone medical/surgical and leadership scenario, care for patient receiving blood transfusion after severe GI bleeding; patient experiences transfusion reaction; students discover wrong blood is hanging	K: Analyze the impact of context (such as access, cost, or team functioning) on improvement efforts. S: Assert leadership in shaping the dialogue about and providing leadership for the introduction of best practices.	*Presimulation:* Identify cases from the same type of systems the learner will be practicing in. *Simulation:* Create a leadership simulation based on the real cases and ask the learners to examine them in light of access, cost, or team functioning. Have student prepare a strategy for providing leadership around best practices.

(Continued)

Table 12.1 (Continued)

QSEN Competency	Prelicensure Knowledge, Skills, Attitudes (KSAs) (Cronenwett et al., 2007)	Simulation Learning Activity	Graduate Knowledge, Skills, Attitudes (Cronenwett et al., 2009)	Simulation Learning Activity
		Postsimulation: Perform root cause analysis of the error, trace through EMR to point of care where error occurred; propose action/ change in policy or procedure to prevent recurrence.	A: Appreciate that continuous quality improvement is an essential part of the daily work of all health professionals.	*Postsimulation:* Have teams of learners present their plan for change to you and other team faculty as though you are the people in the system that can bring about the change.
Safety	K: Describe the benefits and limitations of selected safety-enhancing technologies (such as barcodes, computer provider order entry, medication pumps, and automatic alerts/alarms). S: Demonstrate effective use of strategies to reduce risk of harm to self or others. A: Value the contributions of standardization/reliability to safety.	*Presimulation:* Students complete self-study module on pediatric medication administration and medication calculations (including IV therapy). *Simulation:* In pediatric scenario, students care for 1-year-old with bacterial meningitis. Errors are embedded: ID band is missing; wrong IV fluid is hanging; alarm on IV pump is on silent; parent sitting in chair at bedside, side rail halfway up. IV antibiotic to be given; student must check calculation of dosage for weight of child; dosage is too high; must call HCP, communicate using SBAR, get order changed	K: Describe human factors and other basic safety design principles as well as commonly used unsafe practices (such as workaround and dangerous abbreviations). S: Participate as a team member to design, promote, and model effective use of technology and standardized practice that support safety and quality. A: Appreciate the cognitive and physical limits of human performance.	*Presimulation:* Readings on human factors and the cognitive and physical limits of human performance *Simulation:* Embed confederates in the simulations who consistently use workarounds, inappropriate abbreviations, relying on memory, and other safety issues in the simulation. *Postsimulation:* Debrief the approaches and leadership exemplified by the advanced practice nurse in the scenario. Allow time for the confederate to talk about how the learner's approach felt and their likely response to a long-term change of habits.

Informatics			
K: Identify essential information that must be available in a common database to support patient care. S: Navigate the electronic health record. Document and plan patient care in an electronic health record. A: Value technologies that support clinical decision making, error prevention, and care coordination.	*Postsimulation:* Discuss risks to patient safety identified in scenario and actions that were taken or not taken; how to prevent similar errors in future		
K: Contrast benefits and limitation of common information technology strategies used in the delivery of care. S: Participate in the selection, design, implementation, and evaluation of information systems. A: Value the use of information and communication technologies in patient care.	*Presimulation:* Practice locating information about a patient in the electronic health record (EHR). *Simulation:* Use EHR during handoff report to students; review last vital signs, assessment findings; current MD orders; plan of care. Recorder documents using EHR during scenario. *Postsimulation:* Discuss importance of timely and thorough documentation, including ethical and legal implications.		
	Presimulation: Observe practitioners using common information technology; gather data on positive and negative effects of the technology, such as Alert Fatigue *Simulation:* Design simulation as a panel of the system's personnel making a decision on a point of care technology to bring evidenced-based information to the practitioner. Have the team come to consensus about what system to purchase, including its pros and cons. *Postsimulation:* Discuss roll out of new product, identify concerns about the implementation and its impact on patient safety.		

patient satisfaction; it contributes to safety and improved outcomes (Laird-Fick et al., 2010). It is important to include the patient and/or family in their care decisions. In an effort to do this, nursing educators need to create opportunities for learners to apply patient-centered care approaches.

The patient-centered care competency can easily be incorporated into low- or high-fidelity simulation learning activities. In a medical/surgical nursing course for prelicensure students, a simulation can be created to help students gain a better understanding of what it means to a patient to have an ostomy. Building on ostomy care content from didactic sessions and skills labs, a presimulation exercise helps students consider physical and emotional challenges associated with having an ostomy. Instructions for the students are presented in Textbox 12.1.

This exercise assists students to view an ostomy from a patient's perspective. Learning is enhanced by their reflection about the experience with a focus on patient-centered care. Students report insights about the impact of the ostomy on activities of daily living and gain an awareness of how placement of the stoma and ostomy appliance affects the fitting of clothing. They note discomforts associated with wearing the ostomy bag: the bag is hot, noisy, and bothersome, and there is constant concern about bag leakage. As a result of this exercise, students recognize that the ostomy affects all aspects of the patient's life and affects their family members. They appreciate the importance of optimizing skin care and adhesion of the ostomy bag. Students value patient input for stoma placement and recognize the importance of involving the patient in the care of the ostomy. They acknowledge and appreciate fears associated with having an ostomy and the need to provide quality patient teaching.

Following the presimulation exercise, students participate in a high-fidelity simulation activity to care for a postoperative patient with severe ulcerative colitis following abdominal surgery that resulted in the need for an ostomy. During this acute care, they are prompted to consider how to include the patient and spouse in care and discharge planning. A postsimulation exercise includes developing a discharge plan based on learning needs of the patient and family. In the debriefing, learners reflect on their performance and learning that occurred during the simulation. Providing experiences to assist the

---

Textbox 12.1   Ostomy presimulation exercise

- Students work in pairs.
- Select site for ostomy and draw a stoma.
- Cut ostomy wafer to fit "stoma" and apply ostomy bag.
- Fill ostomy bag with wet brown paper towels with a drop of citrus extract to provide some weight, color, and odor.
- Students wear bag for as long as possible (usual length of time between bag changes for patient is 72 hours).

learners to look beyond the diagnosis and skills to the needs and desires of the patient can assist them in the delivery of patient-centered care.

Patient-centered care includes sensitivity to diversity of cultural, ethnic, and social backgrounds. Educators can intentionally vary the culture and ethnicity of patients and family members in high-fidelity scenarios. For example, in a medical/surgical scenario focused on care of acutely ill elders, the patient is Mr. Gonzalez, a recently widowed 79-year-old male from Mexico with poorly controlled type I diabetes who speaks only Spanish and lives with his daughter.

Teamwork and collaboration

Definition: *Function effectively within nursing and interprofessional teams, fostering open communication, mutual respect, and shared decision making to achieve quality patient care.* (Cronenwett et al., 2007, p. 125)

Simulation provides a venue to allow various health care personnel to collaborate in a patient care scenario to deliver care within a team environment. This experience provides opportunities for learners to communicate and work with other members of the health care team, while also helping them see how their professional role interfaces with other members of the patient care team, described more fully by Disch in Chapter 5, "Teamwork and Collaboration" (2012).

High-fidelity simulation activities most often occur with small groups or teams of learners. In each simulation, learners need to understand their role prior to the start of the simulation. Assigning roles allows the learners to understand what is expected of them within the team and the role of other members of the ream. This allows the students to delegate appropriately, understand with whom to communicate and how best to collaborate. Textbox 12.2 contains an example of team roles and responsibilities in a prelicensure high-fidelity simulation learning activity.

Teamwork and collaboration can easily be incorporated into simulation learning activities using an established, nationally recognized program known as Team Strategies and Tools to Enhance Performance and Patient Safety (TeamSTEPPS). This evidence-based program is designed to improve communication and teamwork skills among health care professionals. There is a national initiative to implement this program to improve the quality and safety of patient care with improved patient outcomes. TeamSTEPPS was developed by the U.S. Department of Defense and the Agency for Healthcare Research and Quality and can be obtained free of charge at http://teamstepps.ahrq. gov/. The authors have used TeamSTEPPS in many different ways and find that it is essential to helping the learner understand the QSEN competency of teamwork and collaboration.

TeamSTEPPS defines teams broadly as either core teams (those you work with daily) or contingent teams (those who come together for a specific purpose or function such as shift work or an emergency code team). Nurses usually recognize that they function within teams, whether nursing or

> **Textbox 12.2 Assigned roles for team members in simulation scenario**
>
> *NOTE: Each team member wears a tag identifying his/her role in the scenario.*
>
> - Primary Nurse: directs the team, delegates tasks, stays at the bedside
> - Secondary Nurse: collaborates with primary nurse in problem solving and care delivery, follows direction of primary nurse, may be assigned specific tasks such as managing IV therapy, administering medications, or starting oxygen
> - Communicator: contacts health care provider, lab, blood bank, pharmacy, or other personnel as needed during scenarios; follows direction of primary nurse; communicates patient care data to primary nurse and team; communicates with patient's family/friends
> - Recorder: documents time and results of assessments, medication administration, and other procedures, calls made to health care provider
> - Observer (used in teams >5): completes scenario-specific form while quietly observing the performance of participants; contributes his/her observations during debriefing; provides thoughtful positive and constructive feedback in a professional manner

interprofessional; however, they may need to be reminded of the significant contributions of nursing assistants, patients, and families as sources of data and input about the plan of care.

Using the TeamSTEPPS model in simulation activities, learners huddle early in the simulation to plan strategies for patient care. During the simulation they apply TeamSTEPPS concepts and terminology. In the debriefing, teamwork and collaboration are discussed.

Schools of nursing and medicine faculty at a large public university collaborated to create interprofessional simulation learning experiences for their students. Nursing students enrolled in the maternal/newborn course and medical students finishing their pediatric course participated in two scenarios involving the birth of a compromised neonate. Nursing students provided care for the laboring mother (using Noelle, the birthing simulator by Gaumard) and assisted her with birth or prepared her for emergency cesarean birth. Medical students were called to assist with a precipitous birth. Once the neonate (Newborn Hal, by Gaumard) was born, medical and nursing students worked together as a team to provide immediate neonatal care and resuscitation. Faculty from both disciplines facilitated the simulations and conducted debriefing sessions where students dialogued about teamwork and collaboration as well as clinical skills and care provided to the neonate.

At the same university, an interdisciplinary course focused on teamwork, communication, and patient safety is offered to nursing, medicine, and pharmacy students. Multiple simulation experiences (simulators and standardized patients) provide opportunities for students from the three professions to work together in patient care scenarios around issues such as medical errors, root cause analysis, error disclosure, teamwork, communication, and challenges associated with power gradients across disciplines.

Evidence-based practice

Definition: Integrate best current evidence with clinical expertise and patient/ family preferences and values for delivery of optimal health care. (Cronenwett et al., 2007, p. 126)

High-fidelity simulation learning activities provide rich opportunities for learners to integrate evidence-based practice into their clinical practice, presented by Tracey and Barnsteiner in the chapter "Evidence-Based Practice" (2012). Research articles can be assigned, applied in the patient care scenario, and then discussed in debriefing.

Examination of research evidence that supports practice is ideally accomplished in presimulation or postsimulation activities. As part of presimulation activities, learners can be asked to find research evidence that supports a specific nursing care policy or protocol. For example, in a maternity scenario, learners may be asked to explore the literature for evidence to support the labor induction or augmentation protocol used in the clinical agency.

During the simulation, the learners can be asked to adopt a spirit of inquiry and make mental notes of things they want to know about or questions generated by the patient care scenario. In debriefing, they may be asked to consider whether or not procedures in the scenario were in accordance with policies, protocols, or research evidence surrounding a particular patient condition or problem. As a postsimulation assignment, learners may be asked to revise a policy, protocol, or procedure based on the latest evidence in the literature.

The authors have used simulation to train long-term care nurses about the latest evidence-based care for elders. The simulators are transported to long-term care facilities where staff in their core teams participate in simulation activities.

Evidence-based practice is key to advanced practice nursing scenarios. For example, nurse practitioner students consider current research evidence as they diagnose and prescribe treatment for a patient with chronic heart failure.

Quality improvement

Definition: Use data to monitor the outcomes of care processes and use improvement methods to design and test changes to continuously improve the quality and safety of health care systems. (Cronenwett et al., 2007, p. 127)

Quality improvement is a challenging competency to incorporate into high-fidelity simulation scenarios that include the knowledge, skills, and attitudes as described by Johnson (2012). Educators may employ out-of-the-box thinking to help students identify aspects of a scenario to search for quality measures and then design an improvement strategy.

Error identification and recovery can be accomplished through high-fidelity simulation scenarios (Henneman et al., 2010). A simulation can be created with embedded errors. The setup of the environment and the manikin allow for incorporating a variety of errors. For example, errors can be as simple as a missing identification or allergy band, an incorrect setting on the IV pump, or the wrong IV fluid infusing. More critical errors can be imbedded in the scenario, such as a transfusion reaction resulting from an incompatible blood transfusion or a severe allergic reaction to a medication. During the course of a high-fidelity scenario, learners can be expected to identify, interrupt, and correct medical errors (Henneman et al., 2010).

During the debriefing session, error identification and recovery are discussed in detail. It is important to assist the learner to recognize the interconnectedness of quality improvement and safety. Consequences of errors and the impact on patient safety are identified. Learners can compare their actions to standards of practice and agency policies/protocols. Recommendations can be made to prevent the errors from occurring in the actual patient care setting. Root cause analysis can be employed to examine an error. Just culture principles can be applied to a discussion of the implications for health care professionals who commit medical errors (Marx, 2001).

As part of an interprofessional course focusing on teamwork, communication, and patient safety, students participate in a scenario in which they discover an overdose of anticoagulant. The medicine, nursing, and pharmacy students must work together to stabilize the patient. The error is documented using the hospital's policies and protocols, and students work with risk management officers to disclose the error to a standardized patient who assumes the role of the patient's family member. Students are equipped to disclose the error through course materials and Harvard School of Medicine's (2006) document *When Things Go Wrong*. Each student receives written feedback from the standardized patient about their communication and skills during the error disclosure. Next, the students participate in a root cause analysis of the event to examine the error through the lens of each profession, discussing the individual and system factors that contributed to the error. These multiple simulated experiences allow the learners to experience the sequence of events following an error from discovery through root cause analysis as they apply the quality improvement QSEN competency and embed other competencies.

Safety

Definition: Minimizes risk of harm to patients and providers through both system effectiveness and individual performance. (Cronenwett et al., 2007, p. 128)

Patient safety is a clear priority for nurses (Barnsteiner, 2012). Safety principles are inherent to all high-fidelity simulation learning activities. Learners are expected to adhere to practices that support safe patient care. Anecdotal evidence suggests that students who are involved in high-fidelity simulation learning activities have an enhanced awareness of patient safety issues in clinical settings (Henneman et al., 2007).

Medication errors are a major source of morbidity and mortality as reported by the IOM in *To Err Is Human* (Kohn et al., 2000). The importance of reducing medication errors was further delineated in the IOM's report *Preventing Medication Errors* (Aspden, Wolcott, Bootman, & Cronenwett, 2007). High-fidelity simulation is an excellent medium for providing novice and experienced practitioners with learning opportunities focused on improving safety in medication administration. Factors associated with common errors include medications that have similar names or are packaged similarly, medications that are rarely used or prescribed, medications that are used often but have a high incidence of patient allergy, and medications that require monitoring therapeutic blood levels. In addition, high-alert medications and those with black box warnings have increased propensity for adverse patient outcomes (Hughes & Blegen, 2008). Nurses across all settings are involved in medication administration. Similarly, high-fidelity simulation scenarios focusing on any area of patient care or nursing specialty can easily incorporate principles of safe medication administration. The six rights of medication administration are imbedded in learning objectives, and learners are expected to strictly follow guidelines in providing medications to their patients. Intentional use of high-alert medications (e.g., insulin, heparin, opiates) can raise awareness of safety concerns. A person assigned as the "resource nurse" in scenarios can utilize a drug reference text or online resource to access information related to medications used in scenarios; during the scenario and in debriefing, the resource nurse provides information to the team about the medications.

Safety related to communication with team members can be easily integrated into simulation scenarios. TeamSTEPPS provides communication strategies that equip students with techniques needed to more effectively address power gradients within patient care settings. For example, when a learner calls the health care provider to report a worrisome change in the patient's condition, the learner is expected to use the C-U-S words to communicate the seriousness of the patient's condition ("I am **C**oncerned that ...", "I am **U**ncomfortable with...", "This is a patient **S**afety issue"; King, Toomey, Salisbury, Webster, & Almeida, 2006). These words empower nurses to express their concerns in a manner that are more likely heard. If the provider dismisses the information, the learner is instructed to use the "two-challenge rule" where they restate the concern (King, Tomey, Salisbury, Webster, & Almeida, 2006). If the provider does not respond to the patient care situation, then the nurse is instructed to go to the next level of command. These communication techniques may seem simple but have a powerful impact on the nurse's ability to be a voice for patient safety.

To help promote safe patient care practices, simulation can be used to allow prelicensure students to rehearse patient care prior to beginning clinical. In a maternal/newborn nursing course, prior to the first day of clinical, students rotate through high-fidelity simulation learning activities to help prepare them for learning experiences in intrapartum, postpartum, and neonatal settings. Students in a nursing fundamentals course complete a basic assessment that incorporates patient communication as an opportunity to "practice" how to interact with their first patient when they enter clinical.

Informatics

Definition: Use information and technology to communicate, manage knowledge, mitigate error, and support decision making. (Cronenwett et al., 2007, p. 129)

Shulman (2010) adeptly describes the significance of informatics in nursing: "One need only spend a few hours with nurses on a hospital floor or in a cancer treatment room, in an individual office or even during a home visit, before being struck by the varieties of technology with which the nurse must competently cope.... And computers are ubiquitous for record keeping, communication, and the monitoring of drugs. All these now fall within the nurse's responsibilities, and he or she is expected to understand what and how to perform in those circumstances" (p. x). The expectations for all health care providers to competently use and adapt to various technologies continues to expand (Warren, 2012). Education has lagged behind in integrating these technologies into their programs due to prohibitive costs, ever-changing models, and lack of preparation. Thus, graduates may lack experience and skill in using informatics as they transition to practice in health care agencies.

Several vendors have developed electronic health records (EHRs) specifically for nursing education. Unfortunately, the costs are prohibitive for many schools. As an alternative, educators may consider purchasing preprogrammed scenarios that include electronic health records. Educators can also develop their own EHRs for use in simulation scenarios; they may select certain components of the EHR with the greatest impact on the scenario and develop electronic forms similar to those used in clinical agencies. Patient data is created and included in the fabricated EHR.

Each simulation should incorporate informatics as appropriate and feasible. Learners should be able to access patient data in an electronic format. In presimulation activities, participants might be assigned a list of data to collect from the electronic health record so that they are aware of the patient's medical history. When possible, point of care information and alerts should be provided to assist learners in the care of the patient in the scenario. Medications can be accessed through an electronic drug dispensing machine. Labs and other reports should be accessed through EHR. Learners should document in the EHR.

In debriefing, informatics issues should be an area for discussion. For example, following a simulation in which a medical error occurs in heparin administration, discussion includes labeling of the heparin vials and placement within the electronic drug dispensing machine as creating potential for errors.

Conclusion

High-fidelity simulation is an effective immersive, learner-centered, experiential instructional strategy that provides learners with opportunities to increase their knowledge, skills, and attitudes related to the quality and safety of patient care. Because the foundations of nursing practice are the same concepts embodied in the QSEN competencies, it is not surprising that many of the KSAs are already imbedded in existing preprogrammed and original nursing scenarios. Educators can map those scenarios using the QSEN competencies and their KSAs. Moving forward, educators can deliberately design quality high-fidelity simulation cases to integrate QSEN competencies. The 2010 Carnegie report states that to do anything less has "grave implications for the extent to which students will develop skills of clinical inquiry and the ability to use knowledge in specific clinical situations" (Benner et al., 2010, p. 65).

References

Ackerman, S. D., Kenny, G., & Walker, C. (2007). Simulator programs for new nurses' orientation: A retention strategy. *Journal for Nurses in Staff Development, 23*(3), 136–139.

Alfes, C. M. (2010). Developing a QSEN competency checklist for simulation experiences. Retrieved from http://www.qsen.org/teachingstrategy.php?id=128

Arocha, O., & Moore, D. Y. (2011). The new Joint Commission standards for patient-centered communication. Retrieved from http://www.languageline.com/main/files/wp_joint_commission_012411.pdf

Aspden, P., Wolcott, J. A., Bootman, J. L., Cronenwett, L. R. (Eds.). (2007). *Preventing medication errors*. Institute of Medicine. Washington, DC: National Academies Press.

Barnsteiner, J. (2012). Safety. In G. Sherwood & J. Barnsteiner (Eds.), *Quality and safety in nursing: A competency approach to improving outcomes*. Hoboken, NJ: Wiley-Blackwell.

Benner, P. (1984). *From novice to expert: Excellence and power in clinical nursing practice*. Menlo Park, CA: Addison Wesley.

Benner, P., Sutphen, M., Leonard, V., & Day, L. (2010). *Educating nurses: A call for radical transformation*. San Francisco: Jossey-Bass.

Berwick, D. M. (2009). What 'patient-centered' should mean: Confessions of an extremist. *Health Affairs 28*(4), w555–w565.

Beyea, S. C., von Reyn, L. K., & Slattery, M. J. (2007). A nurse residency program for competency development using human patient simulation. *Journal for Nurses in Staff Development, 23*(2), 77.

Bremner, M. N., Aduddell, K., Bennett, D. N., & VanGeest, J. B. (2006). The use of human patient simulators: Best practices with novice nursing students. *Nurse Educator, 31*(4), 170–174.

Cronenwett, L., Sherwood, G., Barnsteiner, J., Disch, J., Johnson, J., Mitchell, P., et al. (2007). Quality and safety education for nurses. *Nursing Outlook, 55* (3), 122–131.

Cronenwett, L., Sherwood, G., Pohl, J., Barnsteiner, J., Moore S., Sullivan, D. T., et al. (2009). Quality and safety education for advanced nursing practice. *Nursing Outlook, 57*(6), 338–348.

Disch, J. (2012). Teamwork and collaboration. In G. Sherwood & J. Barnsteiner (Eds.), *Quality and safety in nursing: A competency approach to improving outcomes*. Hoboken, NJ: Wiley-Blackwell.

Durham, C. F., & Alden, K. R. (2008). Enhancing patient safety in nursing education through patient simulation. In R. G. Hughes (Ed.), *Patient safety and quality: An evidence-based handbook for nurses*. Rockville, MD: Agency for Healthcare Research and Quality.

Durham, C. F., & Alden, K. R. (2010). The nuts and bolts of simulation. In L. Caputi (Ed.), *Teaching nursing: The art and science* (2nd ed.). Glen Ellyn, IL: College of DuPage Press.

Gaba, D. M. (2004). The future vision of simulation in health care. *Quality and Safety in Health Care*, *13*(Suppl. 1), i2–i10.

Harvard School of Medicine. (2006). *When things go wrong: Responding to adverse events*. Retrieved from http://www.macoalition.org/documents/responding ToAdverseEvents.pdf

Henneman, E. A., & Cunningham, H. (2005). Using clinical simulation to teach patient safety in an acute/critical care nursing course. *Nurse Educator*, *30*(4), 172–177.

Henneman, E. A., Cunningham, H., Roche, J. P., & Curnin, M. E. (2007). Human patient simulation: Teaching students to provide safe care. *Nurse Educator*, *32*(5), 212–217.

Henneman, E. A., Roche, J. P., Fisher, D. L., Cunningham, H., Reilly, C. A., Nathanson, B. H., & Henneman, P. L. (2010). Error identification and recovery by student nurses using human patient simulation: Opportunity to improve patient safety. *Applied Nursing Research*, *23*(1), 11–21.

Henrichs, B., Rule, A., Grady, M., & Ellis, W. (2002). Nurse anesthesia students' perceptions of the anesthesia patient simulator: A qualitative study. *American Association of Nurse Anesthetists Journal, 70*(3), 219.

Hravnak, M., Tuite, P., & Baldisseri, M. (2005). Expanding acute care nurse practitioner and clinical nurse specialist education. *AACN Clinical Issues, 16*(1), 89–104.

Hughes, R. G., & Blegen, M. A. (2008). Medication safety. In R. G. Hughes (Ed.), *Patient safety and quality: An evidence-based handbook for nurses*. Rockville, MD: Agency for Healthcare Research and Quality.

Ironside, P. M., Jeffries, P. R., & Martin, A. (2009). Fostering patient safety competencies using multiple-patient simulation experiences. *Nursing Outlook, 57*(6), 332–337.

Jarzemsky, P. (2009). A template for simulation scenario development that incorporates QSEN competencies. Retrieved from http://www.qsen.org/teaching strategy.php?id=70

Jarzemsky, P., McCarthy, J., & Ellis, N. (2010). Incorporating quality and safety education for nurses competencies in simulation scenario design. *Nurse Educator*, *35*(2), 90–92.

Johnson, J. (2012). Quality improvement. In G. Sherwood & J. Barnsteiner (Eds.), *Quality and safety in nursing: A competency approach to improving outcomes*. Hoboken, NJ: Wiley-Blackwell.

Kaddoura, M. A. (2010). New graduate nurses' perceptions of the effects of clinical simulation on their critical thinking, learning, and confidence. *The Journal of Continuing Education in Nursing*, *41*(11), 506–516.

King, H. B., Toomey, L. Salisbury, M., Webster, J., & Almeida, S. (2006). TeamSTEPPS® [Team Strategies and Tools to Enhance Performance and Patient Safety], developed by the Department of Defense (DoD) in collaboration with the Agency for Healthcare Research and Quality (AHRQ).

Kohn, L. T., Corrigan, J. M., & Donaldson, M. S. (Eds.). (2000). *To err is human: Building a safer health system*. A report of the Committee on Quality of Health care in America, Institute of Medicine. Washington, DC: National Academies Press.

Laird-Fick, H. S., Solomon, D., Jodoin, C., Dwamena, F. C., Alexander, K., Rawsthorne, L., et al. (2010). Training residents and nurses to work as a patient-centered care team on a medical ward. *Patient Education and Counseling*, June 14.

Larew, C., Lessans, S., Spunt, D., Foster, D., & Covington, B. (2006). Application of Benner's theory in an interactive patient care simulation. *Nursing Education Perspectives, 27*(1), 16-21.

Leigh, G. (2008). Human patient simulation and nursing students' self-efficacy: A review of the literature. *International Journal of Nursing Education Scholarship, 5*(1), 1-16. doi:10.2202/1548-923X.1613.

Marx, D. (2001). Patient safety and the "just culture": A primer for health care executives. Retrieved from http://www.mers-tm.org/support/Marx_Primer.pdf

Miller, K. K., Riley, W., Davis, S., & Hansen, H. E. (2008). In situ simulation: A method of experiential learning to promote safety and team behavior. *Journal of Perinatal and Neonatal Nursing, 22*(2), 105-113.

Nagle, B. M., McHale, J. M., Alexander, G.A., & French, B. M. (2009). Incorporating scenario-based simulation into a hospital nursing education program. *Journal of Continuing Education in Nursing, 40*(1), 18-25.

Nehring, W. M., & Lashley, F. R. (2004). Current use and opinions regarding human patient simulators in nursing education: An international survey. *Nursing Education Perspectives, 25*(5), 244-248.

Paparella, S. F., Mariani, B. A., Layton, K., & Carpenter, A. M. (2004). *Journal for Nurses in Staff Development, 20*(6), 247-252.

Scherer, Y. K., Bruce, S. A., Graves, B. T., & Erdley, W. S. (2003). Acute care nurse practitioner education. *AACN Clinical Issues, 14*(3), 331-341.

Shepherd, I. A., Kelly, C. M., Skene, F. M., & White, K. T. (2007). Enhancing graduate nurses' health assessment knowledge and skills using low-fidelity adult human simulation. *Simulation in Healthcare, 2*(1), 16-24.

Shulman, L. S. (2010). Foreword. In P. Benner, M. Sutphen, V. Leonard, & L. Day (Eds.), *Educating nurses: A call for radical transformation*. San Francisco: Jossey-Bass.

Smith, J. R., & Cole, F. S. (2009). Patient safety: Effective interdisciplinary teamwork through simulation and debriefing in the neonatal ICU. *Critical Care Clinics of North America, 21*, 163-179.

Strouse, A.C. (2010). Multidisciplinary simulation centers: Promoting safe practice. *Clinical Simulation in Nursing*, 6(4), e139-e142. doi: 10.1016/j.ecns.2009.08.007.

Tracey, M. F., & Barnsteiner, J. (2012). Evidence-based practice. In G. Sherwood & J. Barnsteiner (Eds.), *Quality and safety in nursing: A competency approach to improving outcomes*. Hoboken, NJ: Wiley-Blackwell.

Walton, M. K., & Barnsteiner, J. (2012). Patient-centered care. In G. Sherwood & J. Barnsteiner (Eds.), *Quality and safety in nursing: A competency approach to improving outcomes*. Hoboken, NJ: Wiley-Blackwell.

Warren, J. (2012). Informatics. In G. Sherwood & J. Barnsteiner (Eds.), *Quality and safety in nursing: A competency approach to improving outcomes*. Hoboken, NJ: Wiley-Blackwell.

Wilhaus, J. (2010). Interdepartmental simulation collaboration in academia: Exploring partnerships with other disciplines. *Clinical Simulation in Nursing, 6*(6), e231-e232. doi:10.1016/j.ecns.2010.02.011.

Resources

Agency for Healthcare Research and Quality (AHRQ)
This website has a wealth of information and resources, including information on evidence-based practice, relevant research, patient teaching information, and consumer information around quality and safety. http://www.ahrq.gov/

Geriatric Clinical Simulation at the University of North Carolina–Chapel Hill
The purpose of the Center for Geriatric Clinical Simulation is to disseminate innovative, evidence-based clinical simulations involving older adults, focusing on the educational needs of registered nurses, licensed practical nurses, and certified nursing assistants. Simulations cover scenarios ranging from acute exacerbations of chronic conditions to sentinel events, such as falls. Select clinical simulations incorporate interdisciplinary content that facilitates communication between nurses and physicians. http://geroclinsim.org/

Institute for Healthcare Improvement (IHI)
The IHI is a not-for-profit organization leading the improvement of health care throughout the world. IHI website has information about programs, links to patient safety information. http://www.ihi.org/IHI/

Institute of Medicine (IOM)
The IOM is a nonprofit organization that provides science-based information about health and science policy. http://www.iom.edu/
Institute of Medicine Health Care Quality Initiative:
  - *To Err is Human: Building A Safer Health System* (1999)
  - *Crossing the Quality Chasm: A New Health System for the 21st Century* (2001)
  - *Health Professions Education: A Bridge to Quality* (2003)
  - *Keeping Patients Safe: Transforming the Work Environment of Nurses* (2004)
  - *Preventing Medication Errors* (2006)

Institute for Safe Medication Practices (ISMP)
The ISMP is a nonprofit organization that educates healthcare providers and the public about safe medication practices. It has a plethora of resources for safe medication practices. http://www.ismp.org/

The Joint Commission
Accrediting body for many health care organizations, concerned with improving the safety and quality of patient care. http://www.jointcommission.org/

National Patient Safety Foundation (NPSF)
The NPSF is a not-for-profit organization whose mission is to improve the safety of patients. http://www.npsf.org/

Partnering to Heal: Teaming-Up Against Healthcare-Associated Infections
A Virtual Experience Interactive Learning Simulation (VEILS®) with five different roles to allow interactive simulation, with the goal of infection prevention. http://www.hhs.ogove/ash/initiatives/hai/training

Quality and Safety Education for Nurses (QSEN)
The quality and safety competencies are: patient-centered care, teamwork and collaboration, evidenced-based practice, quality improvement, safety, and informatics. Knowledge, skills, and attitudes for prelicensure education are outlined to clarify each competency. This site is a valuable resource because it also offers free downloadable teaching strategies and annotated bibliographies for each of the QSEN competencies. http://qsen.org/

Robert Wood Johnson Foundation Initiative on the Future of Nursing, at the Institute of Medicine. *The Future of Nursing: Leading Change, Advancing Health* (2010). http://www.iom.edu/Reports/2010/The-Future-of-Nursing-Leading-Change-Advancing-Health.aspx

Simulation Innovation Resource Center (SIRC) National League for Nursing
The SIRC is an online e-learning site for nursing educators to learn about simulation and ways to integrate it into their curriculum. It provides various ways for educators to engage with experts and peers. http://sirc.nln.org/

TeamSTEPPS® **(Team Strategies and Tools to Enhance Performance and Patient Safety)** Teamwork and communication curriculum developed by the Department of Defense in collaboration with AHRQ. http://teamstepps.ahrq.gov/

Chapter 13

Interprofessional Approaches to Quality and Safety Education

Shirley M. Moore, PhD, RN, FAAN
Mary A. Dolansky, PhD, RN
Mamta K. Singh, MD, MS

The endpoint of quality and safety education is the ability of health professionals to perform their roles in the provision and improvement of care. It has been well documented that to improve the quality of care, health professionals must work collaboratively—and learning to work collaboratively is facilitated by the use of interprofessional education (IPE) approaches. In this chapter we define interprofessional education as "occasions when two or more professions learn with, from and about each other to improve collaboration and the quality of care" (CAIPE, 1997). This chapter addresses the most recent evidence regarding IPE in quality and safety. It includes exemplar programs that are achieving IPE and provides information on examples of effective pedagogies for planning, implementing, and evaluating learning experiences across disciplines. We address questions such as: *What is the added value of IPE to the learning process? What does it mean to learn with, from, and about another discipline? What are the best-practice considerations to take into account when designing IPE strategies for quality and safety?*

The added value of interprofessional education to the quality and safety learning process

One way to think about the added value of IPE for learning health care quality and safety is to consider the outcomes desired. Thistlethwaite and Moran (2010), on behalf on the World Health Organization (WHO) Study Group on

Quality and Safety in Nursing: A Competency Approach to Improving Outcomes,
First Edition. Edited by Gwen Sherwood and Jane Barnsteiner.
© 2012 John Wiley & Sons, Inc. Published 2012 by John Wiley & Sons, Inc.

Interprofessional Education and Collaborative Practice, conducted a review of the literature on learning outcomes associated with IPE and identified six broad themes: teamwork; roles and responsibilities; communication; learning and reflection; the patient/client (patient-centered care, quality and safety, coordination of care); and ethics and attitudes. Interestingly, these outcomes are consistent with those needed to prepare students for collaborative, patent-centered practice and the improvement of care.

If students are to learn and practice the knowledge and skills associated with quality and safety, they must also learn how to work together. In Cochrane reviews of the literature, IPE was shown to promote interprofessional collaboration (Zwarenstein, Goldman, & Reeves, 2009; Zwarenstein et al., 2001). To consider the added value of IPE to quality and safety education, educators should start by identifying those outcomes that may *only* be achieved through IPE (in either a formal education process or through interprofessional practice in the workplace). In other words, how does the inclusion of other professions enhance learning opportunities because the interactions enhance the chances of achieving outcomes of increased communication skills, teamwork, and collaborative practice? Other learning outcomes include understanding the scopes of practice of other professionals, role negotiation, priority setting, conflict management, and understanding, cooperating, and valuing the contributions of other disciplines.

In addition to interprofessional collaboration, the positive effects of IPE on other professional practice and health care outcomes was shown in a recent literature review (Reeves et al., 2008) in which positive outcomes were found on emergency department culture and patient satisfaction; clinical team behavior and reduction of clinical error rates for emergency department teams; management of care delivered to domestic violence victims; and mental health practitioner competencies related to the delivery of patient care. In their review of these randomized trials of IPE, however, the authors caution that it is not possible to draw generalizable inferences about the key elements of IPE and its effectiveness and call for more rigorous IPE studies to provide better evidence of the impact of IPE on professional practice and health care outcomes.

Learning with, from, and about each other

What does it mean to learn with, from, and about each other? A major goal of IPE is to increase positive attitudes between individuals of different disciplines. Conditions to support this are equal status among participants, positive expectations, a cooperative environment, successful joint work, and a perception that members of the other group are typical (Oandasan & Reeves, 2005a). Specific strategies can be built into education programs to enhance learning with, from, and about. An important strategy is the creation of a nonthreatening learning environment in which learners feel psychologically safe to express themselves freely. This includes the provision of safe places for discussing and dealing with issues of power in education and practice settings. Another approach to promote learning with, from, and about is planning space and time for reflection. Learners need to be able to reflect on their role in a team of equals. Both self- and group reflections are most useful if learners have been exposed to issues that they must grapple with, such as issues related to hierarchy, respect, communication, role delineation, and decision making in groups. These reflections are best when based on subject matter that relates to learners' immediate interests and concerns. Giving learners the opportunity to have input into the teaching design can facilitate this relevance for them. Lastly, learning with, from, and about is facilitated by educators modeling distributive leadership instead of top-down hierarchical models of leadership. Educators need to model and facilitate collaboration and relationship building while reducing professional territoriality and defensive behaviors.

Organizing frameworks for IPE in quality and safety education

In IPE, educators have two purposes—achieving the goals of a particular content area of education, such as quality and safety, as well as achieving the goals associated with learning to collaborate across different disciplines. Either of these two content areas can be the "foreground" or the "background" in a particular learning initiative. When teaching quality and safety in an interprofessional education format, educators can consciously shift quality and safety content and interprofessional collaboration content from the background or implicit learning to the foreground or a more explicit curriculum. The models and competencies described below address IPE for quality and safety and have as their goal to promote competency in the skills of quality and safety improvement and working together in health care teams.

Models of IPE

Several models of IPE have been applied to quality and safety education. Common elements of these models are role clarification, communication, team training (including group process and conflict management skills), and leadership training.

WHO Framework for Action on Interprofessional Education and Collaborative Practice model

A predominant model is the WHO Framework for Action on Interprofessional Education and Collaborative Practice (WHO, 2010). This model calls for the collaboration of local health systems and educational systems to promote processes for shared decision making and governance that support collaboration for the improvement of health.

Canadian Interprofessional Health Collaborative Competency Framework

Another model that guides IPE is the Canadian Interprofessional Health Collaborative Competency Framework, which focuses on role clarification, team functioning, interprofessional conflict resolution, and collaborative leadership to promote interprofessional collaboration (Canadian Interprofessional Health Collaborative, 2010). The model also describes the influence of quality improvement and contextual environmental factors on IPE. The website of the Canadian Interprofessional Health Collaborative contains a particularly rich set of teaching and evaluation strategies and tools for IPE and can be accessed at www.cihc.ca.

The 3P model

The 3P systems model of learning and teaching (Biggs, 1993) has been adapted to address IPE by Freeth and Reeves (2004). This model describes the factors associated with learning to work together (collaborative practice) that are organized in three categories: **P**resage, **P**rocess, and **P**roduct. *Presage* factors make up the context in which a learning experience is conducted and includes the teaching and learning context (e.g., political climate, funding, geography and demography, space and time constraints, competing curricula), teacher characteristics (teacher's expertise, preconceptions of working together, pre-conceptions of learners, enthusiasm), and learner characteristics (prior knowledge and skills, conceptions of collaboration, competing learning needs). *Process* factors consist of the approaches to learning and teaching, such as uniprofessional, multiprofessional, or interprofessional; formal and informal learning; classroom or work-based learning; distance learning; and compulsory or optional experience. *Product* factors consist of both the intended and unintended outcomes of IPE and address collaborative competencies (knowledge, skills, and attitudes) and collaborative working (practice, impact on client care). The 3P model can be particularly helpful to an educators group engaged in planning, conducting, and evaluating IPE in that it illuminates the many interacting factors to be considered in making informed and timely decisions regarding IPE.

TeamSTEPPS

A fourth IPE model that focuses on health care team training for safety and quality improvement is Team STEPPS. Team STEPPS (Strategic Tools to Enhance Performance and Patient Safety) is an evidence-based framework to improve communication and teamwork skills among health care professionals (King et al., 2008). At the core of the framework are four teachable-learnable skills:

- *Leadership* (ability to coordinate the activities of team members by ensuring team actions are understood, changes in information are shared, and that team members have the necessary resources)

- *Situation monitoring* (process of actively scanning and assessing situational elements to gain information, understanding, or maintain awareness to support functioning of the team)
- *Mutual support* (ability to anticipate and support other team members' needs through accurate knowledge about their responsibilities and workload)
- *Communication* (Interaction between the outcomes and skills is the basis of a team striving to deliver safe, quality care.)

Developed by the Department of Defense Patient Safety program in collaboration with the Agency for Healthcare Research and Quality, Team STEPPS provides a source for ready-to-use materials and training curriculum to successfully integrate teamwork principles into all areas of the health care system. Materials are free of charge and can be obtained at http://teamstepps. ahrq.gov. The TeamSTEPPS program consists of a pretraining assessment for site readiness, training tools and modules, an implementation and sustainability plan, and psychometrically validated instruments to measure outcomes. Research testing the effect of the TeamSTEPPS program has demonstrated a relationship to improvement in teamwork skills and outcomes in both operating room (Weaver, Rosen, Salas, Baum, & King, 2010) and trauma teams (Capella et al., 2010).

Core competencies

Interprofessional Education Collaborative competencies

Core competencies also provide organizing frameworks for IPE. Recently, core competencies for interprofessional practice were developed by the Interprofessional Education Collaborative (sponsored jointly by the American Association of Colleges of Nursing, the American Association of Colleges of Osteopathic Medicine, the American Association of Pharmacy, the American Dental Association, the Association of American Medical Colleges, and the Association of Schools of Public Health; Interprofessional Education Collaborative Expert Panel, 2011). These competencies were designed to support the achievement of interprofessional collaborative practice of health professionals toward a vision of safe, high-quality, accessible, patient-centered care. The competencies build on each discipline's expected disciplinary competencies by adding the ability to work effectively as members of clinical teams. The competencies are structured in four interprofessional practice domains: (1) values/ethics for interprofessional practice, (2) roles/responsibilities, (3) interprofessional communications, and (4) teams and teamwork. These competencies represent the most comprehensive set of interprofessional collaboration competences to date and have been distributed to be used and assessed for their usefulness to guide IPE initiatives (Interprofessional Education Collaborative, 2011).

QSEN competencies

Core competencies in quality and safety education for nurses have been defined for undergraduate and graduate nursing students by the Quality and Safety Education for Nurses (QSEN) initiative (Cronenwett et al., 2007; Cronenwett et al., 2009). Described elsewhere in detail in this book, these competencies are displayed in Appendixes A and B and can be accessed at the QSEN website: www.qsen.org. The competencies address six domains related to quality and safety education: patient-centered care, teamwork and collaboration, evidence-based practice, quality improvement, safety, and informatics. Numerous learning strategies related to each domain are provided by learner level, learning setting, and strategy type (classroom, case study, simulation, etc.). Annotated bibliographies, video presentations, and learning modules are also available at this website. The QSEN website is the largest repository of teaching strategies and resources related to quality and safety in nursing; educators are invited to post successful strategies to share with others.

Design of IPE strategies

Key elements of IPE are described in a systematic review of the pedagogical approaches to successful IPE conducted for Health Canada (Oandasan & Reeves, 2005a, 2005b). Textbox 13.1 describes key elements in planning interprofessional learning experiences. In a recent review of team training, Weaver, Lyons, and colleagues (2010) found that team training is being implemented across a wide spectrum of providers and is primarily targeting communication, situational awareness, leadership, and role clarity. Most team training interventions are consistent with best practices from the science of training, adult learning, and human performance. Moreover, a set of core features has been identified that contributes to successful interprofessional learning: cooperative learning, reflective learning, experiential learning, and the promotion of transfer of learning. Each of these core features is expanded upon below.

Cooperative learning

D'Eon (2005) describes five elements of best-practice cooperative learning: (1) positive interdependence, (2) face-to-face promotive interactions, (3) individual accountability, (4) interpersonal and small group skills, and (5) group processing. Textbox 13.2 provides a description of each of these factors. Cooperative learning is best accomplished using experiential learning. One effective way of promoting cooperative learning with experiential learning is to use a series of case studies of increasing complexity. The cooperative learning model matches the teamwork model needed to give and improve care in practice settings. Acknowledgement of the interdependence among health professionals is key to collaborative work. Weaver, Rosen, and colleagues (2010) describe adaptive interdependent performance as consisting of closed-

---

Textbox 13.1   Key factors in planning interprofessional learning experiences

What is driving the development of this program?

What are the opportunities and threats in the current learning environment?

What disciplines will (should) be involved?

What size group?

Where will learning take place?

Are there explicit learning objectives (content and process)?

What content will be included (emphasized)?

What instructional methods will be used (information based, practice based, simulation based)?

How will cooperative learning be built into the program?

How will learner and educator reflections be built into the program?

How will experiences to promote transfer of the skills learned be included?

Who is delivering the educational programming?

How will performance feedback be accomplished?

How will evaluation of training experiences be done?

What is the impact of the training?

    Adapted from Oandasan & Reeves, 2005a, 2005b.

Textbox 13.2   Features of cooperative learning

Positive interdependence means being interconnected. It consists of having roles that complement each other and working together toward shared goals.

Promotive interactions consist of close, purposeful activity, such as discussion, debate, case studies, or patient care that involves joint decision making and where members help each other to succeed.

Individual accountability means each person is held accountable for learning the content and contributing fair share to the group success.

Interpersonal and small group skills refers to team skills, usually involving communication, leadership, group decision making, situation awareness, and management of conflict.

Group processing skills refers to reflecting on the actions of individuals and groups that contribute to the effectiveness of the group process and deciding what to do about it.

 Adapted from D'Eon, 2005.

---

loop communications, shared mental models, and attitudes of trust and belief in collective efficacy.

Small group learning formats have been especially successful to promote cooperative learning. In designing group learning, educators need to consider group balance (an evenly distributed mix of health professionals if possible), group size (8–10 members is desirable), and group stability (extent to which there are established members leaving and new ones joining).

Additionally, problem-based learning and team learning have been found to be effective approaches to making the learning process more meaningful and engaging, while returning the responsibility for learning back to the learners. In problem-based learning, learning occurs in response to learning deficits identified through small-group problem solving (Michaelsen et al., 1984). In team learning, groups of six or seven learners initially progress by preparing for and taking readiness assessment tests and then by building on that foundation through in-class, group application activities. D'Eon (2005) advocates the use of progressively more complex and relevant cases over time in which cooperative groups move from simple classroom-based cases, to simulation cases, to cases in real-life settings.

Reflection

There is wide agreement on the importance of building and promoting mechanisms for reflective learning into IPE. Such skills can be applied to reflective practice (and are inherent in quality and safety processes; Sherwood, 2012). Reflective activities are those activities that assist the learner to "stand back from an experience and make meaning of it." The transformative learning that can result from IPE occurs from the metacognitive insights gained from reflective processes. Specific methods to promote reflection include self-assessments, structured journaling, and written papers based on the journals (Clark, 2009). Self-assessments provide self-knowledge and insights for participants about what they bring to an IPE experience. These self-assessments, in addition to determining strengths and needs regarding a particular content area such as quality and safety, also may assess an individual's skills related to group process, such as learning style preferences, personality type, conflict management style, or leadership abilities. Reflective activities provide opportunities in IPE for learners to engage in reflection of self as well as reflection of how others are the same or different from themselves. Reflective activities, however, must be planned; both space and time for reflection are needed. Specific strategies and tools to promote both individual and group reflection are described on the QSEN website. Last, educators need to "reflect more on reflection" if they are to be effective in ensuring the learning outcomes essential for teamwork and interprofessional practice, including incorporating both theory and practice into the development of interprofessional educational interventions.

Experiential learning

Experiential learning is especially important in IPE. Experiential learning is based on the tenet of learning through action in the real world. John Dewey introduced the "learn by doing" philosophy (Dewey, 1938). He believed that problem solving calls for new responses, especially in situations involving conflict or challenge. Habitual actions and thoughts do not solve these problems, but active experimentation and trying out new processes might. David Kolb introduced the Kolb Experiential Learning Cycle (Kolb, 1984), which is the foundation for current methods of experiential learning. The process of making sense out of experience, learning on a deeper, more integrated level, is articulated in the experiential learning model. Schon described a learning-in-action approach as a way for professionals to reflect on how their practice experiences contribute to professional knowledge acquisition and application (Schon, 1987). Through this structured reflection process, practitioners gain insights that challenge and guide professional practice. Schon later added the reflection-in-action and the reflection-on-action components as important to experiential learning.

In IPE, experiential learning is when learners from two or more health professions schools are given a real-life situation in which they form a plan, implement the plan (with varying levels of supervision), gather observations of the outcomes, and reflect in such a way as to create generalizations about how they would handle similar situations in the future. A positive byproduct of the use of practice-based projects in quality and safety education is the increased attention paid to and recognition of the practitioners in the field. Textbox 13.3 describes a recent IPE project that includes increasing levels of experiential learning over time.

Transfer of learning

Learning activities must prepare participants for the real world in which they will work. Learners must be able to transfer what they have learned in one or more situations to other situations that are not exactly the same. One approach to foster transfer of learning is to expose learners to relevant cases

---

Textbox 13.3   The Interprofessional Learning Exchange and Development (I•LEAD) curriculum and center at Case Western Reserve University

In 2010, The Case Western Reserve University Schools of Medicine and Nursing received a four-year grant from the Josiah Macy, Jr. Foundation to launch the I•LEAD Curriculum and Center. Instead of the traditional episodic interprofessional curriculum that occurs only when the schedule permits, this project took a unique approach by developing collaborative learning experiences or "learning labs" that extended both longitudinally across medical and nursing school curricula and various health care settings (acute, long-term, or community). The goal of these learning labs was to provide the foundation for students in communication, teamwork, and quality improvement skills. Competent in these skills, the learners then progress to work in a collaborative practice setting, such as the Cleveland Free Clinic, where the medical and nursing students work with an underserved population in a student-run clinic.

(Continued)

Textbox 13.3 *(Continued)*

Specific interprofessional learning initiatives planned for this project include the following:

- Interprofessional interface—initial opportunities to learn about the health care system and the multiple roles various providers assume that are unique, complementary, collaborative, and/or congruent.
- TeamSTEPPS (Strategic Tools to Enhance Performance and Patient Safety) program—This model provides a framework for a series of short simulated learning exercises derived from the AHRQ and Department of Defense program that focuses on interprofessional strategies such as team building, communication enhancement, and root cause analysis.
- Community project—Teams of medical and nursing students will engage in a community assessment and collaborate to plan an intervention to meet an environmental health issue.
- Systems (based) Hospital Improvement Plan—Medical and nursing students assess factors that contributed to the hospitalization, evaluate what went well and what could be improved about the inpatient care experience, and collaborate in planning for transitional care upon discharge.
- Student Free Clinic—Medical and nursing students collaborate in the delivery of care to patients using the resources of the Cleveland Free Clinic.

In addition to building a collaborative, comprehensive, and longitudinal interprofessional curriculum, this project helped establish a virtual center to support ongoing educator development related to interprofessional practice and curricular evaluation and enhancement. The I•LEAD Center provides access to evidence supporting interprofessional education and practice, programs and materials developed by the Institute for Healthcare Improvement and the Quality and Safety Education for Nurses initiative, and education and practice evaluation tools.

Principle investigators for this project are Patricia Underwood, RN, PhD, and Daniel Ornt, MD.

that actively challenge them to search for meanings at increasing levels of abstraction with feedback (D'Eon, 2005). Educators need to structure the progression of increasingly complex cases representing learning tasks associated with giving and improving care. Factors that can increase the complexity of learning cases include different comorbidities, more departments involved, more disciplines involved, simulated to real environments, more complex systems, conflicting values, greater number of confounding factors, urgency to make decisions, and data that are more complex. Learning experiences that assist students to identify recurring patterns and salient features of situations requires a conscious effort on the part of the educators.

Evaluation of IPE

Similar to the evaluation of any learning activity, the evaluation of IPE is best accomplished when an overall evaluation framework is used, specific domain competencies to be evaluated are identified, and appropriate measures and methods of assessment of those competencies are employed. Most of the models of evaluation of IPE build on general models of education evaluation, such as that of Kirkpatrick (1994) or the 3P model of learning (Biggs, 1993). Kirkpatrick's framework includes four levels of evaluation: (1) evaluation of reaction, or satisfaction; (2) evaluation of learning, or knowledge or skills acquired; (3) evaluation of behavior, or the transfer of learning to the workplace; and (4) evaluation of results, or the transfer or impact on patient care. Three resources for IPE evaluation are described below, each of which address the Kirkpatrick levels of educational assessment.

A particularly comprehensive model of IPE evaluation has been derived from the 3P model described previously in this chapter. Developed as part of the United Kingdom Higher Education Academy Health Sciences and Practice Network, Freeth, Reeves, Koppel, Hammick, and Barr (2005) adapted the 3P model for evaluation of IPE initiatives. Their useful resource guide, *Evaluating Interprofessional Education: A Self-Help Guide*, is available at www.health.heacademy.ac.uk. This guide uses the 3P framework of presage (context), process, and product to describe sets of assessment domains, measurement approaches, and specific instruments for evaluation of IPE. A thorough review of the literature regarding assessment of IPE education is also provided in this guidebook.

Another comprehensive set of IPE evaluation materials is available from the Canadian Interprofessional Health Collaborative (2010) and can be accessed at www.cihc.ca. Based on the elements of the Canadian Interprofessional Health Collaborative Competency Framework, a set of survey instruments and measurement approaches are provided in the general domains of educational system, learners, educators, institutional factors, administrative processes, educator development, leadership/resources, learning context, and professional beliefs and attitudes. In-depth information on specific IPE instruments and measures is provided, including validity and reliability and details for administration.

Last, a newly developed set of IPE evaluation materials is available at the W(e)Learn website, which describes a model of online interprofessional education (http://ennovativesolution.com/WeLearn/IPE-Instruments.html; see also MacDonald et al., 2010). A toolkit for IPE evaluation includes a set of evaluation tools created by educators from the University of Ottawa. The W(e)Learn Interprofessional Program Assessment is a survey to assess the effectiveness of a program's structure, content, and delivery and serves as a way to measure satisfaction. A measure of changes in attitudes and behaviors that occur as a result of IPE experiences is also provided. A set of qualitative team and learner contracts to assess behavior change is displayed. Further psychometric testing is currently underway for most of these measures.

Continued effort is needed to determine the most effective methods to measure the effectiveness of IPE. Evaluation methods and instruments often are not well validated and the impact of IPE on patient outcomes remains a particular area of needed focus for evaluation. Also, the impact on educators and the overall curriculum is often not included in IPE evaluation efforts. Last, furthering our understanding of the tailoring needed for IPE in quality and safety is critical.

National interprofessional training programs in quality and safety education

IHI Open School

Two national interprofessional training programs stand out as exemplary models of large-scale, comprehensive IPE in health care quality and safety education. Interestingly, both of these programs rely heavily on virtual learning approaches that connect learners across geographical distances. The first of these virtual training programs is the Institute for Healthcare Improvement (IHI) Open School. The IHI Open School for health professions is a virtual school to teach quality improvement skills and patient safety to the next generation in pharmacy, nursing, dentistry, medicine, health management, health policy, and allied health. The IHI Open School is the "other school" that learners attend at their convenience while enrolled in their current educational programs. There are no applications, no admissions requirements, and no fees. Online offerings including courses, case studies, videos, podcasts, and discussions designed to help learners develop competencies in quality improvement and patient safety at beginner, intermediate, and advanced levels. Certification for completion of the online modules is available.

To supplement the IHI Open School's online delivery system (www.ihi.org/OpenSchool), a network of local chapters offers learners the chance to learn and compare notes with learners from different health care professions and to undertake projects with other learners to apply quality improvement knowledge. The IHI Open School encourages organizations (health care and academic institutions) to start local chapters as a way for interprofessional learners to discuss the common goal of increasing quality and safety in health care. Local chapters host a variety of activities from safety conferences to participating in quality improvement activities. Monthly telephone calls are coordinated by IHI and chapters share their activities and work.

VA Quality Scholars Program

Another exemplary model of national interprofessional training programs in quality and safety education is the Veterans Administration National Quality Scholars Program (VAQS). Unlike IHI Open School, which focuses on health professionals in training, the mission of VAQS is to develop leaders who can apply knowledge and methods of health care improvement to the care of veterans and nonveterans, innovate and continually improve health care, teach health professionals about health care improvement, and perform research and develop new knowledge for the ongoing improvement of the quality and value of health care services.

Traditionally a physician-only fellowship program, the 2-year curriculum was recently revised to include pre- and postdoctoral nurses with support from the Robert Wood Johnson Foundation through the QSEN initiative. There are six sites across the United States; each site is located at a VA medical center and partnered with an academic medical center and nursing school. Directed from the Dartmouth Medical School, twice-monthly video teleconferencing is used to provide state-of-the-science information and engage group discussions addressing quality and safety in health care. Local "senior" quality scholars (experienced educators in quality improvement) facilitate the learning activities. Several national face-to-face meetings are held as well, in which scholars from the six sites come together for sharing of experiences and exposure to national leaders in health care quality and safety (Splaine et al., 2009). Additionally, local improvement projects at the respective participating VA centers that are led by the interprofessional team of scholars are an important dimension of this training program. Examples of improvement projects include (1) minimizing the risk of retained sponges after surgery using a failure mode and effect analysis, (2) improving end-of-shift handoffs, (3) implementing evidence-based practice to prevent perioperative hypothermia, and (4) system analysis to improve the red blood cell transfusion process. Most VAQS scholars also participate on local interprofessional Systems Redesign teams conducting quality and safety projects such as lowering acute care beds as a means to improved care and cost savings, evaluating possible solutions to weekend/holiday hospitalizations while waiting for advanced testing to rule out acute myocardial infarction, and improving the mental health 7-day follow-up process. Further information about VAQS can be found at www.vaqs.org.

Educator development for IPE

In this chapter we have described approaches to IPE that have been shown to be successful. Although there are varying levels of evidence regarding their use, they do represent best practices that educators should use in designing IPE for quality and safety. Educators have several roles in IPE for which they must be adequately prepared. First, educators must model collaborative teamwork. This is done in interdisciplinary educator teams during planning, implementing, and evaluating IPE learning experiences. They must demonstrate flexibility and compromise in interactions with educators from other disciplines. This includes reducing professional territoriality and modeling conflict management in constructive ways. To promote effective communication across the "cultural" differences between disciplines, educators need to demonstrate the use of techniques to share their mental models and uncover the mental models of others.

It is highly important that educators understand how power dynamics issues in society related to gender, social class, and race need to be taken into account in IPE, particularly how they affect professional identity formation and power distribution. For example, an understanding of how the historical power and hierarchy differences between physicians and nurses (physicians historically being upper-middle-class men, and nurses historically being middle-working-class women) can affect their respect and regard for the opinions of each other (Ho et al., 2008). This means paying attention to the language that is embedded in the power within communications between learners of different disciplines. Educators who facilitate IPE must be prepared to examine and address these inherent social issues, and learners need to see the desired behaviors modeled by educators. The most effective educators will be those who are able to reflect on these issues with learners as they arise.

Educators also often have the role of being champions of IPE in their organizations. There is wide agreement in the literature that faculty champions are an essential factor of successful IPE programs. Faculty champions make connections with other faculty, make connections with students, and generally promote the program's initiatives (Ho et al., 2008). Formal leaders can use their power to influence structures, promote resources, stimulate interest, and provide reward systems. Faculty champions can also influence governance structures such as bylaws and faculty approval of curriculum to support IPE approaches. Champions play a role in creating a climate for change, cooperation, and flexibility.

Gaining organizational support for IPE is essential for long-term sustainability of this approach to learning. Barnsteiner, Disch, Hall, Mayer, and Moore (2007) propose six criteria that reflect full engagement by an organization in IPE: (1) An explicit philosophy of IPE that permeates the organization; (2) educators from the different professions co-creating the learning experiences; (3) learners having integrated and experiential opportunities to learn collaboration and teamwork and how they relate to the delivery of safe, quality care delivery; (4) IPE learning experiences embedded in the curricula and part of the required caseload for learners; (5) demonstrated competence by learners with a single set of interprofessional competencies; and (6) an organizational infrastructure that fosters IPE, including support for giving educators time to develop IPE options, incentive systems for educators to engage in IPE, and integrated activities across schools and professions for learners and educators.

Summary

In this chapter we present the current evidence for the added value of teaching quality and safety using interprofessional learning approaches. Conceptual frameworks and sets of core competencies relevant to IPE in quality and safety that educators can use to design, implement, and evaluate are described. In particular, the processes of cooperative learning, reflective learning, experiential learning, and transfer of learning are highlighted as key elements of IPE that we believe will promote successful quality and safety education. We also described the need for adequate preparation of educators to facilitate successful interprofessional learning experiences in quality and safety. Cooke, Ironside, and Ogrinc (2011) call for a transformation to quality and safety education that focuses on how the care team's patients fared and how the systems of care were improved. We believe this transformation can best be done using an IPE approach. Never has the need to prepare learners for collaborative, patent-centered practice and the improvement of care been greater.

References

Barnsteiner, J. H., Disch, J. M., Hall, L., Mayer, D., & Moore, S. M. (2007). Promoting interprofessional education. *Nursing Outlook, 55,* 144–150.

Biggs, J. (1993). From theory to practice: A cognitive systems approach. *Higher Education Research and Development, 12,* 73–85.

CAIPE. (1997). Interprofessional education: A definition. *CAIPE Bulletin, 13.*

Canadian Interprofessional Health Collaborative. (2010). A national interprofessional competency framework. Retrieved from http://www.cihc.ca/files/CIHC_IPCompetencies_Feb1210.pdf

Capella, J., Smith, S., Philp, A., Putnam, T., Gilbert, C., Fry, W., et al. (2010). Teamwork training improves the clinical care of trauma patients. *Journal of Surgical Education, 67,* 439–443.

Clark, P. G. (2009). Reflecting on reflection in interprofessional education: Implications for theory and practice. *Journal of Interprofessional Care, 23,* 213–223.

Cooke, M., Ironside, P. M., & Ogrinc, G. S. (2011). Mainstreaming quality and safety: A reformulation of quality and safety education for health professions students. *BMJ Quality and Safety, 20 Suppl 1,* i79–i82.

Cronenwett, L., Sherwood, G., Barnsteiner, J., Disch, J., Johnson, J., Mitchell, P., et al. (2007). Quality and safety education for nurses. *Nursing Outlook, 55,* 122–131.

Cronenwett, L., Sherwood, G., Pohl, J, Barnsteiner, J., Moore, S., Taylor Sullivan, D. T., et al. (2009). Quality and safety education for advanced practice nursing practice. *Nursing Outlook, 57*(6), 338–348.

D'Eon, M. (2005). A blueprint for interprofessional learning. *Journal of Interprofessional Care, 19 Suppl 1,* 49–59.

Dewey, J. (1938). *Experience and education.* New York: Collier Books.

Freeth, D., & Reeves, S. (2004). Learning to work together: Using the presage, process, product (3P) model to highlight decisions and possibilities. *Journal of Interprofessional Care, 18*(1), 43–56.

Freeth, D., Reeves, S., Koppel, I., Hammick, M., & Barr, H. (2005). Evaluating interprofessional education: A self-help guide. Higher Education Academy Health Sciences and Practice Network. Occasional Paper No. 5. Retrieved from http://www.health.ltsn.ac.uk/projects/miniprojects/occp5.pdf

Ho, K., Jarvis-Selinger, S., Borduas, F., Frank, B., Hall, P., Handfield-Jones, R., et al. (2008). Making interprofessional education work: The strategic roles of the academy. *Academic Medicine, 83,* 934–940.

Interprofessional Education Collaborative Expert Panel. (2011). *Core competencies for interprofessional collaborative practice: Report of an expert panel.* Washington, DC: Interprofessional Education Collaborative.

King, H. B., Battles, J., Baker, D. P., Alonso, A., Salas, E., Webster, J., Salisbury, M. (2008). TeamSTEPPS: Team Strategies and Tools to Enhance Performance and Patient Safety. In K. Henriksen, J. B. Batles, M. A. Keyes, & M. L. Grady (Eds.), *Advances in patient safety: New directions and alternative approaches*, Vol. 3. Rockville, MD: Agency for Healthcare Research and Quality.

Kirkpatrick, D. L. (1994). *Evaluation training programs: The four levels*. San Francisco: Berrett-Koehler.

Kolb, D. (1984). *Experiential learning: Experience as the source of learning and development*. Upper Saddle River, NJ: Prentice Hall.

MacDonald, C. J., Archibald, D., Trumpower, D. L., Casimiro, L., Cragg, B., & Jelley, W. (2010). Designing and operationalizing a toolkit of bilingual interprofessional education assessment instruments. *Journal of Research in Interprofessional Practice and Education*, 1(3), 304–316.

Michaelsen, L. K., & Black, R. H. (1994). Building learning teams: The key to harnessing the power of small groups in higher education. In S. Kadel & J. Keehner (Eds.), *Collaborative learning: A sourcebook for higher education, vol. 2* (pp. 65–81). State College, PA: National Center for Teaching, Learning and Assessment.

Oandasan, I., & Reeves, S. (2005a). Key elements for interprofessional education. Part 1: The learner, the educator and the learning context. *Journal of Interprofessional Care, 19*(Suppl. 1), 21–38.

Oandasan, I., & Reeves, S. (2005b). Key elements of interprofessional education. Part 2: Factors, processes and outcomes. *Journal of Interprofessional Care, 19*(Suppl. 1), 39–48.

Reeves, S., Zwarenstein, M., Goldman, J., Barr, H., Freeth, D., Hammick, M. et al. (2008, Jan. 23). Interprofessional education: Effects on professional practice and health care outcomes. *Cochrane Database of Systematic Reviews*, CD002213.

Schon, D. (1987). *Educating the reflective practitioner: How professionals think in action*. London: Jossey-Bass.

Sherwood, G. (2012). The imperative to transform education to transform practice. In G. Sherwood & J. Barnsteiner (Eds.), *Quality and safety in nursing: A competency approach to improving outcomes*. Hoboken, NJ: Wiley-Blackwell.

Splaine, M. E., Ogrinc, G., Gilman, S. C., Aron, D. C., Estrada, C. A., Rosenthal, G. E., et al. (2009). The Department of Veterans Affairs National Quality Scholars Fellowship Program: Experience from 10 years of training quality scholars. *Academic Medicine, 84*, 1741–1748.

Thistlethwaite, J., & Moran, M. (2010). Learning outcomes for interprofessional education (IPE): Literature review and synthesis. *Journal of Interprofessional Care, 24*, 503–513.

Weaver, S. J., Lyons, R., DiazGranados, D., Rosen, M. A., Salas, E., Oglesby, J., et al. (2010). The anatomy of health care team training and the state of practice: A critical review. *Academic Medicine, 85*, 1746–1760.

Weaver, S. J., Rosen, M. A., Salas, E., Baum, K. D., & King, H. B. (2010). Integrating the science of team training: Guidelines for continuing education. *Journal of Continuing Education in the Health Professions, 30*, 208–220.

World Health Organization. (2010). *A framework for action on interprofessional education and collaborative practice*. Geneva, Switzerland: WHO Department of Human Resources for Health, CH-1211.

Zwarenstein, M., Goldman, J., & Reeves, S. (2009). Interprofessional collaboration: Effects of practice-based interventions on professional practice and healthcare outcomes. *Cochrane Database of Systematic Reviews*, CD000072.

Zwarenstein, M., Reeves, S., Barr, H., Hammick, M., Koppel, I., & Atkins, J. (2001). Interprofessional education: effects on professional practice and health care outcomes. *Cochrane Database of Systematic Reviews*, CD002213.

Chapter 14

New Graduate Transition into Practice: Improving Quality and Safety

Nancy Spector, PhD, RN
Beth T. Ulrich, EdD, RN, FACHE, FAAN
Jane Barnsteiner, PhD, RN, FAAN

> I am frightened for my patients and for my own license as I soon will be turned loose with only a resource person and expected to take a full load after only 5 days of orientation in my new assigned unit.
>
> —New graduate (North Carolina Foundation for Nursing Excellence, 2009, p. 35)

The evidence creates a compelling case for all new graduates to have a transition to practice from the student to the professional nurse role. Evidence has linked transition programs to improved safety and quality patient outcomes as well as to the increased retention of new graduate nurses. As a result, the National Council of State Boards of Nursing (NCSBN) has developed a transition to practice (TTP) model that incorporates the Quality and Safety Education in Nursing (QSEN) competencies. This chapter discusses the evidence for TTP programs, describes the NCSBN TTP model and examples of successful TTP programs/residencies, and highlights strategies for educators in preparing the student for transition to practice.

Transition to practice defined

Transition to practice is defined by the NCSBN as a formal program of active learning, implemented across all settings for all newly licensed nurses (registered nurses and licensed practical/vocational nurses), designed to support

---

Quality and Safety in Nursing: A Competency Approach to Improving Outcomes, First Edition. Edited by Gwen Sherwood and Jane Barnsteiner.
© 2012 John Wiley & Sons, Inc. Published 2012 by John Wiley & Sons, Inc.

their progression from education to practice. Transition to practice is a comprehensive program that is integrated throughout the health system and supported from the top down. Orientation, on the other hand, is a separate process that is focused on the hiring institution, and not on transitioning the new nurses to their futures in nursing practice. The American Nurses Association (2000) defines orientation as the process of introducing staff to the philosophy, goals, policies, procedures, role expectations, and other factors needed to function in a specific work setting. Orientation takes place both for new employees and when changes in nurses' roles, responsibilities, and practice settings occur.

The quote at the beginning of this chapter is representative of many new nurses. While some employers provide comprehensive transition to practice programs, transition programs are not required in nursing. Yet many professions such as medicine, pharmacy, pastoral care, physical therapy, and teaching require formalized transition to practice programs for their graduates. Many of these programs receive either federal or state assistance. A recent employer study (Budden, 2011), using the NCSBN and American Nurses Association definitions, found that currently only 9%–31% of employers reported offering a transition to practice program and 1%–8% of employers don't even offer an orientation program to their new graduates.

Evidence linking transition programs to quality and safety

There is evidence linking improved patient care to standardized transition programs in the areas of safety, competence, and retention.

Safety

Research links new nurses to patient safety issues, such as near misses, adverse events, and practice errors (Berens, 2000; Bjørk & Kirkevold, 1999; del Bueno, 2005; Ebright, Urden, Patterson, & Chalko, 2004; Johnstone & Kanitsaki, 2006; Johnstone & Kanitsaki, 2008; Massachusetts Board of Registration in Nursing [MABRN], 2007; NCSBN, 2007; Orsolini-Hain & Malone, 2007). Newly licensed nurses have significant job stresses (Elfering, Semmer, & Grebner, 2006; Fink, Krugman, Casey, & Goode, 2008; NCSBN, 2007; Williams, Goode, Krsek, Bednash, & Lynn, 2007), and this stress has been linked to patient errors (Elfering et al., 2006; NCSBN, 2007). In another study, newly licensed nurses who reported higher stress ratings also reported making significantly more errors than new nurses reporting lower stress levels (NCSBN, 2007). Interestingly, in the NCSBN (2007) national study of newly licensed nurses, the stress levels of new nurses were highest at the 3–6 month period of practice. This is most likely the period when they are no longer in any kind of a transition or orientation program. In the study of the University Health System Consortium/American Association of Colleges of Nursing (UHC/AACN) residency program, stress gradually decreased over the year

(Williams et al., 2007). These results indicate that a comprehensive yearlong transition program may decrease stress, which in turn is related to safe patient care.

Two reports specifically cited reports where nurses were disciplined by the Board of Nursing for violating the Nurse Practice Act (MABRN, 2007; NCSBN, 2009a), and one addressed incident reports (Johnstone & Kanitsaki, 2008). When reviewing discipline data, it should be noted that new nurses are often given the benefit of the doubt. Further, there is quite a leap between discipline and minor errors or near misses; the latter more often is seen with new nurses (Ebright et al., 2004; MABRN, 2007). The NCSBN (2009a) Nursys data on discipline in the boards of nursing over 10 years found that 4.1% of the discipline was with novice nurses. The MABRN's (2007) findings on discipline data from 77 nursing homes had no novice RNs in the analysis. However, of 44 LPNs disciplined, 7 were novices. In the Massachusetts Board of Registration in Nursing study, the researchers concluded that errors with new nurses were linked to inexperience, lack of familiarity, and lack of consistent preceptors. They recommended more supervision and support for new nurses.

A study conducted in Australia (Johnstone & Kanitsaki, 2008) found that incident reporting increased during the novice nurse's first year in a transition program, most likely because they were taught about the importance of reporting errors and near misses for root cause analyses. These nurses were able to integrate patient safety into the system within 3 to 4 months of this 12-month program. The key indicators they used to validate this integration included new graduates' familiarity with the following, and these tie into the above findings from Ebright et al. (2004) and the MABRN (2007):

● hospital layout,
● hospital policies regarding risk assessment tools,
● processes of evidence-based practice, and
● incident reporting.

New nurses often engage in concrete thinking and focus on technology (Benner, 2004; Orsolini-Hain & Malone, 2007), thereby missing the bigger picture. This can be devastating during these complex times in health care (Benner, Sutphen, Leonard, & Day, 2010; del Bueno, 2005; Ebright et al., 2004). With an increasing ratio of novice nurses to seasoned nurses predicted for the future (Orsolini-Hain & Malone, 2007), it is possible that novices are assisting each other, thus putting them in situations where errors in judgment are not corrected by colleagues (Ebright et al., 2004). Indeed, in a prospective study, Bjørk and Kirkevold (1999) found that patient safety can be compromised when there are no effective transition programs in place. They conducted a longitudinal study in Norway, videotaping nursing practice and conducting interviews with nurses and patients. While the nurses reported they had become efficient and rated themselves as better nurses over time, the analysis of their practice revealed that they made the same practice errors (such as contaminating wounds and unsafely removing wound drains) at the end of the study as they made at the beginning. The authors reported that because there were limited opportunities for feedback and reflection, the new nurses did not learn from their mistakes.

Near misses have been cited as a problem for new graduates. Ebright and colleagues (2004) interviewed new nurses and found that of 12 recruited new nurse participants, 7 reported at least one near-miss event, while 1 nurse described two events. Some of the themes identified related to near misses/adverse events, for example, difficulty with first-time experiences, handing off patients, and novices assisting novices, among others. Similar to the Bjørk and Kirkevold (1999) study, if new graduates do not have supportive transition to practice programs, they won't learn from their near misses.

Inexperienced nurses who aren't supported may affect patient safety because of missed nursing care. When nursing care is omitted, patient outcomes could be adversely affected, thus promoting falls, failure to rescue, pressure ulcers, or other adverse events. Using focus groups, Kalisch (2006) identified seven themes as to why care is missed; some of these included the poor use of existing staff resources and ineffective delegation. Further, subthemes included inadequate orientations for new nurses and inconsistent assignments. Without consistent patient assignments and opportunities for follow-through, novice nurses don't have the opportunity to get to know their patients well enough to recognize changes. Similarly, Benner and colleagues (2010) cited student nurses' lack of opportunities for patient follow-up as one reason for implementing transition programs in nursing. Del Bueno (2005), for example, found when new nurses were given patient scenarios, 50% would miss life-threatening changes. Further, 65%–76% of inexperienced RNs did not meet the expectations for entry-level clinical judgment, and the majority had difficulty translating knowledge and theory into practice. Yet, Ashcraft (2004), in presenting three cases, discussed how crucial pattern recognition is when patients are in prearrest states. Since novice nurses take longer to "put the pieces together," they need support from experienced nurses in these critical situations. A standardized transition program would assist new nurses to identify subtle changes and avoid practice errors.

An NCSBN (2007) national study found that when transition programs in hospitals addressed specialty care, new nurses reported making significantly fewer practice errors. Similarly, when nurses perceived they were more competent, they reported making significantly fewer practice errors, and this was especially true when they reported more competence in clinical reasoning abilities and communication and interpersonal relationships.

Novice nurses who do not take part in transition programs have a high turnover rate. When these nurses leave, they are often replaced by temporary nurses who tend to make more errors. Berens (2000), after reviewing Illinois state disciplinary data, reported that temporary nurses were the increased focus of investigations and their reasons for errors were most often linked to lack of knowledge of hospital procedure and unfamiliarity with patients. Unfamiliarity with patients and units and first- time experiences have been cited as reasons for near misses or errors by others (MABRN, 2007; Ebright et al., 2004). In addition, Duffield, Roche, O'Brien-Pallas, and Catling-Paull (2009) found that downstream effects of turnover (which they termed "churn") included adverse outcomes for patients, a lack of continuity of care, additional time required to manage employees, and loss in staff productivity.

Competence

Keller, Meekins, and Summers (2006) provide insight as to why new nurses need continued support for the first year, even though they graduated from a Board of Nursing–approved nursing program and passed the NCLEX. They state that nursing education cannot prepare new graduates for acculturating into their workplaces and for using a recently acquired new vernacular, which differs across specialties. New graduates, the authors assert, are expected to become skilled in a wide range of absolutely necessary skills and to gain a sense of the wider world of their organization and health care. They describe some of these necessary skills as being self-aware and learning about team dynamics, leading teams, coordinating care, managing conflict, understanding the psychological effects of change and transition, communication, evidence-based practice, systems thinking, and financial pressures. Neophyte nurses become overwhelmed and stressed with all of these expectations (Elfering et al., 2006; NCSBN, 2007; Williams et al., 2007), and stress in the first year of practice has been significantly related to practice errors (Elfering et al., 2006; NCSBN, 2007).

Employers report new graduates are not ready to practice. NCSBN studies found that fewer than 50% of employers reported "yes definitely" when asked if new graduates are ready to provide safe and effective care (NCSBN, 2002; NCSBN, 2004a). Similarly, Berkow, Virkstis, Stewart, and Conway (2008), from the Nursing Executive Center, conducted a survey of more than 5,700 frontline nurse leaders, asking about employer perceptions of new graduates on 36 competencies. Improvement was needed across levels of education (ADN and BSN). For example, 53% of employers were satisfied with the top-rated competency (utilization of information technologies), while only 10% were satisfied with the last-rated competencies, such as delegation of tasks. Berkow and colleagues (2008) noted that the bottom-rated competencies would be better taught in an experiential environment, such as a transition to practice program.

There is evidence linking competence to the need for effective transition programs (Benner et al., 2010; Beyea, Slattery, & von Reyn, 2010; Bjørk & Kirkevold, 1999; del Bueno, 2005; NCSBN, 2007; NCSBN, 2009b; Orsolini-Hain & Malone, 2007; Williams et al., 2007). NCSBN (2007) reported that new graduates were significantly more likely to self-report practice errors when they also perceived themselves to have decreased competence and increased stress. In this study, 3 to 6 months after hire was the vulnerable period where nurses reported more stress and less competence and therefore were at risk for practice breakdown. Other research has shown this "V-shaped" pattern, showing declines in novice nurse variables at mid-program, with subsequent gains (Halfer, Graf, & Sullivan, 2008; Williams et al., 2007), though in these studies the decline began at the 6-month level. This evidence supports the vulnerable period of new graduates as occurring from 3 to 9 months after employment.

In the Bjørk and Kirkevold (1999) study, there were no opportunities for feedback or reflective practice, which likely would have improved the competence of these nurses. This is excellent empirical data about what can happen when new nurses do not have supportive transition programs.

Beyea and others (2010) studied an experiential transition program using simulation, measuring confidence, competence, and readiness to practice, all of which significantly increased after their program. This program uses simulation vignettes that highlight high-risk and low-frequency events (such as cardiac arrests), as well as commonly occurring clinical situations. According to this study, a transition program incorporating active learning is a highly effective way of developing competency and confidence in new graduates.

Retention

Some might argue whether job retention is a fair measure of quality and safety in patient care because, while nurses may leave one job during the first year, they generally move to another position. The first workplace, however, is challenged with recruiting and orienting a new nurse, and often the employer must fill the nurse's position with a temporary nurse. Job satisfaction is a predictor of anticipated turnover and it has been linked to adverse health care outcomes (Beecroft, Hernandez, & Reid, 2008). Other evidence links the use of temporary nurses to adverse health outcomes (Alonso-Echanove et al., 2003; Berens, 2000; MABRN, 2007), though the findings are conflicting. For example, Aiken (2007) did not find that temporary nurses affected quality and safety, while Bae, Mark, and Fried (2010) found that there were significantly more falls on units with high levels of temporary nurses, but there were significantly fewer medication errors on those units, compared to those without temporary nurses. More research is needed to better understand the relationship between turnover and safety and quality outcomes.

Do new graduates leave nursing altogether? Kovner and Djukic (2009) report that 98% of nurses who pass the NCLEX are working in nursing 2 years later. Yet, Orsolini-Hain and Malone (2007), reviewing national data from the U.S. Department of Health and Human Services, report that 4.5% of nurses were employed outside of nursing in the late 1980s, whereas in 2004 it was 16.8%. Additional research in this area is needed. The literature reports moderate to high turnover rates during new graduates' first year of practice. Turnover rates are not reported the same across studies, and thus it is difficult to compare. Turnover rates have been reported as high as between 35% and 60% for 1 year in practice (Advisory Board Company, 2006; Halfer et al., 2008; Pine & Tart, 2007; Ulrich et al., 2010; Williams et al., 2007). Kovner and

Djukic (2009) report a 26% turnover rate in 2 years using unpublished raw data from the RN Work Project. Ulrich and others (2010), in analyzing new graduate turnover data from hospitals prior to implementing the Versant RN Residency, found an average new graduate turnover of 27% in the first 12 months and 30% in the second 12 months, resulting in a cumulative 24-month turnover of 49%. Comprehensive transition programs, however, are associated with significantly decreased turnover rates after the programs are implemented (Beecroft, Kunzman, & Krozek, 2001; Halfer et al., 2008; Pine & Tart, 2007; Ulrich et al., 2010; Williams et al., 2007).

A variable currently affecting turnover rates may be the economy. For example, Budden (2011), in a survey conducted in 2009–2010, found that 61% of hospital employers reported low turnover rates for new nurses, though it is unclear if this could be due to the economic downturn during that time period. It appears that across the United States, nurses are not leaving their positions until the job climate improves (Randolph, 2010).

Data indicate that temporary nurses, who are often hired when a new nurse resigns, have an increased number of disciplinary complaints filed at state boards of nursing (Berens, 2000) compared with nurses hired on a permanent basis. Similarly, errors made by novice LPNs in nursing homes (MABRN, 2007) and near misses reported by RNs (Ebright et al., 2004) are linked to unfamiliarity with the workplace setting. Further, every study examined found that increased retention resulted from a formal transition program (Beecroft et al., 2001; Halfer, 2007; Keller et al., 2006; Mississippi Office of Nursing Workforce, 2010; NCSBN, 2007; Pine & Tart, 2007; Ulrich et al., 2010; Vermont Nurses in Partnership [VNIP], 2010; Williams et al., 2007).

The solution: a standardized model

A committee of NCSBN's membership, with a representative of the Association of Nurse Executives at each meeting, spent a year reviewing the evidence to develop a standardized transition model. The model was designed to be flexible in that any program (independently developed or in partnership with other institutions) that meets the requirements of this model can be used. It is robust because it is intended to be used across all settings and with all levels of education, from practical nursing to master's entry nursing.

At each meeting, members had collaborative conference calls with nursing and health care organizations to gain input, and many changes were made after communicating with more than 35 nursing and health care organizations. For example, the model was recategorized to highlight the QSEN competencies so that it would be in line with national nursing initiatives. NCSBN's TTP model was designed as a "no-blame" model. That is, it was assumed that education programs are adequately preparing our nurses for practice and that practice settings are not unfairly expecting new nurses to move immediately into skilled practice. Instead, NCSBN believes there is a missing piece in nursing: no standardized transition to practice program.

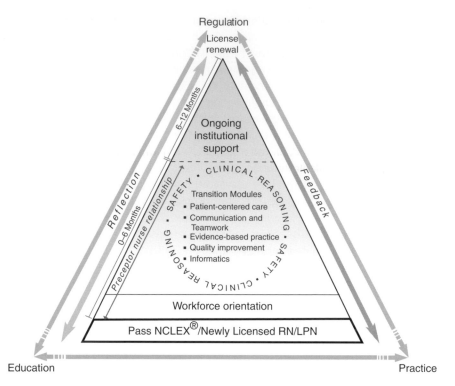

Figure 14.1 Transition to practice model.
Reprinted with permission from the National Council of State Boards of Nursing.

Elements of the model are described below. A visual description of the model is shown in Figure 14.1.

Preceptorship for 6 months followed by institutional support for 6 months

NCSBN's model is dependent on a well-developed preceptor-nurse relationship, in which preceptors are trained for the role, either in face-to-face or online courses. Preceptors work with the new graduates throughout the 6-month transition program, though the level of oversight decreases as the newly licensed nurse becomes more experienced, thus fostering independence.

The evidence supports that preceptors must be skilled in the role. Often, preceptors feel unprepared and unsupported for the preceptorship role. For example, in one study of 86 preceptors, researchers found preceptors reported they were unprepared to precept new graduates and they needed more support and recognition (Yonge, Hagler, Cox, & Drefs, 2008). While many transition programs incorporate preceptor training, Vermont Nurses in Partnership (2010) is an exemplary model of preceptor education that has been well developed. There are also other preceptor models available in the literature (Nicol & Young, 2007). Phillips (2006) describes the pros and cons of online preceptor education and what to consider when planning a successful online training program. Additionally, there is evidence that team preceptorships are successful (Beecroft et al., 2008), and therefore team preceptoring would be an acceptable strategy in the NCSBN model. When preceptors are not available, a national website could be designed to connect preceptors, through a remote interface, to novice nurses. This innovative approach has been successfully implemented in Scotland's Flying Start program (Roxburgh et al., 2010) and could provide new nurses with opportunities for feedback, reflection, and support, even when preceptors are not geographically available.

During the last 6 months of NCSBN's TTP model, the institution provides ongoing institutional support. This includes allowing the new nurse to evaluate any processes that could be done differently and being empowered to make some changes. During this period, the new nurses reflect on what lessons were learned from specific situations. In order to facilitate feedback, there should be a discussion of the performance appraisal, including any strengths or weaknesses. In addition, this is a good time for the institution to provide new nurses with opportunities to review any sentinel events or near misses that have occurred so that they can develop an understanding of problem solving methods. The institution will encourage the new nurse to participate in committee work or grand rounds in order to engage the new nurse with the institution. Finally, there will be a celebration of the end of the program (whether individual or hospital-wide) in order to formally recognize the new nurse's transition period.

NCSBN TTP: experiential learning—five modules

Transition programs, in order to be effective in promoting safe and quality patient outcomes, must incorporate the broad concepts from the QSEN initiative (Cronenwett et al., 2007), allowing experiential learning. Johnstone and Kanitsaki (2006, 2008) have found that, particularly related to safety and quality education, experiential learning is essential. In their undergraduate programs, students often are not able to actively learn the concepts they are taught because of the limitations of clinical education (Benner et al., 2010).

Therefore, these five transition modules, supported by the evidence, are based on the Institute of Medicine (Greiner & Knebel, 2003) competencies and the QSEN initiative (Cronenwett et al., 2007). A sixth module trains preceptors for the role.

- Patient-centered care
- Communication and teamwork
- Evidence-based practice
- Quality improvement
- Informatics

Safety, clinical reasoning, and feedback and reflection are threaded through-out all the modules. The content of the modules should be incorporated into the new nurses' experiences so they continue to learn experientially, interac-tively, and from preceptor role modeling how to "think like a nurse." This dis-cussion provides a broad scope of the modules; specific competency content is in other chapters.

Patient-centered care

Patient-centered care emphasizes specialty content and prioritizing/organiz-ing care around the needs of the patient and family (Walton & Barnsteiner, 2012). Specialty content in a transition program has been linked significantly to self-reports of lower practice errors (NCSBN, 2007). Other research sup-ports integrating specialty practice into transition programs (Beecroft et al., 2001; Benner et al., 2010; Beyea et al., 2010; Halfer, 2007; Joint Commission, 2002; Keller et al., 2006; Pine & Tart, 2007; Roxburgh et al., 2010; VNIP, 2010). The preceptor should be trained on the importance of assisting new gradu-ates to identify and learn from experts in the new nurse's specialty.

Prioritizing and organizing is a part of clinical practice that is often a weak-ness for novice nurses (Berkow et al., 2008; Halfer, 2007; NCSBN, 2004b; NCSBN, 2006b; Williams et al., 2007), most likely because of lack of experi-ence. Specifically, the UHC/AACN residency program measured ability to organize and prioritize before and after their program and found significant increases at the end of the program (Williams et al., 2007). While none of the transition programs reviewed specifically identified boundary issues (bound-ary crossings, violations, misuse of social media, etc.) as a topic, boards of nursing have identified this as an important area to stress in the TTP model.

Communication and teamwork

Communication and teamwork are essential in any transition model. The 2003 IOM report on health professions education (Greiner & Knebel, 2003) stressed the importance of teaching health care students to collaborate across profes-sions. McKay and Crippen (2008) report that in hospitals where collaboration occurs, there is a 41% lower mortality rate than would be predicted. In other hospitals, McKay and Crippen (2008) report, where collaborative communica-tion is not emphasized (or not part of the culture), mortality rates were 58% higher than would be predicted. Similarly, enhanced communication in hospi-tals has been linked to nurse satisfaction, lower costs, and greater responsive-ness of health care providers (McKay & Crippen, 2008). One NCSBN (2007) study found that new nurses perceived they made significantly fewer practice errors when they reported being more competent in communication and interpersonal relationships. Yet Benner et al. (2010) report that prelicensure nursing programs provide their students with few opportunities for interpro-fessional communication. Most of the reports of transition programs reviewed recommended a purposeful integration of communication, including interpro-fessional relationships, into transition programs (Beecroft et al., 2001; Beyea et al., 2010; Halfer, 2007; Keller et al., 2006; Pine & Tart, 2007; Roxburgh et al., 2010; Williams et al., 2007).

The communication and teamwork module also includes role socialization, which is a very important concept for new nurses. They must have a good understanding of their scope of practice, as well as that of others on the health care team (Disch, 2012). Closely related to role socialization is the need for new nurses to develop a better understanding of delegating and supervising. NCSBN studies of new nurses, since 2002, have consistently found that new nurses report a lack of understanding of delegation (NCSBN, 2004b; 2006a, b; 2007; 2009a, b), as do others (Berkow et al., 2008). Transition programs should be incorporating delegation/supervising into their curricula, though not many specifically indicate that.

Evidence-based practice

Another essential experiential module is evidence-based practice, because nurses are expected to base their practice on the evidence (Cronenwett et al., 2007; Greiner & Knebel, 2003, Tracey & Barnsteiner, 2012). Yet NCSBN research (NCSBN, 2006a, b) has shown that new nurses are weak in this area. Evidence-based practice is integral to most of the TTP programs. In the Launch into Nursing program in Texas, for example, new nurses participate in an evidence-based project and present the results to the hospital unit on which they work (Keller et al., 2006). The international and national programs support incorporating evidence-based practice into transition programs (Beecroft et al., 2001; Roxborgh, 2010; Williams et al., 2007), as do individual programs (Pine & Tart, 2007; Bratt, 2009).

Quality improvement

With health care institutions focusing on safety and improving their systems, novice nurses need experiential learning related to quality improvement processes, such as Six Sigma (Johnson, 2012; Pocha, 2010). Berkow et al. (2008) surveyed educators and practice leaders about the emphasis of 36 competencies taught in nursing programs, compared to how prepared new nurses were in those competencies. They found that quality improvement, priority setting, and delegation were not emphasized enough in nursing education and concluded they are best learned in a practice setting with experiential learning, such as a TTP program. Additionally, Barton, Armstrong, Preheim, Gelmon, and Andrus (2009) conducted a national Delphi study to determine the progression of quality and safety competencies and identified quality improvement knowledge and skills to be included in TTP programs (Appendix C).

Informatics

As electronic health records become more pervasive in health care, nurses need informatics skills (Warren, 2012). Yet nursing students have little, and sometimes no, opportunity to learn these skills as students in the workplace.

Newly licensed nurses, therefore, will learn how to identify the electronic information at the point of care and learn how to access information that isn't readily available but is needed. The TIGER initiative (Technology Informatics Guiding Educational Reform; 2010) is a valuable resource in this module.

Threads throughout the curriculum

Safety

Teaching safety is an essential part of a transition to practice regulatory model, and this is threaded throughout all the modules. Johnstone and Kanitsaki (2006, 2008) in Australia have reported on the importance of experientially teaching risk management to new nurses. Cronenwett and colleagues (2007), using the expertise of national health care leaders across disciplines, have described safety as a competency in detail, and this could be used in transition programs (Barnsteiner, 2012). The resulting consensus opinion document, QSEN, can be considered excellent evidence for this transition model (see Appendixes A and B). The MABRN (2007) findings on nursing home errors called attention to addressing safety issues in transition programs, based on their review of discipline of new practical nurse graduates. Likewise, an NCSBN study (2007) found that, according to self-reports, practice errors made by new graduates were prevalent. Many of the successful transition programs focus on safety (Beecroft et al., 2001; Beyea et al., 2010; Bratt, 2009; Halfer, 2007; Pine & Tart, 2007; Roxburgh, 2010; Williams et al., 2007).

Clinical reasoning

Clinical reasoning, sometimes referred to as critical thinking or clinical judgment, is a second essential thread integrated throughout all the TTP modules. The Carnegie study on nursing education points out this is a critical point in which nurses learn to "think like a nurse" (Benner et al., 2010). Many transition programs specifically report integration of clinical reasoning/critical thinking (Beecroft et al., 2001; Bratt, 2009; Halfer, 2007; Keller et al., 2006; Mississippi Office of Nursing Workforce, 2010; Molinari, Monserud, & Hudzinski, 2008; Pine & Tart, 2007; VNIP, 2010; Williams et al., 2007). The Dartmouth program (Beyea et al., 2010) provides an exemplary model in the use of simulation to assist novice nurses in actively making decisions in simulated experiences.

Feedback and reflection

Feedback and reflection are a third thread in the TTP model and should be formally maintained during the 6-month transition program as well as during the 6 months that follow. New nurses need feedback on their practice, along with an opportunity to reflect, to improve their practice. Consistent with Bjørk and Kirkevold's (1999) study, without those opportunities, new graduates are at risk of making the same mistakes time and time again. It is very important for preceptors to be taught how to provide constructive feedback and how to foster reflective practice. Many of the transition programs included in this review did provide opportunities for feedback and reflection (Beyea et al., 2010; Bratt, 2009; Halfer, 2007; Keller et al., 2006; Pine & Tart, 2007; Roxburgh, 2010; Williams et al., 2007). Horton-Deutsch and Sherwood (2008) show how fostering reflection, particularly through journaling and personal inventories, is a successful leadership development strategy.

A multisite, randomized study of the model

NCSBN, in collaboration with a Research Advisory Panel of experts in safety and quality research of new graduates, is conducting a longitudinal, multisite, randomized study to evaluate its TTP model. It is the first study to examine patient outcomes in standardized nursing transition programs compared with sites that use their traditional programs. The primary objective of this study is to determine whether newly licensed nurses' participation in NCSBN's TTP model improves patient safety, leads to higher quality outcomes, and improves nurse retention. The secondary objectives are (1) to determine whether NCSBN's preceptor module adequately prepares nurses for the preceptor role, (2) to identify the challenges and potential solutions of planning and implementing the transition model within the organization and across the state/jurisdiction, and (3) to determine the cost-benefit analysis to implement the TTP model at a health care organization by evaluating the return on investment based on new nurse turnover rates. To establish whether the primary objective has been achieved, this study will examine the differences between the experimental group and the control group across the variables highlighted in Table 14.1. The final results of the study will be reported in May of 2014. If the study finds that a standardized transition program improves quality and safety, the state boards of nursing may decide to require new graduates to complete a transition program before renewing their license after the first year in practice.

Transition to practice programs: examples

Two programs that have demonstrated success in TTP are the University Health System Consortium/American Association of Colleges of Nursing (UHC/AACN) Nurse Residency Program (begun in 2002) and the Versant RN Residency (begun in 1999). The use of the Benner novice-to-expert model is central to both programs as a foundation, an evidence-based curriculum, preceptor-guided clinical experiences, supportive components (i.e., mentoring),

Table 14.1 Outcome measures for phase I of NCSBN's transition to practice study

Outcomes	Measurement (collected per unit of new nurses and per hospital)
Patient safety: infection rates, decubiti, post-op thrombosis, falls with and without injury	National Database of Nursing Quality Indicators data
Adverse events: failure to rescue, medication errors	Reports from institution
Patient satisfaction	System organization uses, such as Press Ganey
Length of stay	Report from institution
Competence of the new nurse	Surveys of new nurse and preceptor
Experiential knowledge of the new nurse	Knowledge assessment pre- and postprogram
Stress perceived by the new nurse	Report of new nurse
New nurse job satisfaction	Use of established tool (Brayfield & Rothe, 1951)
Retention	Actual turnover rates and reports by new nurses of intent to leave

celebrations and recognition, a dedicated residency coordinator/manager, and the measurement of outcomes.

The UHC/AACN Nurse Residency Program began as a joint venture task force between UHC Chief Nursing Officers and AACN deans to develop a postbaccalaureate residency program (Goode & Williams, 2004). A central tenet of the UHC/AACN Nurse Residency Program is collaboration between the academic hospital and its affiliated school of nursing (Krugman et al., 2006). The program is presented in two phases. The first phase, which occurs in the first 6 months, includes the hospital's orientation, the incorporation of a 1:1 baccalaureate-prepared clinical preceptor, clinical specialty training, and monthly resident seminars with an emphasis on mentoring and professional development. The second phase, in the second 6 months, includes monthly seminars with a resident facilitator. Two key components are the cohort groups and their relationships, clinical narratives to promote reflective inquiry, and standardized evidence-based residency curriculum (Krugman et al., 2006). Outcomes of the UHC/AACN Nurse Residency Program found improved retention and increased graduate perceptions that they grew in terms of organizing and prioritizing, communicating, and providing clinical leadership. New graduates also report significantly decreased stress (Williams et al., 2007).

The Versant RN Residency began in 1999 at Children's Hospital of Los Angeles and has since expanded nationwide. The Versant RN Residency is designed to meet the needs of all new graduate nurses. It is a structured, evidence-based residency that consists of an 18-week clinical immersion using

1:1 preceptors and standardized competencies and curricula (which have been crosswalked to the QSEN recommendations). Residents also have targeted experiences in units and departments related to their home units ("looping").

Real-time information about resident progress is shared between residents, preceptors, educators, and other individuals involved in the Versant RN Residency via a web portal. Supportive components (i.e., mentoring and debriefing) are an integral part of the residency. Data is collected at various points throughout the RN residency and for the first 5 years of the new graduate's practice as well as from organizational comparison groups. Outcomes of the Versant RN Residency include accelerated development of new graduate competence and confidence, a significant increase in new graduate retention, improved engagement of new graduates during and after the residency, and positive organizational transformation (Ulrich et al., 2010).

Both the UHC/AACN Nurse Residency Program and the Versant RN Residency have demonstrated the need for dedicated organizational commitment and resources when implementing a TTP program. The evidence from both programs demonstrates that TTP programs can have beneficial results for individual new graduate nurses and health care organizations.

Implications for nursing education programs

This chapter has presented the case for a postgraduate transition program for all newly licensed nurses as one aspect of improving quality and safety. Partnerships between clinical settings and schools of nursing are critical links to successful new graduate transition (Sherwood & Drenkard, 2007). Educators should be an integral part of transitioning new nurses to practice, both in preparing their students for practice and also in collaborating with practice as they plan and implement transition programs.

But what else can educators do to facilitate the transition to practice? Many already have designed excellent immersion courses, with preceptors, at the end of the program. This is highly recommended. Some worry about preceptor burnout if educational programs were to all have immersion programs at the same time that a standardized model was implemented. This would probably be the case for the first few years. However, as nurses become acclimated to being preceptored in their first year of practice, they will see the importance of "giving back" and will themselves become preceptors. After a standardized preceptor model has been implemented for a few years, it is expected that preceptors will be readily available.

Educators are strongly encouraged to develop practice partnerships where practitioners and educators can work together to design clinical and simulation experiences that will foster a more seamless transition to practice. Participating in dedicated education units is an innovative way some nursing programs collaborate with practice partners. In this model, nurse executives, faculty, and staff nurses partner to transform patient care units into supportive environments for nursing students and staff nurses, while continuing to provide quality care to patients (Mulready-Shick, Kafel, Banister, & Mylott, 2009).

There is a movement in nursing education to transform clinical experiences from the frequent randomness that we now have to more focused learning experiences. Gabrud-Howe and Schoessler (2008) outline some new ways of delivering clinical education, including

- focused direct client care experience,
- concept-based experience,
- case-based experience,
- intervention skill-based experience, and
- integrative experience.

Berkow et al. (2008) developed 36 mutually agreed-upon competencies essential for safe and effective nursing practice. To be included on the list, the competencies had to be specific, actionable, and reflective of current hospital demands. After extensive surveys with employers and educators, the competencies (shown in Textbox 14.1) were identified as areas "needing improvement" with new graduates; at the same time, educators have reported giving these areas less emphasis. Educators and those planning transition programs, therefore, should focus on how to best incorporate those elements into their curricula. Some of them have been supported by other national research.

Textbox 14.1   Research-supported elements for transition programs. These seven competencies were cited in Berkow, Virkstis, Stewart, and Conway's (2008) research as being weaknesses of new graduates. Others have documented these competencies as being important to integrate into transition to practice programs.

- Follow-up in patient care (Benner, Sutphen, Leonard, & Day, 2010, also cited this in nursing education)
- Taking initiative
- Understanding quality improvement (Cronenwett et al., 2007, cited this as needing more emphasis)
- Completion of tasks within expected timeframes (NCSBN, 2006b, also supports this)
- Track multiple responsibilities
- Conflict resolution (Benner et al., 2010, also cites this as a weakness in nursing programs)
- Delegation (NCSBN, 2006a, cited this as needing more emphasis)

The Advisory Board Company (2008) has outlined some exemplars in clinical instruction where educators and practice partners have collaborated, and have illustrated how partnerships have helped to design outstanding clinical experiences. The exemplars presented were in the broad categories of targeted clinical rotations, expert clinical instruction, and exceptional student experiences. It makes sense for educators and nurses in practice to collaborate when educating nurses because they both have the same goal: to provide safe and high-quality patient care.

Conclusion

The evidence is increasingly clear that TTP programs are a critical element in the success of individual nurses, their organizations, and patient quality, safety, and outcomes. As a result, the support for these programs is growing (Benner et al., 2010; IOM, 2010; NCSBN, 2007). Using the NCSBN TTP model to provide guidance and direction, organizations in all health care settings can establish TTP programs. Quality and safety can only be assured if TTP programs become the expectation for every new graduate nurse.

References

Advisory Board Company. (2006). *Transitioning new graduates to hospital practice: Profiles of nurse residency program exemplars*. Washington, DC: Author.

Advisory Board Company. (2008). *Bridging the preparation-practice gap: Volume II. Best practices for accelerating practice readiness of nursing students*. Washington, DC: Author.

Aiken, L. H. (2007). Study: Temporary nurses not a threat to quality. *Healthcare Benchmarks and Quality Improvement*, 14(11), 128–130.

Alonso-Echanove, J., Edwards, J. R., Richards, M. J., Brennan, P., Venezia, R. A., Keen, J., et al. (2003). Effect of new nursing staffing on antimicrobial-impregnated central venous catheters on the risk of bloodstream infections in intensive care units. *Infection Control and Hospital Epidemiology*, 24(12), 916–925.

American Nurses Association. (2000). *Scope and standards of practice for nursing professional development*. New York: Author.

Ashcraft, A. S. (2004). Differentiating between pre-arrest and failure-to-rescue. *Medsurg Nursing*, 13(4), 211–216.

Bae, S. H., Mark, B., & Fried, B. (2010). Use of temporary nurses and nurse and patient safety outcomes in acute hospital units. *Health Care Management Review*, 35(3), 333–344.

Barnsteiner, J. (2012). Safety. In G. Sherwood & J. Barnsteiner (Eds.), *Quality and safety in nursing: A competency approach to improving outcomes*. Hoboken, NJ: Wiley-Blackwell.

Barton, A. J., Armstrong, G., Preheim, G., Gelmon, S. B., & Andrus, L. C. (2009). A national Delphi to determine developmental progression of quality and safety competencies in nursing education. *Nursing Outlook*, 57, 313–322.

Beecroft, P., Hernandez, A. M., & Reid, D. (2008). Team preceptorships: A new approach for precepting new nurses. *Journal for Nurses in Staff Development*, 24(4), 143–148.

Beecroft, P. C., Kunzman, L., & Krozek, C. (2001). RN internship: Outcomes of a one-year pilot program. *Journal of Nursing Administration, 31*(12), 575–582.

Benner, P. (2004). Using the Dreyfus model of skill acquisition to describe and interpret skill acquisition and clinical judgment in nursing practice and education. *Bulletin of Science, Technology & Society, 24*(3), 188–199.

Benner, P., Sutphen, M., Leonard, V., & Day, L. (2010). *Educating nurses: A call for radical transformation*. San Francisco: Jossey-Bass.

Berens, M. J. (2000, September 10). Nursing mistakes kill, injure thousands: Cost-cutting exacts toll on patients, hospital staffs. [First of three-part series: Dangerous care: Nurses' hidden role in medical error]. *Chicago Tribune, p.* 20.

Berkow, S., Virkstis, K., Stewart, J., & Conway, L. (2008). Assessing new graduate nurse performance. *Journal of Nursing Administration, 38*(11), 468–474.

Beyea, S. C., Slattery, M. J., & von Reyn, L. J. (2010). Outcomes of a simulation-based residency program. *Clinical Simulation in Nursing, 6*(5), 169–175.

Bjørk, I. T., & Kirkevold, M. (1999). Issues in nurses' practical skill development in the clinical setting. *Journal of Nursing Care Quality, 14*(1), 72–84.

Bratt, M.M. (2009). Retaining the next generation of nurses: The Wisconsin Residency Program provides a continuum of support. *Journal of Continuing Education in Nursing, 40*(9), 416–425.

Brayfield, A. H., & Rothe, H. F. (1951). An index of job satisfaction. *Journal of Applied Psychology,* 35, 307–311.

Budden, J. S. (2011). A survey of nurse employers on professional and practice issues affecting nursing. *Journal of Nursing Regulation, 1*(4), 17–25.

Cronenwett, L., Sherwood, G., Barnsteiner, J., Disch, J., Johnson, J., Mitchell, P., et al. (2007). Quality and safety education for nurses. *Nursing Outlook,* 55, 122, 131.

del Bueno, D. (2005). A crisis in critical thinking. *Nursing Education Perspectives, 26*(5), 278–282.

Disch, J. (2012). Teamwork and collaboration. In G. Sherwood & J. Barnsteiner (Eds.), *Quality and safety in nursing: A competency approach to improving outcomes.* Hoboken, NJ: Wiley-Blackwell.

Duffield, C., Roche, M., O'Brien-Pallas, L., & Catling-Paull, C. (2009). The implication of staff "churn" for nurse managers, staff, and patients. *Nursing Economic, 27*(2), 103–110.

Ebright, P. R., Urden, L., Patterson, E., & Chalko, B. (2004). Themes surrounding novice nurse near-miss and adverse-event situations. *Journal of Nursing Administration, 34*(11), 531–538.

Elfering, A., Semmer, N. K., & Grebner, S. (2006). Work stress and patient safety: Observer-rated work stressors as predictors of characteristics of safety-related events reported by young nurses. *Ergonomics, 49*(5/6), 457–469.

Fink, R., Krugman, M., Casey, K., & Goode, C. (2008). The graduate nurse experience: Qualitative residency program outcomes. *Journal of Nursing Administration, 38*(7/8), 341–348.

Gabrud-Howe, P., & Schoessler, M. (2008). From random access opportunity to a clinical education curriculum. *Journal of Nursing Education, 47*(1), 3–4.

Goode, C. J., & Williams, C. A. (2004). Post-baccalaureate nurse residency program. *Journal of Nursing Administration, 34*(2), 71–77.

Greiner, A. C., & Knebel, E. (Eds.). (2003). *Health professions education: A bridge to quality.* Institute of Medicine. Washington, DC: National Academies Press.

Halfer, D. (2007). A magnetic strategy for new graduates. *Nursing Economic, 25*(1), 5–11.

Halfer, D., Graf, E., & Sullivan, C. (2008). The organizational impact of a new graduate pediatric mentoring program. *Nursing Economic*, *26*(4), 243-249.

Horton-Deutsch, S., & Sherwood, G. (2008, December 16). Reflection: An educational strategy to develop emotionally competent nurse leaders. *Journal of Nursing Management*, *8*, 946-954.

Institute of Medicine. Committee on the Robert Wood Johnson Foundation Initiative on the Future of Nursing. (2010). The future of nursing: Leading change, advocating health. Washington, DC: National Academies Press. Retrieved from http://www.nap.edu/catalog.php?record_id=12956

Johnson, J. (2012). Quality improvement. In G. Sherwood & J. Barnsteiner (Eds.), *Quality and safety in nursing: A competency approach to improving outcomes*. Hoboken, NJ: Wiley-Blackwell.

Johnstone, M. J., & Kanitsaki, O. (2006). Processes influencing the development of graduate nurse capabilities in clinical risk management: An Australian study. *Quality Management in Health Care*, *15*(4), 268-278.

Johnstone, M. J., & Kanitsaki, O. (2008). Patient safety and the integration of graduate nurses into effective organizational clinical risk management systems and processes: An Australian study. *Quality Management in Health Care*, *17*(2), 162-173.

Joint Commission (2002). Health care at the crossroads: Strategies for addressing the evolving nursing crisis. Chicago: Author. Retrieved from http://www.jointcommission.org/NR/rdonlyres/5C138711-ED76-4D6F-909F-B06E0309F36D/0/health_care_at_the_crossroads.pdf

Kalisch, B.J. (2006). Missed nursing care: A qualitative study. *Journal of Nursing Quality Care*, *21*(4), 306-313.

Keller, J. L., Meekins, K., & Summers, B. L. (2006). Pearls and pitfalls of a new graduate academic residency program. *Journal of Nursing Administration*, *36*(12), 589-598.

Kovner, C., & Djukic, M. (2009). The nursing career process through the first 2 years of employment. *Journal of Professional Nursing*, *25*(4), 197-203.

Krugman, M., Bretschneider, J., Horn, D. B., Krsek, C. A., Moutafis, R. A., & Smith, M. O. (2006). The national post-baccalaureate graduate nurse residency program: A model for excellence in transition to practice. *Journal for Nurses in Staff Development*, *22*(4), 196-205.

Massachusetts Board of Registration in Nursing, Division of Health Professions Licensure, Massachusetts Department of Public Health. (2007). *A study to identify evidence-based strategies for the prevention of nursing errors*. Massachusetts: Author.

McKay, C. A., & Crippen, L. (2008). Collaboration through clinical integration. *Nursing Administration*, *32*(2), 109-116.

Mississippi Office of Nursing Workforce. (2010). Mississippi Nurse Residency Program. Retrieved from http://www.monw.org/residency/

Molinari, D. L., Monserud, M., & Hudzinski, D. (2008). A new type of rural residency. *Journal of Continuing Education in Nursing*, *39*(1), 42-46.

Mulready-Shick, J., Kafel, K. W., Banister, G., & Mylott, L. (2009). Enhancing quality and safety competency development at the unit level: An initial evaluation of student learning and clinical teaching on dedicated education units. *Journal of Nursing Education*, *48*(12), 716-719.

National Council of State Boards of Nursing. (2002). *Report of findings from the 2001 employers survey*. Chicago: Author.

National Council of State Boards of Nursing. (2004a). *Report of findings from the 2003 employers survey*. Chicago: Author.

National Council of State Boards of Nursing. (2004b). *Report of findings from the 2003 practice and professional issues survey: Spring 2003*. Chicago: Author.

National Council of State Boards of Nursing. (2006a). *Evidence-based nursing education for regulation (EBNER)*. Chicago: Author. Retrieved from https://www.ncsbn.org/Final_06_EBNER_Report.pdf

National Council of State Boards of Nursing. (2006b). *A national survey on elements of nursing education*. Chicago: Author.

National Council of State Boards of Nursing. (2007). *The impact of transition experience on practice of newly licensed registered nurse*. Data presented at February 2007 Transition Forum, Chicago, IL.

National Council of State Boards of Nursing. (2009a). *An analysis of Nursys® disciplinary data from 1996–2006*. Retrieved from https://www.ncsbn.org/09_AnalysisofNursysData_Vol39_WEB.pdf

National Council of State Boards of Nursing. (2009b). Post-entry competence study. Retrieved from https://www.ncsbn.org/09_PostEntryCompetenceStudy_Vol38_WEB_final_081909.pdf

Nicol, P., & Young, M. (2007). Sail training: An innovative approach to graduate nurse preceptor development. *Journal for Nurses in Staff Development*, *23*(6), 298–302.

North Carolina Foundation for Nursing Excellence. (2009). *Progress report: Phase I study of North Carolina evidence-based transition to practice initiative project*. Retrieved from http://ffne.org/file_library/Phase%20I%20Findings%20Summary.pdf

Orsolini-Hain, L., & Malone, R. E. (2007). Examining the impending gap in clinical nursing expertise. *Policy, Politics, & Nursing Practice*, *8*(3), 158–169.

Phillips, J. M. (2006). Preparing preceptors through online education. *Journal for Nurses in Staff Development*, *22*(3), 150–156.

Pine, R., & Tart, K. (2007). Return on investment: Benefits and challenges of a baccalaureate nurse residency program. *Nursing Economic*, *25*(1), 13–18.

Pocha, C. (2010). Lean six sigma in health care and the challenge of implementation of six sigma methodologies at a Veterans Affairs medical center. *Quality Management in Health Care*, 19(4), 312–328.

Randolph, P. K. (2010). What happened to the nursing shortage? *Leader to Leader*, Spring. Retrieved from https://www.ncsbn.org/L2L_Spring2010.pdf

Roxburgh, M., Lauder, W., Topping, K., Holland, K., Johnson, M., & Watson, R. (2010). Early findings from an evaluation of a post-registration staff development programme: The Flying Start NHS Initiative in Scotland, UK. *Nurse Education in Practice*, *10*(2), 76–81.

Sherwood, G., & Drenkard, K. (2007). Quality and safety curricula in nursing education: Matching practice realities. *Nursing Outlook*, *55*(3), 151–155.

Technology Informatics Guiding Education Reform. (2010). *The TIGER initiative*. Retrieved from http://www.tigersummit.com/Home_Page.php

Tracey, M. F., & Barnsteiner, J. (2012). Evidence-based practice. In G. Sherwood & J. Barnsteiner (Eds.), *Quality and safety in nursing: A competency approach to improving outcomes*. Hoboken, NJ: Wiley-Blackwell.

Ulrich, B., Krozek, C., Early, S., Ashlock, C. H., Africa, L. M., & Carman, M. L. (2010). Improving retention, confidence, and competence of new graduate nurses: Results from a 10-year longitudinal database. *Nursing Economic*, 28(6), 363–376.

Vermont Nurses in Partnership. (2010). *Vermont Nurses in Partnership*. Retrieved from http://www.vnip.org/

Walton, M. K., & Barnsteiner, J. (2012). Patient-centered care. In G. Sherwood & J. Barnsteiner (Eds.), *Quality and safety in nursing: A competency approach to improving outcomes.* Hoboken, NJ: Wiley-Blackwell.

Warren, J. (2012). Informatics. In G. Sherwood & J. Barnsteiner (Eds.), *Quality and safety in nursing: A competency approach to improving outcomes.* Hoboken, NJ: Wiley-Blackwell.

Williams, C. A., Goode, C. J., Krsek, C., Bednash, G. D., & Lynn, M. R. (2007). Postbaccalaureate nurse residency 1-year outcomes. *Journal of Nursing Administration, 37*(7/8), 357-365.

Yonge, O., Hagler, P., Cox, C., & Drefs, S. (2008). Listening to preceptors. *Journal for Nurses in Staff Development, 24*(1), 21-26.

Chapter 15
Leadership to Create Change
Joanne Disch, PhD, RN, FAAN

"Leadership is a critical function in promoting high quality, safe health care" (Joint Commission, 2009, para. 1). What evidence exists to support the belief that it makes a difference? Are particular forms of leadership better than others? Who should lead the quality/safety journey? What can the leader do to engage others in improving patient safety and quality? In Chapter 6, Johnson (2012) examines the role of nurses in quality improvement. This chapter will review research findings on the relationship between leadership and quality/safety; offer a new way to think about leadership, particularly as it relates to quality and safety; and provide a framework for creating change. A basic premise of this chapter is that all nurses are leaders at some level, if the definition of leadership is the one used by this author when working with nursing students, staff nurses, managers, and nurse executives: *working with and through people to improve something*. This underscores the fundamental responsibility that *all* nurses have, for example, working with patients to better manage their pain, communicating clearly with other members of the health care team to revise the plan of care, and developing a better staffing plan. We work with and through others to improve patient health, health care delivery, the education of our students, and our interventions. While much of the research that will be reported highlights the role of nurses as leaders in formal roles, which has been the focus for most of the research conducted, the principles and concepts apply to all nurses.

The evolution of leadership

A visit to a bookstore or the Amazon website will illustrate the explosive growth in approaches to leadership. While decades ago, leaders were categorized as authoritarian, laissez-faire, or democratic, today's leader is more likely to be called authentic (George, 2003), resonant (Boyatzis & McKee,

Quality and Safety in Nursing: A Competency Approach to Improving Outcomes, First Edition. Edited by Gwen Sherwood and Jane Barnsteiner.
© 2012 John Wiley & Sons, Inc. Published 2012 by John Wiley & Sons, Inc.

2005), exceptional (Dye & Garman, 2006), value (Harris, 1998), quantum (Porter-O'Grady & Malloch, 2007), servant (Schwartz & Tumblin, 2002), courageous (Hybels, 2002), or quiet (Rock, 2006). A few years ago, the *New York Times* reported on green-thumb leadership: "a future-oriented management style that understands, and even encourages, taking risks" (Rae-Dupree, 2008, p. 4).

Northouse (2010) describes leadership as a "process whereby an individual influences a group of individuals to achieve a common goal" (p. 3). He notes that there are four components central to the concept: (1) leadership is a process; (2) leadership involves influence; (3) leadership occurs in a group context; and (4) leadership involves goal attainment. This author suggests a similar definition with an important distinction: "working with and through others *to improve something*." Using a framework of generative leadership, generative leaders are "individuals who create new options or new approaches to old problems, and work with and through others to effect needed change" (Disch, 2009, p. 173). The goal is change for the purpose of improvement and, in the context of this chapter, working with and through others to improve quality and patient safety. These individuals are

> intellectually curious and never satisfied with the status quo; they are resilient and optimistic, seeing opportunities where others see insolvable problems ... [they] recognize there are multiple ways of knowing, and surround themselves with other thought leaders, including those with whom they disagree. They use a holistic, systems perspective in their thinking and move beyond perceived limitations of time, space, traditional thought, and their own views of the world. (Disch, 2009, p. 173)

A related concept is whole-systems leadership, a systemic, participative, and emergent approach to help navigate to a collective vision of a preferred future (Center for Spirituality & Healing, 2010). This involves deep listening, an awareness of systems and self, seeking diverse perspectives, embracing uncertainty, and taking adaptive action.

The relationship between leadership and safety

The role of leadership in promoting safety has been a focus in the occupational setting for years (Cooper, 2001; Geller, 2000; Grubbs, 1999). In a comprehensive review of the topic, Hofmann and Morgeson (2004) differentiated safety-specific leader behaviors from general leader behaviors. They found that when supervisors engaged in more safety-related behavior, such as undergoing training (Zohar, 2002b), developing positive-negative contingencies, and demonstrating safe practices (Tomas, Melia & Oliver, 1999), followers engaged in more safety-related behavior. When leaders had cooperative relationships with their employees, safety compliance was also enhanced. Several researchers (Hofmann, Morgeson, & Gerras, 2003; Zohar, 2000a) posited that leadership and safely are actually independent of each other and found support for safety being positively related to leadership when the supervisor clearly valued safety as a priority. Alternatively, when there was a poor safety climate (little value for safety) and positive leader/member exchange, employees engaged in safety behaviors less frequently. This suggests that leadership alone is not enough, but a culture of safety must also be created and expectations conveyed. Furthermore, Mullen and Kelloway (2009) found that leaders' safety attitudes (and employees' ratings of leader safety-specific behaviors) were highest when the leaders received safety-specific leadership training, as compared to when they received general leadership training.

In health care, it is becomingly increasingly clear that leaders throughout the organization have to be accountable for safety and quality, depending on their particular roles. This responsibility is increasingly complex due to the dynamic nature of health care, competing demands for resources, the escalating pressure for achieving quality and safety goals, and the proliferation of criteria that must be monitored and reported. Increasingly, physicians are becoming actively involved (Oliva & Totten, 2007; Prybil et al., 2009), as are boards of directors of health care systems (Caldwell, Butler, & Grah, 2008; Joshi & Hines, 2006; Prybil et al., 2009). However, there is relatively little research on the impact of leadership on safety and quality. Hoff, Jameson, Hannan, and Flink (2010) came to the conclusion that there is "little evidence for asserting the importance of any individual, group, or structural variable in error prevention or enhanced patient safety at the present time" (p. 3). What has been the focus of most of the research is studies on intermediate activities, tools, or initiatives that clinical or managerial leaders have put in place, for example, rapid response teams (Jones, Bleyer, & Petree, 2010), rounds (Frankel et al., 2008), patient safety audits (Ursprung et al., 2005); checklists (Tanner, 2010), and patient safety officers (Frankel, Gandhi, & Bates, 2003).

Wong and Cummings (2007) conducted a systematic review of 7 studies that examined the relationship between nursing leadership and patient outcomes. They found a significant positive relationship between leadership behaviors, styles and/or practices, and patient satisfaction, and a negative relationship between leadership behaviors, styles and/or practices, and adverse patient outcomes in nursing home residents. Jennings, Disch, and Senn (2008) reviewed two studies, chosen because they looked at measurable outcomes: one linking chief nurse officer leadership to a decline in patient falls and nosocomial bloodstream infections (Burritt, 2005), and another to communication, staffing, and leadership (Scott-Cawiezell et al., 2004). A number of other studies were mentioned but not reported in detail since they were narrative or descriptive of leadership styles or key executive characteristics. The authors concluded, "Ironically, although leadership is a topic of tremendous interest, little empirical evidence [to its effectiveness] exists" (Jennings et al., 2008, pp. 2-18). More recently, Richardson and Storr (2010) examined 11 studies, consisting of a systematic review, a cohort study, qualitative studies (4), cross-sectional studies (3), a survey, and an evaluation. They also commented that the quality of the papers was variable and provided limited evidence of nursing leadership, collaboration, or empowerment on nursing care and quality outcomes.

A general consensus is emerging that suggests that the leader possibly indirectly influences patient safety and quality of care. The two principal ways by which leaders are hypothesized to influence quality and safety are by creating a culture of safety (Krause & Weekley, 2005; Pronovost et al., 2003; Ruchlin, Dubbs, & Callahan, 2004) and by giving their employees the knowledge, skills, and attitudes to practice safely (American Association of Colleges of Nursing, 2008; Cronenwett et al., 2007). The two are interrelated.

The role of the chief nurse officer (CNO) in quality and safety

In a chapter in an Agency for Health Care Research and Quality text on quality and safety, Disch (2008) answers the question "Who should lead the patient quality/safety journey?" with a simple answer–the CNO. This person is a logical recommendation for several reasons:

- The nursing profession has been at the forefront of assuring quality and safety for decades.
- Nurses are at the patient's side 24/7 as care provider, integrator, and/or coordinator.
- Nurses understand what the issues are.
- Nurses have workable solutions.
- CNOs have the background, perspective, and platform to help.

Draper, Felland, Liebhaber, and Melichar (2008) noted that "nurses are the key caregivers in hospitals [and] significantly influence the quality of care provided and, ultimately, treatment and patient outcome" (p. 1). Wong and Cummings (2007) have noted that nursing leaders fill a vital responsibility in administering the context, staffing, and financial resources needed to provide effective care The Institute of Medicine report (2004) *Keeping Patients Safe* asserted that "the vigilance function often thrusts nurses into a role that has been described as the 'front line' of patient defense" (p. 35). Mason (2008) adds that this is a moral imperative: "Anything less violates the patient advocacy mantle that we claim as a core nursing role" (pp. 2-39).

The Gallup Poll's report (Institute of Medicine, 2010) titled *Nursing Leadership from Bedside to Boardroom: Opinion Leaders' Perceptions* identified nurses as being "one of the most trusted sources of health information," yet predicted they would have the least amount of influence on health care reform. A large majority of the opinion leaders would like nurses to have much more influence in reducing medical errors, increasing quality of care, and promoting wellness. The Institute of Medicine's 2011 report on the future of nursing advocated, "Leadership from nurses is needed at every level and across all settings. ... Nurses must understand that their leadership is as important to providing quality care as is their technical ability to deliver care at the bedside in a safe and effective manner" (p. 225).

Although there is much support for nurses leading the way, a recent study by Disch, Dreher, Davidson, Sinioris, and Wainio (2011) found that the specific role of the CNO in promoting quality and safety was unclear, and that physician leaders were often unaware of the CNO's participation in quality and safety initiatives. The eight CNOs in the study usually attended board meetings, but none were voting members of the board. One CNO gave a report on patient care at each meeting while several others periodically provided updates on relevant topics. Fortunately, there is increasing pressure to actively include CNOs and other community nursing leaders in board member roles. In a major report on governance in high-performing community health systems, a key recommendation was that "community health system boards and their CEOs should re-examine their current size and composition ... [and] consider the appointment of highly-respected and experienced nursing leaders as voting members of the board to complement physician members and strengthen clinical input in board deliberations" (Prybil et al., 2009, p. 41).

Creating a culture of safety

Everyone associated with an organization is responsible for promoting safety. In 2002, the Minnesota Alliance for Patient Safety (2002) developed a manifesto on patient safety, clarifying the roles of all stakeholders in promoting safe health care. Stakeholder groups include the board of trustees, senior leadership, middle managers, employees, physicians, patients, and families. Within organizations, there are formal and informal leaders who can influence care processes, communication channels, systems, and structures. A culture of safety is evident throughout an organization in the values, beliefs, attitudes, words, and actions of its stakeholders.

Cultures of safety possess three essential elements: (1) environmental structures and processes, (2) safety-promoting attitudes and perceptions, and (3) safety-related behaviors of individuals, both leaders and followers (Cooper, 2000). Rather than just focusing on the behavior of individuals, leaders know that safety is based in the culture and the system. In organizations that are highly reliable in being safe ("high-reliability organizations"), there is a continual drive toward the goal of maximum attainable safety, and there is recognition that the goal is not to eliminate errors but to prevent harm to the patient (Bagian, 2005). In these organizations, everyone is aware of the interconnected and dynamic nature of daily operations, and that a change in one area or process can ripple out to other areas within the organization. Reason and Hobbs (2003) caution that a safety culture should be "a wary one" with a "collective mindfulness" of the things that can go wrong. Safe clinical environments rely on leaders and staff to connect frequently, through such mechanisms as daily check-ins and huddles, to learn from and update each other on how things are going and what might be safety threats. Leaders who are committed to safety talk directly with frontline caregivers, through opportunities such as executive rounds and open forums, and keep the focus on what the employees and medical staff need to provide safe care to patients and families. Leaders who are committed to safety demonstrate this on a daily basis through their questions, decisions, and priorities. In an organization where concerns for patient safety are paramount, members of the board of directors know the key quality indicators as well as the financial metrics, and the board agenda often starts with the quality/safety content rather than being covered at the end of the meeting when time allows.

The Joint Commission (2009) developed a set of recommendation for leaders in assuring quality and safety in their Sentinel Event Alert #43, "Leadership Committed to Safety." This clarifies the behaviors expected of leaders and thus provides a consistent focus for leadership and a direction for research on the impact of leadership on patient outcomes.

A growing body of evidence suggests that there is a relationship between having a safe culture and a productive organization (Hofmann & Morgeson, 1999; Krause, 2004; Tansky & Cohen, 2001). Krause and Weekley (2005, p. 37) summarize these nine cultural characteristics predictive of successful organizational outcomes:

(1) Teamwork: the effectiveness of workgroups in meeting targets and deadlines
(2) Workgroup relations: the degree to which workers respect each other
(3) Procedural justice: the level at which workers rate the fairness of first-level supervisors
(4) Perceived organizational support: the level at which employees feel the organization is concerned for their well-being
(5) Leader/member exchange: the strength of relationship that workers feel they have with their supervisors
(6) Management credibility: the perception of consistency and fairness of management in dealing with workers
(7) Organizational value for safety: the perceived level of the organization's commitment to safety
(8) Upward communication: the adequacy of upward messages about safety
(9) Approaching others: the probability that workers will speak to each other about performance issues

Creating and sustaining change

Kotter, creator of a well-known model for change, notes that "leaders who successfully transform businesses do eight things right (and they do them in the right order)" (2010, p. 81). The eight steps of this model are are (1) establishing a sense of urgency, (2) forming a powerful guiding coalition, (3) creating a vision, (4) communicating the vision, (5) empowering others to act on the vision, (6) planning for and creating short-term wins, (7) consolidating improvements and producing still more change, and (8) institutionalizing new approaches.

However, as Bridges (1993) has noted, there is a difference between change and transition. Change occurs "when something new starts or something old stops, and it takes place at a particular point in time" (p. 17). Transition is more diffuse, "the gradual psychological process through which individuals and groups reorient themselves so that they can function and find meaning in a changed situation" (p. 17). Transition is the process by which the change is accepted and embedded within an organization. A change can be announced; the transition can take months or years. This distinction is important because it recognizes the extensive effort and time that may need to go into helping an organization accept a particular change. It is especially important when addressing quality and safety issues in an organization because efforts to change how one practices can evoke defensive reactions and resistance. It is also known that individuals can drift from adhering conscientiously to policies and practices, unless these are reinforced and strongly embedded within an organization (Just Culture Community, 2008).

Silversin and Kornacki (2000) have developed a pragmatic and helpful process for helping health care leaders deal with change and transition. Originally developed as a method for engaging physicians in working with hospital administrators to address quality and cost issues, it provides a blueprint for action with five areas for attention by leaders as they intentionally introduce a change into an organization.

Tension and remedy

This step requires the leader to identify why the change needs to be made, and pose possible remedies or solutions to the problem. Put another way, the leader has to create a tension between *what is* and *what could be* or *what needs to be*. Possible reasons for change can arise from answers to a variety of questions: Has a root cause analysis identified a major safety threat? Has a review of patient satisfaction data indicated an unacceptable level of performance? Are there societal or demographic reasons for the change? Is there a competitive reason for the change? Is new technology being introduced for which people need to be trained? Is there an exciting new approach to patient care that people want to try? In other words, why is the change necessary? What is apparent is that some changes are exciting, eagerly anticipated, and supported, while others may be resisted or rejected, and still other changes supported by some and not others. The change agent has to create the business, legal, or quality case for the change through whatever data would be compelling to those needing to change. This can include statistics, compelling stories, appreciative inquiry, benchmarking data, or regulatory mandate. The needed change should be clearly defined and then linked to the proposed remedy, for example, a practice change for catheter care, the introduction of bedside rounds, a patient/advisory council, or reporting requirements for serious reportable events. A compelling, well-stated vision of a preferred future with the change fully embedded in the organization is a powerful motivator for change.

Aligned leadership

Change requires strong, aligned leadership and committed, engaged followers. For successful change, there are several key roles that must be identified, and the leader must adequately consider who is in what role, whether they are clear in their role(s), and how their participation can be optimized in support of the change. The roles include the following:

(1) The sponsors, those individuals who have the power to launch and give approval to the change. These individuals usually have formal authority and the responsibility for holding people accountable. The initiating sponsor starts the change and authorizes it to happen, while the sustaining sponsor is the one who will assure that it gets carried out.

(2) The agents of change, those responsible for making the change happen. These individuals may or may not have line authority over those expected to change. Their role is to develop a plan to accomplish the change, diagnose any anticipated problems or reinforcing strategies, work with and through others to accomplish it, and acquire resources.

(3) The advocates or champions who lack formal authority in this situation but can support the change occurring. They are the cheerleaders. It's important to note, however, that advocates can also be those who advocate against a change and for the status quo.

(4) Those expected to change are all those who will have to do something different as a result of the change. This group of individuals can be found far away from the original change but be affected nonetheless

(5) Healthy skeptics, those individuals who pose questions about the need for the change, the way in which it's being proposed, or the benefits. While sometimes challenging to deal with, these people can be helpful in identifying potential weaknesses in the need for or plan of change. Asking "under what conditions could X change be made to work?" can sometimes elicit helpful suggestions.

The human dynamics

It is well known that individuals possess different levels of tolerance for change. In his landmark work on the diffusion of innovation, Rogers (2003) noted that people range from being active adopters of change to laggards who reluctantly come along when the vast majority of individuals have accepted the change. Bridges (1993) observed that people adapt to change differently, and that many factors enter into a person's ability to change.

There are many reasons why people resist change: earlier change attempts that failed, a sense that "this too shall pass," comfort with the status quo, inadequate communication about the benefits of the change, or too many initiatives at once. Given the current dynamic state of the health care industry, the phenomenon of change fatigue is understandable. Change fatigue "refers to impairments in an individual's and organization's abilities to cope with the ever-increasing scope and pace of change" (Valusek, 2007, p. 355).

In preparing to mount a change initiative, leaders need to assess their organization's change tolerance. What else is occurring at the present time? How could a particular change be connected to something else already going on in the organization? How could it be framed so that it is seen as a helpful adjunct rather than a burdensome interruption? Valusek (2007) advocates implementing a change calendar to manage the timing of changes and using a weekly time line to identify and coordinate the multitude of changes occurring across an organization.

Culture and compact

In their work with physicians, Silversin and Kornacki (2000) noted that "the culture defines normative behavior and typically is a barrier to physicians' embracing changes that call for new behaviors" (p. xvii). They go on to describe the implicit compact that organizational leaders have had with physicians, that is, admit patients, provide quality care, and we'll leave you alone. Today, that compact is no longer adequate for physicians, nurses, and other employees. All are called to deliver quality care in a cost-effective manner while providing a positive patient experience. This may be particularly challenging for nurses because of the close relationship and extended length of contact that they experience with patients and their families, often during a health care episode that is difficult in itself. Silversin and Kornacki (2000) describe culture as being "made up of individual and collective values, attitudes, and beliefs that translate into unwritten rules of behavior. These rules, or norms, clue us in to what others in the organization expect of us, and they allow us to predict their behavior" (p. 45). In introducing change and facilitating transitions, leaders have to take the organization's culture into serious consideration and assess a number of factors:

- What gets rewarded?
- Who is respected and admired?
- How are decisions made?
- How are they communicated?
- Whose input is vital?
- Whose support is essential?
- How is conflict dealt with?
- Are diverse ideas encouraged?
- Can you disagree with your department head?
- What motivates and excites people?

Measurement, incentives and rewards

Finally, for a change to take hold, tangible results have to be achieved, measured, and communicated. As an early step in the process, a desired vision or preferred future should be created and shared, preferably with input by those who will be affected by the change. Kouzes and Posner (2007) describe the importance of a vision and the leader's role in envisioning the future in a way that inspires others. "They see something out ahead, vague as it might appear from a distance, and they imagine that extraordinary feats are possible and that the ordinary could be transformed into something noble" (p. 105). Leaders also must be able to pragmatically envision better ways of doing immediate tasks, or tackling more mundane challenges. The leader has an idea, and then co-creates it with others to garner their ideas, support, and energy. This can be enjoyable when the change is widely embraced. It can be more difficult when introducing change that is difficult or imposed. During those times, according to Disch (1998), the leader's role may be "taking people on a journey in which nobody wants to go."

Identifying the specific goal to be achieved, developing concrete, measurable outcomes, and measuring the progress toward the goal are key stems in achieving change. Nelson, Batalden, and Godfrey (2007) have produced a rich compendium of resources in their book *Quality by Design*. This resource provides useful tools, case studies, references, and recommendations to help formal and informal leaders, students, and educators strengthen their competency in leading change to improve quality and safety.

Implementation strategies for education and practice

In addition to the strategies covered above in structuring change, several specific assignments are offered here to help nurses develop leadership skills for improving quality and safety.

- Partner a student nurse with a practicing leader involved in some aspect of operational quality and safety in health care to examine the leader's role
- Conduct an environmental assessment to identify a threat to quality and safety in the organization, and design a plan for change using Silversin's model
- Participate in a quality/safety committee meeting and analyze the formal and informal leadership roles displayed by members
- Conduct a review of articles on leadership's impact on quality/safety over the last 5 years in the *Joint Commission Journal on Quality and Patient Safety*
- Contrast the standards from the Joint Commission and the American Organization of Nurse Executives regarding the leader's role in quality and safety

- Attend a root cause analysis of a serious reportable event to (1) identify factors contributing to the event stemming from the culture, environment, and educational needs of staff; and (2) develop plans for their improvement
- Read *Wall of Silence* (Gibson & Singh, 2003) and identify leadership deficiencies
- Watch the video by Helen Haskell on her son's death (http://www.icvclients.com/ehcca/quality_2007/1_1045/) and reflect on the following questions: (1) Could this happen in your facility? (2) Why or why not? (3) What would be the leadership reaction? (4) What would be the staff's reaction?
- Conduct an assessment of your organization's safety culture
- Read about high-reliability organizations at (http://www.ahrq.gov/qual/hroadvice/hroadvice.pdf) and reflect on how closely your organization matches the description
- Read pages 221–254 and 269–284 of the Institute of Medicine's *Future of Nursing* report, identifying one course of action that you would like to undertake and three interested parties or stakeholders who would share your interest in change
- Write an issue brief (a compelling letter of 1–2 pages about an issue threatening quality or safety, using evidence to support its impact) with a recommended action to persuade an individual to take specific, concrete action

Conclusion

As the Institute of Medicine (2011) proclaims in its Key Message #3 in the *Future of Nursing*: "Nurses should be full partners, with physicians and other health care professionals, in redesigning health care in the United States" (p. 221). The tagline for this groundbreaking report is *Leading Change, Advancing Health*. Nursing leaders must be actively involved with others in transforming care delivery, nursing education, and the public's perception of nursing's role if the full impact of the report is to be realized. Nurses have long been known as the frontline of defense in the safety movement. Now nurses at all levels, and in all organizations, are equipped to also be the logical partners in leading this quality and safety journey (Robert Wood Johnson Foundation, 2010). Nurses as leaders, whether in formal or informal roles, must raise their voices in identifying the threats to quality and patient safety and in proposing the solutions to make health care safe for all.

References

American Association of Colleges of Nursing. (2008). *The essentials of baccalaureate nursing education for professional nursing practice*. Washington, DC: Author.

Bagian, J. P. (2005). Patient safety: What really is at issue? *Frontiers of Health Services Management, 22*(1), 3–16.

Boyatzis, R., & McKee, A. (2005). *Resonant leadership*. Boston, MA: Harvard Business School Press.

Bridges, W. (1993). Surviving corporate transition. Mill Valley, CA: William Bridges & Associates.

Burritt, J. E. (2005). Organizational turnaround: The role of the nurse executive. *JONA, 35*(11), 482–489.

Caldwell, C., Butler, G., & Grah, J. (2008). Breakthrough quality: What the board must do. *Trustee, 61*, 32–33.

Center for Spirituality and Healing. (2010). Whole systems leadership. Retrieved from http://www.csh.umn.edu/wsh/Leadership/index.htm/

Cooper, M. (2000). Towards a model of safety culture. *Safety Science, 36*, 111–136.

Cronenwett, L., Sherwood, G., Barnsteiner, J., Disch, J., Johnson, J., Mitchell, P., et al. (2007). Quality and safety education for nurses. *Nursing Outlook, 55*(3), 122–131.

Disch, J. (1998). Keynote presentation, Third Annual State of the Art Nursing Conference. Omaha, NE: Nebraska Health System.

Disch, J. (2008). Who should lead the patient safety/quality journey? In R. Hughes (Ed.), *Patient safety and quality: An evidence-based handbook for nurses* (pp. 2-41-2-43). AHRQ Publication No. 08-0043. Rockville, MD: Agency for Healthcare Research and Quality.

Disch, J. (2009). Generative leadership. *Creative Nursing, 15*(4), 172–177.

Disch, J., Dreher, M., Davidson, P., Sinioris, M., & Wainio, J. (2011). The role of the chief nurse officer in ensuring patient safety and quality. *JONA, 41*(4), 179–185.

Draper, D. A., Felland, L. E., Liebhaber, A., & Melichar, L. (2008). *The role of nurses in hospital quality improvement*. Research Brief #3. Washington, DC: Center for Studying Health System Change.

Dye, C. F., & Garman, A. N. (2006). *Exceptional leadership: 16 critical competencies for healthcare executives*. Chicago, IL: Health Administration Press.

Frankel, A., Gandhi, T. K., & Bates, D. W. (2003). Improving patient safety across a large integrated health care delivery system. *International Journal for Quality in Health Care, 15* (issue supplement), i31–i40.

Frankel, A., Grillo, S. P., Pittman, M., Thomas, E. J., Horowitz, L., Page, M., & Sexton, B. (2008). Revealing and resolving patient safety defects: The impact of leadership WalkRounds on frontline caregiver assessments of patient safety. *Health Services Research, 43*(6), 2050-2066.

Geller, E. S. (2000). 10 leadership qualities for a total safety culture. *Professional Safety, 45*, 38–41.

George, B. (2003). *Authentic leadership: Rediscovering the secrets to creating lasting value*. San Francisco, CA: Jossey-Bass.

Gibson, R., & Singh, J. P. (2003). *Wall of silence*. Washington, DC: LifeLine Press.

Grubbs, J. R. (1999). A transformational leader. *Occupational Health and Safety, 68*, 22–26.

Harris, M. C. (1998). Value leadership: *Winning competitive advantage in the information age*. Milwaukee, WI: ASQ Quality Press.

Hoff, T., Jameson, L., Hannan, E., & Flink, E. (2004). A review of the literature examining linkages between organizational factors, medical errors, and patient safety. *Medical Care Research Review, 61*(1), 3-37.

Hofmann, D. A., & Morgeson, E. P. (1999). Safety-related behavior as a social exchange: The role of perceived organizational support and leader-member exchange. *Journal of Applied Psychology, 84*, 286-296.

Hofmann, D. A., & Morgeson, F. P. (2004). The role of leadership in safety. In J. Barling & M. Frone (Eds.), *The psychology of workplace safety* (pp. 159–180). Washington, DC: American Psychological Association.

Hofmann, D. A., Morgeson, E. P., & Gerras, S. J. (2003). Climate as a moderator of the relationship between LMX and content specific citizenship behavior: Safety climate as an exemplar. *Journal of Applied Psychology, 88,* 170–178.

Hybels, B. (2002). *Courageous leadership*. Grand Rapids, MI: Zondervan.

Institute of Medicine. (2004). *Keeping patients safe: Transforming the work environment of nurses*. Washington, DC: National Academies Press.

Institute of Medicine. (2010). *Groundbreaking new study finds that diverse opinion leaders say nurses should have more influence on health systems and services*. Retrieved from http://www.rwjf.org/pr/product.jsp?id=54488

Institute of Medicine. (2011). *The future of nursing: Leading change, advancing health*. Washington, DC: National Academies Press.

Jennings, B. M., Disch, J., & Senn, L. (2008). Leadership. In R. Hughes (Ed.), *Patient safety and quality: An evidence-based handbook for nurses* (pp. 2-11–2-33). AHRQ Publication No. 08-0043. Rockville, MD: Agency for Healthcare Research and Quality.

Johnson, J. (2012). Quality improvement. In G. Sherwood & J. Barnsteiner (Eds.), *Quality and safety in nursing: A competency approach to improving outcomes*. Hoboken, NJ: Wiley-Blackwell.

Joint Commission. (2009). *Leadership committed to safety*. Sentinel Event #43, Retrieved from http://www.jointcommission.org/assets/1/18/SEA_43.pdf

Jones, C. M., Bleyer, A. J., & Petree, B. (2010). Evolution of a rapid response system from voluntary to mandatory activation. *Joint Commission Journal on Quality and Patient Safety, 36*(6), 266–270.

Joshi, M. S., & Hines, S. C. (2006). Getting the board on board: Engaging hospital boards in quality and patient safety. *Joint Commission Journal on Quality and Patient Safety, 32*(4), 179–187.

Just Culture Community. (2008). *Patient safety and the just culture: Overview*. [Booklet]. Plano, TX: Outcome Engineering.

Kotter, J. P. (2010). Leading change: Why transformation efforts fail. In *HBR's 10 must reads: The essentials* (pp. 137–152). Boston: Harvard Business Review Press.

Kouzes, J. M., & Posner, B. Z. (2007). *The leadership challenge* (4th ed.). San Francisco: Jossey-Bass.

Krause, T. R. (2004, June). Influencing the behavior of senior leadership: What makes a great safety leader? *Professional Safety,* 29–33.

Krause, T. R., & Weekley, T. (2005, November). Safety leadership. *Professional Safety,* 34–40.

Mason, D. J. (2008). Transforming health care for patient safety: Nurses' moral imperative to lead. In R. Hughes (Ed.), *Patient safety and quality: An evidence-based handbook for nurses* (pp. 2-35–2-40). AHRQ Publication No. 08-0043. Rockville, MD: Agency for Healthcare Research and Quality.

Minnesota Alliance for Patient Safety. (2002). Retrieved from http://www.mnpatientsafety.org/files/pdfs/A%20Call%20to%20Action.pdf

Mullen, J. E., & Kelloway, E. K. (2009). Safety leadership: A longitudinal study of the effects of transformational leadership on safety outcomes. *Journal of Occupational and Organizational Psychology, 82*(2), 253–272.

Nelson, E. C., Batalden, P. B., & Godfrey, M. M. (2007). *Quality by design: A clinical microsystems approach*. San Francisco: Jossey-Bass.

Northouse, P. (2010). *Leadership: Theory and practice* (5th ed.). Thousand Oaks, CA: Sage.

Oliva, J., & Totten, M. (2007). *A seat at the power table: The physician's role on the hospital board*. Chicago: Center for Health Care Governance.

Porter-O'Grady, T., & Malloch, K. (2007). *Quantum leadership: A resource for health care innovation* (2nd ed). Sudbury, MA: Jones and Bartlett.

Pronovost, P. J., Weast, B., Holzmueller, C. G., Rosenstein, B. J., Kidwell, R. P., Haller, K. B., et al. (2003). Evaluation of the culture of safety: Survey of clinicians and managers in an academic medical center. *Quality and Safety in Health Care*, *12*(6), 405–410.

Prybil, L., Levey, S., Peterson, R., Heinrich, D., Brezinski, P., Zamba, G., et al. (2009). *Governance in high-performing community health systems: A report on trustee and CEO views*. Chicago: Health Research and Educational Trust.

Rae-Dupree, J. (2008, November 2). It's no time to forget about innovation. *New York Times*, p. 4.

Reason, J., & Hobbs, A. (2003). Safety culture. In J. Reason & A. Hobbs, *Managing maintenance error: A practical guide* (pp. 145–158). Hampshire, England: Ashgate.

Richardson, A., & Storr, J. (2010). Patient safety: A literature review on the impact of nursing empowerment, leadership and collaboration. *International Nursing Review, 57*(1), 12–21.

Robert Wood Johnson Foundation. (2010). Nursing leadership from bedside to boardroom: Opinion leaders' perceptions. Retrieved from http://www.rwjf.org/pr/product.jsp?id=54350

Rock, D. (2006). *Quiet leadership: Six steps to transforming performance at work*. New York: HarperCollins.

Rogers, E. M. (2003). *Diffusion of innovations* (5th ed). New York: Free Press.

Ruchlin, H. S., Dubbs, N. L., & Callahan, M. A. (2004). The role of leadership in instilling a culture of safety: Lessons from the literature. *Journal of Healthcare Management*, *49*(1), 47–58.

Schwartz, R. W., & Tumblin, T. F. (2002). The power of servant leadership to transform health care organizations for the 21st-century economy. *Archives of Surgery*, *137*, 1419–1427.

Scott-Cawiezell, J., Schenkman, M., Moore, L., Vojir, C., Connolly, R. P., Pratt, M., & Palmer, L. (2004). *Journal of Nursing Care Quality*, *19*(3), 242–252.

Silversin, J., & Kornacki, M. J. (2000). *Leading physicians through change: How to achieve and sustain results*. Tampa, FL: American College of Chest Physicians.

Tanner, K. (2010). Checklists and teamwork lower number of surgery deaths. Retrieved from http://www.huffingtonpost.com/2010/10/20/study-lives-saved-by-surg_n_769421.html

Tansky, J. W., & Cohen, D. J. (2001). The relationship between organizational support, employee development and organizational commitment: An empirical study. *Human Resource Development Quarterly*, *12*, 285–300.

Tomas, J. M., Melia, J. L., & Oliver, A. (1999). A cross-validation of a structural equation model of accidents: Organizational and psychological variables as predictors of work safety. *Work and Stress*, *13*, 49–58.

Ursprung, R., Gray, J. E., Edwards, W. H., Horvar, J. D., Nickerson, J., Plsek, P., et al. (2005). Real time patient safety audits: Improving safety every day. *Quality and Safety in Health Care*, *14*, 284–289.

Valusek, J. R. (2007). The change calendar: A tool to prevent change fatigue. *Joint Commission Journal on Quality and Patient Safety*, *33*(6), 355–360.

Wong, C. A., & Cummings, G. G. (2007). The relationship between nursing leadership and patient outcomes: A systematic review. *Journal of Nursing Management*, doi: 10.1111/j.1365-2834.2007.00723.x

Zohar, D. (2002a). The effects of leadership dimensions, safety climate and assigned priorities on minor injuries in work groups. *Journal of Organizational Behavior*, *23*(1), 75–92.

Zohar, D. (2002b). Modifying supervisory practices to improve sub-unit safety: A leadership-based intervention model. *Journal of Applied Psychology*, *87*, 156–163.

Chapter 16

Creating Cultures of Excellence: Transforming Organizations

Pamela Klauer Triolo, PhD, RN, FAAN

The research is clear. The business case for quality has been made. The pathways, tools, and strategies for performance improvement have been in existence for well over fifty years. There are research-driven models for organizational improvement with demonstrated results. Then why is it that a recent *New England Journal of Medicine* article (Landrigan et al., 2010) reported that there has been little improvement in quality in U.S. hospitals over the past decade? Why is it so difficult to create cultures of quality and safety? Why is it that some institutions achieve it and others do not? How do hospitals and other care settings operate as high-reliability organizations so that every patient receives the best quality care every time? Why does it take so long for changes to occur in health care practice, some say as many as twenty years (Bohmer, 2010)?

While quality improvement (QI) and performance improvement (PI) are sometimes used interchangeably, both QI and PI are constantly developing, and there is no discrete boundary between them. Although QI and PI grew from different origins, they both take a systems view. Fundamentally, PI addresses human performance in organizations at three levels: individual, process, and organization. Since this chapter focuses on culture and takes a comprehensive view, the term *performance improvement* is used. PI is used as the organizing framework for a variety of federal agencies as well as professional organizations, from the National Institute of Standards and Technology in the Baldrige Award to the American Medical Association in the Physician Consortium for Performance Improvement (http://www.nist.gov/baldrige/publications/criteria.cfm, http://www.ama-assn.org/resources/doc/cqi/pcpi-brochure.pdf).

Our challenge in nursing is to understand that using one tool, strategy, or model will not leverage organizational change. As Albert Einstein wisely said,

Quality and Safety in Nursing: A Competency Approach to Improving Outcomes, First Edition. Edited by Gwen Sherwood and Jane Barnsteiner.

"Doing the same thing over and over again achieves the same results." If we have not prepared clinicians and leaders for not only practicing nursing but doing so with a mindset that their role is to continuously improve the quality of care and the environment by continuously learning and evolving themselves, then change will never happen. If we have not prepared all nurses with some of the basic understanding of how organizations work like living systems, then it is impossible for a nurse to see how reluctance to change a practice, or impairment from sleep deprivation or other human factors, creates a ripple effect across the unit that can result in practice stagnation, and in some cases, commit errors that kill. The Quality and Safety Education for Nurses (QSEN) project specified knowledge, skills, and attitude objectives (Appendix A and B) designed to help transform nursing practice so that quality and safety are part of every nurse's role identity and responsibility (Cronenwett et al., 2007; Cronenwett et al., 2009). Knowing how quality improvement and safety awareness fit within the organizational culture lays the critical foundation for organizational excellence as described in this chapter; it begins from an organizational philosophy lived out in each employee's application to their own work.

The following analogy will illustrate the ingredients required to transform organizations. One tool from the tool box will not build a home. The creative journey of home building, the transformation of a piece of land into a home, begins first with a vision—seeing the right house on a mountain slope or green space. With the right leader (builder) who has the right "stuff" in every way, blueprints, the clear aligned plan, are developed. Then the team of electricians, carpenters, plumbers, and tile layers is formed. The team members have not only essential but high-quality skills, a sense of the art and science of their trade, a commitment to excellence, and a fundamental awareness of building codes to protect the people doing the building as well as guarantee the safety of the future occupants. The blueprints are designed so that every trade knows the direction and their unique role in transforming this space into a home. A continuous cycle of feedback is built into the process as blueprints are adapted, quality is evaluated, and changes are made along the way. Every tool in the tool box is used; the synergistic strength and talents of many, guided by the leadership of the builder and the interests of the stakeholder (the homeowner), culminate in the achievement of the goal.

Health care is one of the most complex businesses in the world. The business, economic, and social case for quality has been made, beginning with Deming, continuing with Donabedian (2005), through Berwick with the Institute for Health Care Improvement (www.ihi.org), and the Institute of Medicine (www.iom.edu). The "missing link" to achieving breakthroughs may be integrating the importance of the focus on quality and safety into the preparation of clinicians. Cultures of excellence are not possible without an organization embracing a focus on quality and safety from the point of care through the board room. This chapter will provide an overview of how organizations work and change, supply some guiding principles for organizational development, and describe how, using blended tools and strategies, a committed group of the right people can create a culture of excellence, a level of achievement that demonstrates the highest level of quality and safety.

Global formula for creating cultures of excellence

The fundamental unit of every organization is people. People come to work with their hopes and dreams, values, skills, needs, and expectations. Organizations are living and breathing biological systems. Using Systems Thinking, a vital tool for organizational development, people are like the red blood cells of the circulatory system. The quality of the cell influences the system's ability to oxygenate tissue and organs. Oxygen is a fundamental unit of life. The same is true of people in organizations. The opportunity to leverage high quality is firmly based on the caliber of the people hired, their willingness to continuously learn, and their values about life and work. Systems that value quality and safety must demonstrate those attributes at every level of the organization. Attention to quality and safety are fundamental to cultures of excellence.

Culture is often described as "the way we work." Each college, university, hospital, or business has not only an overarching culture but hundreds of subcultures. Each culture is integrated by a set of values, attitudes and beliefs, social and professional norms, systems, and structures. Safety and quality must be imbedded into the culture as values. In order to leverage lasting change, the values of safety and quality must be aligned and woven through everything from job descriptions to policies and procedures to performance evaluations. Communication, from websites, to e-mailed bulletins, to nursing publications, must consistently repeat the values to the community. Changing a culture, moving it from mediocrity to excellence, or from chaos to stability, takes years because it involves adjustments in every aspect of the structure and function.

Since the organization is a system, change in one area creates a cascading impact on the rest of the organization. The following are two examples; in the first, the change does not consider organizational improvement while the second does. Example 1: A 10% across-the-board budget cut applied uniformly across cost centers can affect the speed, service, programs, and people in a destructive manner. How will this decision and the one below impact safety and quality of the organization? An alternative approach of budget adjustments based on supporting key priorities, consolidation of services, and eliminating non-value added programs, may disrupt the system less and lead to a goal of more efficient service. Example 2: A hospital with the goal of achieving Magnet recognition decides to increase the number of BSN prepared RNs. Though positive, this will also impact the system, but it is managed with planning. For example, by hiring only new graduates with a BSN, the hospital creates an infrastructure to collaborate with schools of nursing to provide BSN classes on site or through online learning supported by tuition assistance to assist in-house staff to meet the goal. Expectations without infrastructure are at risk for failure. Finally, expectation must be built into performance evaluations and career ladders. This will be examined later in the chapter.

People development is crucial to increasing organizational capacity for change and growth essential to sustaining a focus on safety and quality. If people are not learning about safety science and their quality improvement metrics, they cannot perform at new levels. Great football teams are not formed by picking players randomly out of grocery stores. Prospective players are carefully screened, their performance in action is observed, and they compete against other candidates for starting roles on the team. Once selected, the player, who has already demonstrated his commitment to successful performance by studying plays, working out with a rigorous training schedule, eating to maintain the proper weight for the position, and then practicing his role, is continuously evaluated for performance.

Yet often we, the practitioners, or we, the managers in health care, act as if we do not need to improve our performance by tending to our physical health or to our intellectual strength by continuous learning and self-care. The number one job of leaders is the creation of the infrastructure and expectations for a vital, learning organization. Developing others, while teaching through role modeling, is essential to a culture of excellence.

To create a learning organization, it is important to consider how people learn. The Center for Creative Leadership reports that leaders primarily develop their skills from experience (Pulley & Gurvis, 2004; Yip, 2009). Development needs to be planned, not happen haphazardly. The continual change that comes with a focus on quality and safety is built on three components: leadership, performance improvement and models of guiding principles. Changes that may be both system level and unit level require coordination with the various types of staff to direct the pace of change as well as the data management that drives initiation of change. The focus on safety requires leaders to provide the resources to avoid the danger of work-arounds, assure safe medication administration, and manage safe staffing.

Leadership

Leadership is the first component in the transformational model and the fundamental currency of cultures of excellence (Figure 16.1). Leadership is the driver for organizational change and is the common element in models from the Burke-Litwin Model (Burke, 2002) through the National Quality Award Baldrige (see Figure 16.2) through ANCC Magnet Recognition (Figure 16.3). Leadership has been defined in many ways. An effective definition is described by Kouzes and Posner (2002): Leadership is everyone's business; it is built on relationships and is composed of a learnable set of practices and a visible set of behaviors. Leadership in cultures of excellence is found at all levels of the organization from the point of care, through middle management to senior administration. Leadership is a "choice," not a position (Covey, 2004).

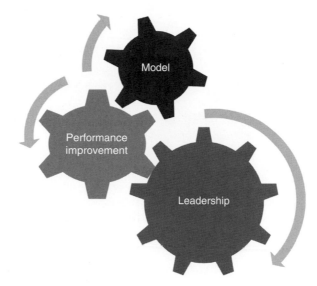

Figure 16.1 Global formula for creating cultures of excellence.

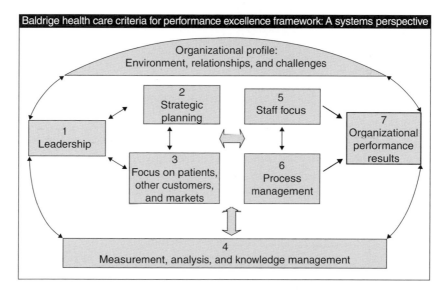

Figure 16.2 Baldrige systems model.
Reprinted from 2011–2012 *Health Care Criteria for Performance Excellence* with permission from the Baldrige Performance Excellence Program at the National Institute of Standards and Technology in Gaithersburg, MD.

Leadership at all levels of the organization is essential to creating a culture of quality and safety (Disch, 2012). The ingredients for leading successful change and managing the emotional transition response of people are clear but varied. Leadership begins with a respectful environment, then the creation of

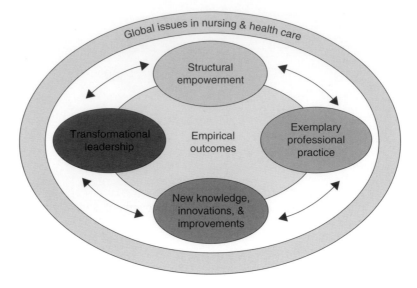

Figure 16.3　ANCC Magnet Recognition Program magnet model.

trust that create the potential for relationships. It is through relationships that we influence behavior. Leaders who are invisible, who do not respect and trust their followers, cannot lead them (O'Toole, 1995).

Performance improvement

The second major component of creating a culture of excellence, beyond leadership and people, is embedding a process for continuous performance improvement into the culture. The steps of the nursing process provide a formula for advancing an organization, not only its processes, but its people. The performance improvement cycle is assess, prioritize/plan, implement/execute, and evaluate discussed in the next section.

Models and guiding principles

The third component in the model for building excellence is using models and guiding principles. There are effective organizational development models for excellence, such as the Baldrige Performance Excellence Program and the Magnet Recognition Program, that consider the dynamic flow of organizations. Criterion-based programs provide a map for the journey. These programs with their integrated models can be used as templates, applied to, or assessed against. The Baldrige and Magnet models have demonstrated results that provide a business case for their use. In addition, many professional organizations are producing guidelines for practice rooted in research. The evidence-based leader is constantly scanning the literature for new findings to translate to the work setting.

To sum up, the overarching model for organizational excellence has three major components: leadership, performance improvement, and a model to chart the way. These three components work together synergistically. One component alone cannot achieve results. In management science, the concept of duality means that the leader focuses on multiple courses of action. Duality can mean pursuing multiple pathways, but it also can mean the synergy that comes from the alignment of strategies. Leadership is discussed in Chapter 15 of this book (Disch, 2012); hence, the remainder of this chapter will focus on performance improvement and models for performance excellence.

Performance improvement

Taking the concept of duality one step further, the continuous improvement process must be imbedded in a goal to actually drive the organization to quality (see Figure 16.4). The goal could be as simple as reducing wait time for everything in a hospital. Or it could be as complex as a school's achieving the Baldrige National Quality Award using the education criteria or becoming accredited by one of the national accreditation agencies. Capturing the hearts and minds of people to align the workforce to achieve transformation requires a clear, value-driven, and measureable goal that is communicated through all tiers of the organization in a consistent fashion. The four components are assessment, plan and prioritize, implement, and evaluate.

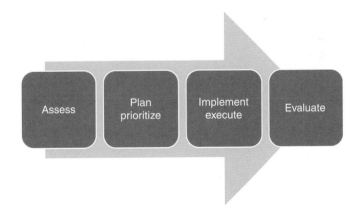

Figure 16.4 Duality: goal imbedded in process improvement.

Assessment

The performance improvement cycle begins with assessment, both macro and micro, local and global (Johnson, 2012). The good clinician always begins with assessment, taking a good history, evaluating through a physical, and reviewing lab results, before beginning care or treatment. Leaders must begin with assessment, thinking globally (national) and locally (internal). There are three major categories of assessment: people, core business, and financial. Since this chapter focuses on people and how they develop and change, this section will provide a brief overview of the types of assessment related to people. Figure 16.5 illustrates layers of assessments: global, population or stakeholder, and individual. The transformational leader will use at least one assessment strategy or tool from each of these layers and usually several to get a good picture of the issues and challenges they face. Assessment is the first step in health care, and the great leader remembers that he or she is a clinician first. Successful leaders assess frequently and take the pulse of all areas of the organization they hope to lead to excellence.

Assessment instruments can be qualitative or quantitative or both and can be created or purchased. Assessment can be as simple as looking at the existing data, such as turnover or student satisfaction, to see if there are issues. If there is high turnover, root cause analysis will determine factors and the actions that need to follow. It is vitally important to address the root cause and not only the presenting data (turnover, satisfaction). Below is an example.

In 1998, the chief nursing officer council of the Texas Medical Center in Houston met on a monthly basis to discuss issues and concerns together. This coalition of nurse leaders from diverse hospital types, including tertiary acute care, which also included children's hospitals and cancer centers, found one thing in common: nurses were leaving the Texas Medical Center to work in

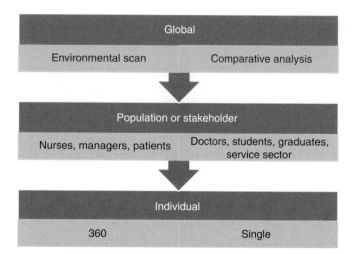

Figure 16.5 Layers of assessment.

community hospitals. This exodus of intellectual currency had a great impact on the quality and safety of the work environment. Although they thought they knew why nurses were leaving, they never anticipated the reason they found. The chief nursing officer council hired a marketing company to conduct focus groups on nurses who left. They suspected that parking, the commute, and gas prices might be the reason; however, the primary reason for the turnover was perceived physician abuse. Following this finding, they created a coalition with the CEO council who aligned the boards, medical staff leadership, and administration at each hospital in a series of strategies that focused on creating respectful cultures with consequences for physicians who were not respectful. Research and experience tell us that healthy nurse-physician relationships are essential to a culture of quality and safety. Chapter 13 discusses interpersonal relationships as related to quality and safety (Moore, Dolansky, & Singh, 2012).

In the above case, action based on speculation could have created new marketing campaigns to win nurses back and increased salaries to attract nurses. Yet the underlying problem would not have been addressed, wasting millions of dollars.

The second example is at the individual level in which assessment is an effective learning tool for the individual as well as the leader. Assessments can include a 360 model in which an individual completes a self-assessment and then is assessed by their boss, peers, and any direct reports. There are research-driven assessment instruments that measure values, leadership potential, leadership competencies, employee engagement, trust, emotional intelligence, spiritual intelligence, personality style, learning agility, and learning style, to name a few. These knowledge, skills, and attitudes are also reflected in the six quality and safety competencies defined by the QSEN project (Cronenwett et al., 2007; Cronenwett et al., 2009). Examples of their application are reflected in the tool kit used at the University of Pittsburgh Medical Center. The Leadership Development Intensive designed by the author to develop high-performing executives both nationally and internationally used a suite of assessments that included Emergenetics, DiSC, Emotional Intelligence through the Emotional Competency Index, Benchmarks, the MBTI, and the Hogan Leadership Forecast Series. Knowledge of self is the first step in becoming a successful leader, and assessments provide clear feedback. Knowledge of self creates the potential for understanding others and forging teams. These could also be folded into transition-to-practice programs in clinical settings or used by nurse faculty in helping students develop leadership capacity.

Performance improvement is a cycle that never ends. The assessment results become the foundation of a dynamic plan. The most effective strategy requires flexibility, with the leader constantly recalibrating the plan based on new data, priorities, and the readiness for change. Ralph Waldo Emerson said, "The voyage of the best ship is a zigzag line of a hundred tacks." A great leader, like a great sailor, is making constant adjustments to the plan that considers new data or issues.

Plan and prioritize

Plan and prioritize, the second phase of organizational continuous improvement, works best when imbedded in a model. In the science of organizational development, organizations are described as having transformational factors and transactional factors (Burke, 2002). These concepts are important to the understanding of how change actually occurs during the planning process as well as fundamental to the structure of models that leverage change. The concept of transformation is based on Burns's (1978) comparison of two types of leadership.

Transformational leaders bring about sustainable change. The imprint of a transformational leader is long-standing. Transactional leaders, on the other hand, view the leader-follower relationship as a transaction: if you do this you will be rewarded. Transformational factors, those that have the potential to transform an organization toward excellence, include leadership, strategic planning, organizational culture, mission and strategy, individual and organizational performance, and external environment. The transactional factors, those that managers often seem to focus on, are structure, management processes, policies and procedures, task requirements, and so forth.

Models that recognize quality

Organizations that have embraced the significance of a culture of quality pursue models integrated into national recognition programs rooted in research. The model supports the organizational goal and provides a blueprint, a clear strategy or process for action. Models that support excellence are dynamic versus static. Three models designed to drive an organization toward excellence are briefly described in this section: The Baldrige Performance Excellence Program, The Magnet Recognition Program, and Great Places to Work. Each of these models includes transformational and transactional factors. These three models are national and/or international awards for quality and business results.

The Baldrige National Quality Award is a U.S. Presidential Award given annually to one organization in each of three sectors: education, health care, and business. The Baldrige Performance Excellence Program is described as a management framework based on results in which excellence is viewed as a journey and not a destination. The mission is to improve the competiveness and performance of U.S. organizations. The Baldrige Criteria for Performance Excellence (Figure 16.2) provide the framework as well as an assessment tool for analyzing organizational strengths and opportunities for improvement. Performance excellence as defined by the Baldrige Performance Excellence Program is an integrated approach to organizational management that results in delivery of ever-improving value to customers and stakeholders, contributing to organizational sustainability; improvement of overall organizational effectiveness and capabilities; and organizational and personal learning.

Performance management framework
scoring 2011–2012

1. Leadership (120)
2. Strategic planning (85)
3. Customer focus (85)
4. Measurement, analysis and knowledge
   management (90)
5. Workforce focus (85)
6. Operations focus (85)
7. Organizational performance results (450)

Figure 16.6 Baldrige criteria.

Analyzing the components of the Baldrige scoring (Figure 16.6), one sees Donabedian's (2005) triad: structure, process, and outcome, the foundation of quality. The Baldrige Award scoring criteria balance structure and process with a heavy weight in outcomes. The transformational factors of leadership and strategic planning are also heavily weighted in the scoring process. In addition, Baldrige criteria are scored based on a variety of factors including deployment, integration, and learning, as well as comparisons and trends in results (Baldrige, 2011).

Baldrige criteria assist the three sectors in achieving human, financial, and stakeholder world-class results. For example, the education criteria are designed to assist educational organizations achieve and sustain the highest levels of student learning outcomes, customer satisfaction and engagement, product and service outcomes, financial and market results, and social responsibility.

The Magnet Recognition Program, established 25 years ago to recognize nursing excellence, is the highest level of recognition that the American Nurses Credentialing Center can give to health care organizations that employ registered nurses. The original components of the Magnet Program were based on research published by McClure, Poulin, Sovie, and Wandelt (1983) that identified 14 factors that when embedded into the culture created cultures of excellence. The Forces of Magnetism focused on development of the nursing workforce and building environments for the highest quality patient care.

In 2007, the Magnet Commission launched a dynamic new model based not only on the recommendations for change made during Magnet Program redesign but through expert panels and research (Drenkard, Wolf, & Morgan, 2011; Triolo, Scherer, & Floyd, 2006; Wolf, Triolo, & Reid Ponte, 2008). This model (Figure 16.4) illustrates an evidence-based program built to incorporate transformational factors that mirror Baldrige and incorporate a greater focus on outcomes. Like Baldrige, the Magnet goal of excellence is ongoing, not an end point.

Analysis of the research on Magnet facilities (Drenkard, 2010; Drenkard, Wolf, & Morgan, 2011) describes an extensive return on investment: increased

RN retention and lower burnout, reduced use of agency RNs, increased patient satisfaction, increased RN satisfaction, decreased mortality rates, decreased pressure ulcer rates, and decreased falls, to name a few. Many research studies describe a strong link between using the Magnet model to create the infrastructure and develop the capacity to create a culture of excellence. Organizations must be redesignated on a regular cycle. In early 2011, there were over 380 Magnet-designated hospitals. Unlike Baldrige, there is no limit on the number of health care organizations that can be designated.

The Great Places to Work model is the foundation for the Fortune "100 Best Companies to Work for in America" list. The model is: a Great Place to Work is one in which you "trust the people you work for, have pride in what you do, and enjoy the people you work with" (Great Places to Work, 2011). The model has five dimensions: credibility, respect, fairness, pride, and camaraderie. The mission of Great Places to Work is to help companies transform their workplace, much like high-reliability organizations focused on cultures of safety. Congruent with the principles of teamwork and collaboration (Disch, 2012), this company believes that trust-based relationships are the foundation of every great workplace and that any place can be a great place to work. Relationships are at the heart of transformational leadership founded on the concepts of emotional intelligence. Leadership is at the core of creating cultures of quality and safety in which the environmental context is so critical.

Great Places to Work surveys employees with a 15-minute, 58-item trust survey that assesses cultures and identifies best companies. Research on the 100 Best Companies to Work for in America has demonstrated that these companies receive more qualified job applicants, have lower turnover, have higher customer satisfaction and loyalty, and the cultures foster greater innovation, creativity, and risk taking. All of these are demonstrated in cultures of excellence. People with the knowledge, skills, and attitudes use a model to plan and guide the work, and create alignment with organizational direction and goals with a clear path to quality outcomes.

Implementation and execution

Successful performance improvement is a partnership between staff, middle management, and senior leadership. This partnership is possible when values are aligned; there are trusting relationships, clear communication, and willingness to learn. Creating the potential for such relationships is a lot of work, and the job of senior leadership is to set the tone and example.

While there are many assets and barriers to change that range from financial to political, organizational psychology develops three areas: development, readiness, and response to change. Every organizational culture has a predominant learning style that may be introverted, constantly looking within for answers, or extroverted, scanning the environment for new initiatives, or benchmarking against other like organizations. Senge (1990) also describes how organizations usually have some form of learning disability. An organizational learning disability, like a classic individual learning disability, means that a culture is growth challenged and limited by mental models.

Learning is essential for individual performance to improve. Yet to be open to learning, the individual must have commitment, courage, and energy, and must feel accountable for development. There are many personal barriers to learning: anxiety, fear of taking risks, arrogance, lack of commitment, and unwillingness to feel discomfort, to name a few. Management is accountable for developing the infrastructure and unit culture for formal and informal learning. Encouraging pursuit of advanced degrees is a desired goal; the evidence indicates that the higher the percentage of BSN-prepared staff, the lower patient morbidity and mortality (Aiken, Clarke, Cheung, Sloane, & Silber, 2001). As important, each work area unit should be a living laboratory, where mentoring, discovery, practice, and research foster the growth of the team and drive performance improvement. A learning organization operationalizes the value of learning in job descriptions and performance appraisals.

Readiness for change is perhaps the most difficult goal to achieve but is essential for successful quality and safety transformation. In order for change to happen, the workforce's will and motivation must align with the goal and the process. Readiness depends on a culture of learning. The foundation of readiness is willingness to learn, trusting, and a perception of a fair transparent process. Emotionally, people seek recognition of their value; intellectually, they want their ideas to be considered. The marriage of trust, productivity, buy-in, and engagement drives change (Kim & Mauborgne, 2005).

Change is a continuous process, and leaders have many forces to consider. Change is the event: marriage, divorce, birth of a baby, merger, downsizing. The psychological response to change is called transition (Bridges, 2009). Transition mimics the stages of grief. It is a unique experience for each person, and the response can be compounded if many changes are occurring in a person's life. For example, the staff nurse who has just had a baby and moved into a new house resists when the manager asks her to support a new initiative. She is overloaded with the emotion of transition.

Transition has three stages: (1) ending (letting go of the old identity), (2) neutral zone (the stage between when the old is gone and the new is not in place), and (3) beginning (Bridges, 2009). The neutral zone is a dangerous place where old weaknesses return, historical resentments flourish, and an increase in errors, illness, and absenteeism occurs. During this period of time, organizational performance slides and it is vitally important to be clear about the process, communicate constantly and supportively, and keep the neutral zone as short as possible. Although staff may be resistant to change, an example may be implementing an electronic health record, organizational performance may deteriorate, but it is important to have additional resources in place, constant communication from leadership regarding the status, and opportunities to voice concerns. Having adequate processes in place insures patient safety.

Change initiatives often fail because of execution errors. Sustaining change requires following three important steps: (1) setting a clear, realistic, and measureable goal; (2) creating a compelling scorecard to measure progress; and (3) deployment. Deployment means that the high-level goal is translated into specific tactics or actions. The tactics are then assigned to individuals or teams that are accountable for results within the timeline. Flawless execution requires that new behaviors are expected and consequences developed. Another example: a hospital in the interest of achieving greater supply cost containment develops an online ordering system with specific vendors versus a paper and pencil system with multiple vendors. Just communicating this, without training staff in using the system and creating consequences for work-arounds, the change will not be sustained or it will be implemented inconsistently.

Successful execution requires goal clarity, commitment, translation, development and readiness, infrastructure, and engagement of the workforce. Leaders who successfully drive an organization to performance improvement juggle multiple tasks while attending to the needs of employees.

Communication is not only a factor in safety, it is also important for trust between providers. Communication patterns within an organization reflect the culture and should be planned versus allowed to randomly occur. There should be a strategy in place for cascading communication from senior administration to middle management to staff. Staffs want regular communication from their supervisor rather than hearing it through the grapevine or reading about it in the newspaper first, which breaks trust not easily won back. Routine communication needs to include 24/7 rounds, staff meetings, town hall meetings, websites, and letters to staff.

The communication medium must match the message. That means the initial news of a major shift, such as closing part of the hospital, should not be sent by e-mail. Senior administration should hold meetings with workers on all shifts, deliver the message with compassion, describe the process and timeline, and explain the "why" behind the "what."

Finally, if leaders are to transform organizations, they must have discipline, passion, and conscience (Covey, 2004). They must have the discipline to forge vision with commitment and face the facts about what really needs to happen and what it will take to reach the outcomes. They must have the passion, the fire, to maintain the vision over time. Leaders are guided by an ethical framework with a moral sense of what is right and wrong, of timing and pace reflecting the importance of their employees, and of managing the stress of transition. Decisions and actions are driven from the spirit and not the ego.

Evaluation

While there are many forms of evaluation, one of the first principles of organizational development is that people are the fundamental unit of an organization. It is important to focus on people who must learn, grow, and change in order for an organization to change. Performance evaluation is an area most often neglected in considering all of the factors that must be implemented into an organization for it to grow to excellence.

Change initiatives fail when management neglects to provide rewards and consequences for individual performance. Position descriptions must be updated to match the values and goals of the organization to assure the right people are hired and retained; they must have feedback consistent with the goals and values of the organization. There must be a consistent message on performance, consequences, and rewards to maintain trust between management and employees. Employees must have feedback consistent with the goals and values of the organization. Stellar plans, terrific communication, and research-driven models do not change an organization. Staffs suffer cognitive dissonance when the leadership says they value one thing and then behave differently, shattering trust.

The ABC model is known to improve individual performance (Daniels & Daniels, 2004). The ABC model for performance management is built on shaping behavior through three components that must be present and work together to shape performance. The *A* refers to antecedents, anything that prompts people to act. Examples of antecedents are communication platforms such as websites or other forms of information sharing, position description, career ladders, educational programs, and interviewing processes. The *B* refers to behaviors, which is what a person says or does. The new career ladder includes an expectation that only nurses with a BSN can advance to Level II. One nurse goes back to school to achieve a BSN. Another nurse decides not to go back to school. The *C* stands for consequences that happen to a person as a result of the behavior. Consequences can be both positive and negative. For the nurse who achieves the BSN, positive consequences such as the potential for advancement on the career ladder are possible. The nurse who does not choose to go back to school will not advance and may be confined to the same pay grade for the remainder of his or her career. The ABC model fits well with the focus on quality and safety so that behaviors link with consequences.

In an organization that values the ABC model of performance management, job descriptions, infrastructure for development, career ladders, and performance evaluations align with the goals and values of the organization. If education is valued, it is seen in both the job description and performance evaluation. Aligned systems achieve results.

Conclusion

Creating a culture of excellence by learning and applying new quality and safety competencies is challenging work. Yet it is some of the most important work in health care. In this chapter, we described the synergy that must happen between leadership, performance improvement, and a model or models. We described the complexities of organizations and that change is not possible if people do not learn and grow. Excellence in health care requires a commitment on the part of everyone in the organization to grow and develop, and mindfully engage to improve patient care outcomes. It is this mindful engagement that builds an organizational culture based on quality and safety.

References

Aiken, L., Clarke, S. P., Cheung, R. B., Sloane, D. M., & Silber, J. H. (2003) Educational levels of hospital nurses and surgical patient mortality. *Journal of the American Medical Association, 290*(12), 1617-1623.

Bohmer, R. M. J. (2010). Fixing health care on the front lines. *Harvard Business Review, 88*(4), 62-73.

Baldrige Performance Excellence Program. (2011). Retrieved March 10, 2011, from http://www.baldrige21.com/Baldrige%20Scoring%20System.html

Bridges, W. (2009). Transitions: Making the most of change (3rd ed.). Philadelphia: Da Capo Press.

Burke, W. W. (2002). Organization change: Theory and practice. Thousand Oaks, CA: Sage.

Burns, J. (1978). *Leadership*. New York: Harper and Row.

Covey, S. R. (2004). *The 8th habit: from effectiveness to greatness*. New York: Free Press.

Cronenwett, L., Sherwood, G., Barnsteiner, J., Disch, J., Johnson, J., Mitchell, P., et al. (2007). Quality and safety education for nurses. *Nursing Outlook, 55*(3), 122-131.

Cronenwett, L., Sherwood, G., Pohl, J., Barnsteiner, J., Moore, S., Taylor Sullivan, D. T., et al. (2009). Quality and safety education for advanced practice nursing practice. *Nursing Outlook, 57*(6), 338-348.

Daniels, A. C., & Daniels, J. E. (2004). Performance management: changing behavior that drives organizational effectiveness. Atlanta: Performance Management.

Disch, J. (2012). Leadership to create change. In G. Sherwood & J. Barnsteiner (Eds.), *Quality and safety in nursing: A competency approach to improving outcomes*. Hoboken, NJ: Wiley-Blackwell.

Donabedian, A. (2005). Evaluating the quality of medical care. *Milbank Quarterly, 83*(4), 691-729.

Drenkard, K. (2010). The Business Case for Magnet. *Journal of Nursing Administration, 40*(6), 263-271.

Drenkard, K., Wolf, G., Morgan, S. H. (Eds.). (2011). Magnet: The next generation–nurses making the difference. Silver Springs, MD: American Nurses Credentialing Center.

Great Places to Work. (2011). Retrieved March 7, 2011 from http://www.greatplacetowork.com/who_we_are/index.php

Johnson, J. (2012). Quality improvement. In G. Sherwood & J. Barnsteiner (Eds.), *Quality and safety in nursing: A competency approach to improving outcomes*. Hoboken, NJ: Wiley-Blackwell.

Kim, W. C., & Mauborgne, R. (2005). *Blue ocean strategy*. Boston: Harvard Business Review Press.

Kouzes, J. M., & Posner, B. Z. (2002). *The leadership challenge* (3rd ed.). San Francisco: John Wiley & Sons.

Landrigan, C. P., Parry, G. J., Bones, C. B., Hackbarth, A. D., Goldman, D. A., & Sharek, P. J. (2010). Temporal trends in rates of patient harm resulting from medical care. *New England Journal of Medicine, 363*(22), 2124-34.

McClure, M., Poulin, M., Sovie, M., & Wandelt, M. (1983). *Magnet hospitals: Attraction and retention of professional nurses*. Kansas City, MO: American Nurses Association.

Moore, S. M., Dolansky, M. A., & Singh, M. K. (2012). Interprofessional approaches to quality and safety education. In G. Sherwood & J. Barnsteiner (Eds.), *Quality and safety in nursing: A competency approach to improving outcomes*. Hoboken, NJ: Wiley-Blackwell.

O'Toole, J. (1995). *Leading change*. San Francisco: Jossey-Bass.

Pulley, M. L., & Gurvis, J. P. (2004, July/August). The ultimate learning experience. *Across the Board*, 42–46.

Senge, P. (1990). *The fifth discipline: The art and practice of the learning organization*. New York: Doubleday.

Triolo, P. K., Scherer, E. M., & Floyd, J. M. (2006). Evaluation of the Magnet recognition program. *Journal of Nursing Administration, 36*(1), 42-48.

Wolf, G., Triolo, P., & Reid Ponte, P. (2008). Magnet recognition program: The next generation. *Journal of Nursing Administration, 38*(4), 200-204.

Yip, J. (2009). Return on experience: A mind-set for learning leadership at work. *Leadership in Action, 29*(4), 13-17.

Chapter 17

Quality and Safety: Global Issues and Strategies

Gwen Sherwood, PhD, RN, FAAN

Patient safety and health care quality are significant global health issues. Agencies in nearly every country report quality and safety issues, and health care systems are seeking solutions to the increasing awareness of the need for system improvements. There is growing recognition of the link of quality and safety across borders as well as the myriad ways that shared information of local solutions can help in seeking broader, even global applications. Health care is a complex combination of processes, technologies, and human interactions that have an inevitable risk of adverse events, whether in hospitals, physicians' offices, pharmacies, or other outpatient settings; this ongoing risk can contribute to a complacency that makes poor quality and adverse events unavoidable. The commitment to identify and reduce the risks in health care requires a change in mindset on the part of all health professionals in all types of settings. Culture changes, improved education and training, and organizational commitment are necessary to create high-reliability organizations that focus on improvement. High-reliability industries that have a perceived higher risk, such as aviation and nuclear plants, have a much better safety record than health care. In fact, travelers have a one in 1,000,000 chance of being harmed while in an aircraft, but patients have a 1 in 300 chance of being harmed while receiving health care (World Health Organization [WHO], n.d.-a; www.who.int).

Preventable adverse and sentinel events occur with startling frequency, affecting ten percent of patients worldwide (WHO, n.d.-a). Unsafe medical care affects tens of millions of patients worldwide whose medical care is prolonged or results in disabling injuries, suffering, or even death. The economic benefits of improving patient safety are compelling. Studies show that additional hospitalization, litigation costs, hospital-acquired infections, lost income, disability, and medical expenses have cost some countries between $6 billion and $29 billion a year. The United States reports the national cost of preventable adverse health care events is between $17 billion and $29 billion, including

Quality and Safety in Nursing: A Competency Approach to Improving Outcomes,
First Edition. Edited by Gwen Sherwood and Jane Barnsteiner.
© 2012 John Wiley & Sons, Inc. Published 2012 by John Wiley & Sons, Inc.

lost income, disability, and added medical expenses (Institute of Medicine [IOM], 2000). In the United Kingdom, the National Health Service estimates adverse events cost £2 billion annually in extended hospital costs alone (World Health Professions Alliance, 2002).

Differences between developed and developing countries reported by the World Health Organization (WHO) are equally unsettling (www.who.org). As many as 1 in 10 patients in developed countries are harmed by the care they receive by a range of errors or adverse events. The number is even higher in developing countries, particularly the risk of health care–associated infection, which can be as much as 20 times higher. At any given time, WHO estimates that 1.4 million people worldwide suffer from hospital-acquired infections. Hand hygiene is the most essential measure for reducing health care–associated infection, yet having a clean, reliable water supply remains a public health problem in many areas. Surgical safety is complex, and problems associated with surgery account for half of the avoidable adverse events that result in death or disability in developing countries.

The data have significant implications in a world that is increasingly interconnected. These reports have stimulated practice changes in many health care systems that are implementing a new accountability for quality and safety for which nurses and other disciplines may not be prepared to work in or lead. To address emerging roles and responsibilities for nurses and other health professionals in quality and safety worldwide, WHO and the International Council of Nursing (www.icn.ch) have each issued position statements, recommendations, and guidelines for improving quality and safety as well as global standards for nursing and midwifery education (WHO, 2009). To improve health care outcomes requires education in the new quality and safety science for all health care providers through changes in academic curricula and clinical education programs to assure a workforce skilled in leading the improvements demanded by regulatory agencies, consumers, and professional organizations (Sherwood, 2012). There continues to be a need for research to determine best practice, impact of reporting systems, and other areas still untested in the new quality and safety science. This chapter will describe quality and safety from a global perspective, examining it from the tripartite mission of practice (health care delivery), education needs and competencies, and research methods and priorities in patient safety relevant to all health professions.

Why global matters: globalization of health and health care

Globalization has profoundly changed how we address patterns of disease and the supply and availability of health care workers worldwide, as well as the environments in which they work. In recent years, countries have increasingly recognized the importance of shared solutions that contribute to quality and safety improvements. Mobility has direct effects on diseases; health care workers and patients move frequently around the world, so there is consideration of how differences in workforce standards, language, and culture affect health care quality and safety. Additionally, global agreements, politics, and various institutions affect how governments as well as health care systems meet population health needs. Global health was the focus of two reports from the U.S.-based Institute of Medicine (IOM) in 2009 outlining recommendations to address the U.S. Commitment to Global Health (IOM, 2008, 2009). For the first time, the U.S. National Institutes of Health has made global health one of its top five priorities (www.nih.gov), opening the way for global collaborations in quality and safety research. Quality and safety are urgent global health priorities for developing a global research platform that could include universal health regulations, global chronic disease management, environmental protection, and international treaties on counterfeit drugs and devices.

We can learn from global cooperation. The United States has one of the most expensive health systems in the world yet underperforms on most quality measures. In the United States, the Institute of Medicine issued one of the most comprehensive analyses of the depth and breadth of safety and quality data through its Quality Chasm series (Sherwood, 2012). The IOM (2001) cited six measures to determine the quality of health care using the acronym STEEEP: care delivered in a Safe, Timely, Effective, Efficient, Equitable, and Patient-centered way. A 2007 Commonwealth Fund report shows the United States ranked last on indicators of patient safety, efficiency, and equity when compared with New Zealand, Australia, the United Kingdom, and Germany (Davis et al., 2007). The United States had mixed scores in each of the four categories measuring quality: care that was right (effective), safe, coordinated, and patient centered. The United States lags in implementing information technology and national policies that promote quality improvement. While many health care systems in the United States are working to improve quality and safety processes, there is opportunity to learn from innovations and best practices in other countries, particularly from areas of success such as public reporting of quality data, payment systems based on quality outcomes, and a team approach for managing chronic conditions.

Global health also brings up differing perspectives on human rights and social justice in differing locales and how that influences an ethical framework in practice. Ethical practice protects human rights and cultural and linguistic sensitivity that is foundational in quality and safety, especially in professional practices based on patient-centered care. Working to improve quality and safety outcomes not only addresses our moral commitment to do no harm, it also contributes to a healthy work environment that increases worker satisfaction and retention. Workers with the training and opportunities to contribute to improving quality and safety report more satisfaction, which in turn lends to a positive work environment.

Recognizing the need to improve quality and safety

Patient safety is a universal, fundamental principle of health care, yet every point in the process of caregiving contains a certain degree of inherent safety risk. Adverse events may result from problems in practice, health care products, treatments, or procedures, or in the health care system itself. Although human errors do happen, there is most often a deeper systemic set of factors that, if addressed earlier, could have prevented the error from occurring. Patient safety improvements demand a complex systemwide effort involving a wide range of actions in performance improvement, environmental safety, and risk management, including infection control, medication and equipment safety, safe clinical practice, and safe environment of care. Human resources are one component in the health care system that affects quality and safety; workforce roles and responsibilities, shortages, and surpluses are considerations in quality and safety outcomes. Growing evidence links inadequate staffing to an increase in adverse events such as falls, bed sores, medication errors, and nosocomial infections (World Health Professions Alliance, 2002).

Global responses to quality and safety concerns

A number of programs and projects have been initiated to address quality and safety globally. The World Alliance for Patient Safety (WHO, 2004), an affiliate of WHO, was formed in response to a World Health Assembly resolution in 2002 that asked WHO member states to focus on patient safety. It has facilitated and promoted patient safety policies and practices around the world in focused areas: safety solutions, global patient safety challenge, patients for patient safety, reporting and learning, taxonomy, research, safety in action, and technology. For example, in 2007–2008, the focus was "Safe Surgery Saves Lives." The cooperative alliance among WHO member states allows faster progress than any one single member can achieve alone.

The International Classification for Patient Safety is another World Alliance for Patient Safety initiative that developed a conceptual framework to provide a common language and conceptualization around patient safety (www.who.int). Grouping patient safety concepts into an internationally agreed-upon classification enables learning about patient safety across systems throughout the world. Standardized sets of concepts provide patient safety definitions and terms as well as the relationships between them so that scholars and clinicians have a common language for sharing information and solutions across borders. The International Classification for Patient Safety is a convergence of international perceptions of the main issues related to patient safety. It facilitates the description, comparison, measurement, monitoring, analysis, and interpretation of information to improve patient care, and it is applicable in regional and national settings. The ten high-level classes identified are as follows:

(1) Incident type
(2) Patient outcomes
(3) Patient characteristics
(4) Incident characteristics
(5) Contributing factors/hazards
(6) Organizational outcomes
(7) Detection
(8) Mitigating factors
(9) Ameliorating actions
(10) Actions taken to reduce risk

Each of the 10 conceptual classes has subdivisions of concepts to allow for regional dialects, different languages, different clinical disciplines, and/or provider or patient preferences. The classification can guide educational programs, practice applications, and research to determine evidence base.

The World Alliance for Patient Safety also works with 40 champions who have suffered due to the health care they received to improve safety in health care worldwide, through the Patients for Patient Safety initiative. Consumers consistently rank quality and safety as top concerns in their care. Their experience and health are the foundation driving the patient safety movement. Patients for Patient Safety (PFPS or P4PS) recognizes the contributions that patients and consumers can have in health care improvement and safety through their work with agencies in advisory roles. Patients for Patient Safety works with a global network of patients, consumers, caregivers, and consumer organizations that supports patient involvement in patient safety programs, both within countries and globally (WHO, 2004).

The International Society for Quality in Healthcare (http://www.isqua.org) is a leading organization promoting quality with members that include quality health providers and agencies in more than 70 countries. The society has formal affiliate status with WHO to be able to assist with sharing technical and policy advice based on evidence and best practices.

WHO has developed comprehensive resources for improving quality and safety (www.who.int). Many of the practice, education, and research materials will be further discussed in this chapter. Textbox 17.1 offers examples of the patient safety program areas sponsored by various groups and member states within WHO.

Global applications of quality and safety: practice, education, and research

The complex range and subtleties of the knowledge, skills, and attitudes essential to quality and safety improvements creates challenges in advancing practice, education, and research. Organizational culture, whether a learning organization or a blaming culture, is a critical variable in the development of sustainable improvements. Practice improvements, educational transitions,

> **Textbox 17.1 Examples of the WHO Patient Safety Program areas (www.who.int/patient/about/programmes/en/index.html)**
>
> - Clean Care is Safer Care focuses on health care–associated infection with emphasis on hand hygiene.
> - Safe Surgery Saves Lives develops the WHO Safe Surgery Checklist with three phases of safety checks: preanesthesia, before skin incision, and before the patient leaves the operating room; checklists for other hospital areas are now being developed.
> - Patients for Patient Safety involves patients and consumers in a global network of patients and patient organizations to champion patient safety.
> - Research for Patient Safety established a multifaceted global approach to research in patient safety including education, assessments, and safety measures.
> - International Patient Safety Classification defines patient safety concepts with an internationally agreed-upon classification system.
> - Reporting and Learning generates best practice guidelines for reporting systems.
> - Solutions for Patient Safety explores interventions and actions that prevent patient safety problems from occurring and thus reduce patient risk.
> - Education for Safer Care developed a model for medical student education in patient safety.

and research priorities suffer from complacency that complications are a normal part of health care, that errors will happen, and that traditional education methods are sufficient. Florence Nightingale first observed in the 1800s that quality care was dependent on consistent reliable care and that poor patient outcomes may be due to variability or lack of attentiveness from staff; results were influenced by factors other than the patient's underlying illness. Now in the 21st century, we have the opportunity to address the issues Nightingale identified a century and a half ago by exploring global responses to innovations, applications, and responses for improving quality and safety.

Applying quality and safety in health care delivery (practice)

Health professionals all over the world have increasing pressure to improve health care outcomes. Working in systems that focus on quality and safety can increase awareness of adverse and sentinel events. Applying knowledge from other high-performance industries has helped analyze the depth and breadth of the issues as well as potential practice solutions. Most health professionals have not been taught systems for identifying, reporting, and systematically analyzing a near miss or adverse events. Health care systems are beginning to create a culture that focuses on quality improvement and safety. New approaches for identifying and reporting errors and near misses have changed from one that collects reports for establishing blame on an individual worker to one in which there is an organizational reporting system. In the new culture of quality and safety, organizations encourage the disclosure of near misses as well as mistakes through a reporting system in which trained health care providers examine the patient safety incident to learn how to prevent future occurrences (Barnsteiner, 2012).

A long-standing issue, however, is the lack of centralized reporting beyond the single health care setting. Some countries and regions are developing reporting systems to have a more analytic approach to data collection so that aggregated reports can identify gaps in how health care is delivered, identify care interventions for which we need evidence to support, and identify when organizations lack a climate to support quality and safety initiatives. Formal reporting requirements aggregate data on errors, near misses, and poor outcomes from across the industry so that repeated system issues can be detected, analyzed, and changed to establish new evidence-based procedures that may build in a checks and balance to prevent occurrences. There is increasing interest in sharing data across countries. In health care, adverse and sentinel events and near misses usually occur one at a time. Lack of aggregate reporting has enabled process and system issues to remain undetected, sometimes repeating the same errors.

System issues, equipment failures, or high-risk drug packaging may be detected more quickly with aggregate reporting. Systems can be analyzed for reducing work-arounds that health care personnel develop to overcome resource shortages or hindrances in completing a task. Using shortcuts to standard methods to complete their work may compromise safety and quality, or may be an indication a process needs to be changed. Other high-performance industries such as aviation, nuclear power, and railway have used aggregate reporting as one key aspect of dramatically improving safety outcomes.

Cheng and others (2011) compared incidence reporting systems for health care risk management in the United Kingdom, United States, Canada, Australia, and Taiwan to be able to develop health care risk management policy in China. According to the study, reporting systems have expanded from medication errors and hospital-acquired infections to all patient safety incidents. Reporting systems were grouped as led by governmental agencies or by regulatory nongovernmental organizations. The United Kingdom has a government Sentinel Events (SIRL) (death or serious injury) database. The United States maintains a database of health care–associated infections and was the first country to have any kind of reporting system, though for a limited range of incident types. Canada and Australia modeled their system after the United States'. The Taiwanese system is the most comprehensive. Management of incidents has become more reliable with increased application of laws, regulations, and reporting standards.

Medication errors are another example of a universal issue. The International Council of Nurses (www.icn.ch) has focused on medication errors as a major patient safety and quality concern. Medication errors are attributed to human errors as well as system failures and are considered preventable. However, medication errors are rarely the result of a single action; rather, there is usually a series of events or decisions that progressed to the error. Having a nonpunitive reporting system can allow errors to be analyzed to determine the steps in the process that can be improved to reduce the possibility of future error.

Another WHO initiative is the development of checklists to detect potential errors before harm occurs or to outline the steps to be followed to prevent an error from occurring. Checklists assume human error in the complex world of modern medicine is inevitable but can be avoided. Complex pathways of care function with high reliability when users apply a checklist to pause and take stock of their actions before proceeding to the next step. The WHO surgical safety checklist and other checklists for labor and delivery, neonatal, and trauma care have improved reliability and helped to standardize care globally (www.who.int).

Butterworth, Jones, and Jordan (2011) reported on two examples of innovative programs for improving quality and safety at the point of service in England. Working in partnership with the Institute for Healthcare Improvement in the United States, teams of staff from various health care delivery settings were trained in the knowledge, skills, and attitudes needed for quality and patient safety improvements with successful results. A systematic organizational change is the second example that was led by nurses and modeled after the U.S. project *Transforming Care at the Bedside* (Sherwood, 2012). Four themes were emphasized, based on the premise that all four must operate simultaneously to achieve care transformation: safe and reliable care, vitality and teamwork, patient-centered care, and value-added care processes. Butterworth and colleagues (2011) postulate that staff are thus prepared and empowered to develop innovations in practice that can make a difference. For example, nurses who are administering medications may wear signs that ask not to be interrupted; interruptions are associated with a higher risk of errors. Staff are required to participate in shift handovers that use Situation, Background, Assessment and Recommendation (SBAR), a standardized communication strategy that is concise and clear to all health professionals.

To achieve changes in practice, solutions that redesign care processes can prevent errors that are likely to happen. The World Alliance for Patient Safety issued nine universal patient safety solutions that can help avoid mistakes. These have been translated into Arabic, Chinese, German, and Spanish (WHO, n.d.-b).

- Confusing drug names that sound/look alike
- Confirming patient identification
- Performing correct procedure, correct site
- Control of concentrated drug solutions

- Assuring medication accuracy during transitions
- Avoiding catheter and tubing misconnections
- Single-use injection devices
- Improved hand hygiene
- Communication during patient handovers (handoffs)

Other examples of multinational practice improvements are reported in the literature. For example, Hellings, Schrooten, Klazinga, and Vleugels (2010) measured a patient safety culture improvement project in five Belgian hospitals using an adaptation of the Hospital Survey on Patient Safety Culture translated into Belgian. The survey measured 12 dimensions pre- and postimprovement effort, lasting 18 to 26 months. Findings included teamwork within hospital units scored highest in both pre- and post- surveys, improving safety culture is complex, hospital workers demonstrate high motivation to improve, transfers between units needs improving, and a nonpunitive response to error and staffing is important.

Sharing quality improvement work can help expand practice improvements across countries and speed innovation. Groene and colleagues (2010) report the DUQuE project: Deepening our Understanding of Quality Improvement in Europe to determine effectiveness of quality improvement strategies used in eight European countries. The project investigates the relationship of organizational quality improvement systems, patient empowerment, organizational culture, and professionals' involvement with hospital care quality based on clinical effectiveness, patient safety, and patient involvement. The sample includes patients diagnosed with stroke, acute myocardial infarction, hip fracture, and delivery to develop a set of instruments and tools for health care systems to measure and improve quality.

Several studies report findings from the Methods of Assessing Response to Quality Improvement Strategies (MARQuIS) project to examine quality improvement strategies to improve patient safety structures and mechanisms in 389 hospitals in eight European countries. Patient safety management was well developed, but there was variation across sites for electronic ordering systems; guidelines to avoid wrong patient, wrong site, and wrong surgical procedure; and adverse events reporting systems (Suñol et al., 2009). Many hospitals failed to use basic safety principles such as patient identification bracelets and correct medication labeling. Another report from the MARQuIS project found that up to 85% of the study hospitals had implemented policies for patients' rights, informed consent, strategies to involve patients, and ways to learn from patients' experiences (Groene et al., 2009). Hospitals with a well-developed quality improvement system were more likely to have patient centeredness at the institution level but less likely at the ward level where it is applied. Lombarts, Rupp, Vallejo, Klazinga, and Suñol (2009) used a web-based questionnaire to measure seven domains of quality improvement maturity in the study hospitals: organizational quality management programs, systems for obtaining patient views, audit and internal assessment of clinical standards, clinical practice guidelines, performance indicators, and external assessment. External assessment was the most often implemented domain, and systems for obtaining patient views was the least (Lombarts, Rupp, Vallejo, Suñol, & Klazinga, 2009). No one country (*N* = 8) implemented all the domains at all hospitals, leaving considerable scope for progress, but the study does serve as benchmark data as well as identify areas for future application and study of hospital policies compared to actual implementation and performance.

Education and core competencies

Nurses are challenged to create educational approaches so nurses have the necessary skills and leadership opportunities. Around the world, nurses, midwives, and all health professionals are developing new roles and responsibilities for improving health care. Health professions education must be transformed to address quality and safety competencies needed for the new roles. In the United States, the IOM (2003) identified the goals for 21st-century health care as being (competencies are italicized) *patient-centered* based on *evidence-based standards*, delivered collaboratively by *interprofessional teams*, within systems focused on continuous *quality improvement* and *safety* science, enhanced by *informatics* (Appendixes A and B). There are new knowledge, skills, and attitudes defining these six competencies that expand traditional definitions. Patient-centered care has been a foundation on which nursing care is based, but it now includes the patient and his or her family as valuable team members and safety allies to help identify and prevent errors. Complex care requires teamwork and collaboration among physicians, pharmacists, and others involved in a patient's care to communicate through briefings (planning), huddles (problem solving), and debriefings (process improvement). Competence in informatics enables nurses to search literature and other sources to determine best practices that establish evidence-based standards to guide practice, implement quality improvement strategies, manage and design electronic health records, and utilize decision support resources.

What are educational strategies and content for applying these competencies into nursing educational programs in both clinical and academic settings? What content is included in nursing education to address quality and safety? The U.S.-based Quality and Safety Education for Nurses (QSEN) project is an exemplar (Cronenwett et al., 2007; Cronenwett et al., 2009; Cronenwett, 2012). QSEN defined the quality and safety competencies for both prelicensure (Appendix A) and graduate education (Appendix B) to transform nursing curricula and educational standards. Results of a survey of schools of nursing combined with faculty focus group data helped define the gap between changes in health care systems and nurses' educational preparation to be able to initiate the educational changes required. The goal is to enable nurses to practice from the framework of asking questions about the care they deliver for evidence-based practice, seek quality improvements to close gaps, and address patient safety from a system perspective.

Butterworth and colleagues (2011) describe nursing curriculum revision in England for nurses and physicians in both academia and clinical areas in which clinical mentors help with skill development. Working with more than 30 universities, more than 10,000 undergraduate and postgraduate students have completed the curriculum. As in most academic programs, finding time in crowded curricula is a major constraint.

Another curriculum approach was developed by the U.S. government-funded Agency for Healthcare Research and Quality. The Patient Safety Education Project is a core curriculum with practice improvement tool kits to implement patient-centered, systems-based care (Emmanuel et al., 2008). By partnering with professional organizations in the United States and Australia, the project uses a train-the-trainer approach.

Health care educators in all settings must be prepared to achieve the goals for quality and safety if they are to be able to lead integration across hospital education programs, continuing education offerings, and academic curricula. Innovative partnerships between practice settings and schools of nursing can design human patient simulation exercises and redesign clinical learning opportunities that facilitate mastery of the competences. Collaboration across global regions for research and evaluation studies can help determine applicability in varied settings to assess the universality of the six competencies defined by the IOM and QSEN project.

An Expert Working Group with broad representation of experts from the six WHO regions began a revision of the WHO Curriculum Guide to expand from medical students to include a multiprofessional edition (www.who.int). The International Confederation of Midwives, International Council of Nurses, International Pharmaceutical Federation, International Pharmaceutical Students Federation, World Dental Federation, and World Medical Association also participated. And the International Council of Nurses (2008) issued an information and action tool kit, *Positive Practice Environments for Health Care Professionals: Quality workplaces for Quality Care* to influence the nurse working environment.

Research methods and priorities in patient safety and quality

The complexities of quality and safety, the contextual variables, and the iterative quality improvement process (Plan Do Study Act) make traditional empirical research methods a challenge to apply in quality and safety measures (Johnson, 2012). But to transform health care, there must be a scholarly basis to undergird quality and safety education, practice, and systems applications. To achieve large-scale results in reducing patient harm requires sustained efforts for research that addresses local problems in quality and safety and then shared across institutions and even countries. There is insufficient scientific evidence to understand why adverse events occur, how and to what extent patients are harmed, how these issues could be reduced and the related patient harm minimized. Because research needs are so vast with scarce resources, setting priorities, particularly in transitional and developing countries, could speed shared information toward solutions.

Expanding research capacity

Patient safety research is an emerging field requiring some understanding of the field to manage the complexities. Researchers need skills and preparation in the methods that will help determine the extent of issues and create ways to aggregate data in order to seek solutions to correct. To develop quality and safety research requires a basic understanding of knowledge around patient safety issues, particularly in developing and transitional countries; it also requires developing researcher skills in methods and measure and identifying research questions.

The scarcity of research evidence on how to solve the global issue of quality and safety is compounded by a lack of trained researchers in many areas, particularly in developing regions. Andermann and others (2011) developed a research framework for patient safety through three processes that (1) reviewed the existing literature on competencies in patient safety research, (2) consulted with end users and international experts, and then (3) conducted a global consensus discussion. They found three themes from the literature review and proposed competencies for each: patient safety, research methods, and knowledge translation. WHO (2011) issued these recommendations as *Core Competencies to Carry Out Patient Safety Research* to help strengthen research capacity, particularly useful in locales where there is little data on quality and safety issues. The core competencies document identifies the set of knowledge, skills, and attitudes necessary for patient safety researchers and patient safety officers to effect change through three core competency areas:

- Describe the fundamental concepts of the science of patient safety, in their specific social, cultural, and economic context.
- Design and conduct patient safety research.
- Contribute to the process of translating research evidence to improve the safe care of patients.

WHO has further demonstrated its leadership in advancing quality and patient safety through a variety of other guides, curricula, and strategies designed to improve patient safety and quality globally with open access on its website, www.who.int/patientsafety/research/online_course. The research development curriculum uses a case study approach to facilitate the spread and use of research findings to inform safer health care in all WHO member states. Modules include the concept of patient safety and research methods followed by components of the research cycle: measure patient safety adverse events to determine priority areas, understand underlying causes of the priority areas, explore solutions, evaluate effectiveness of solutions, and translate findings into practice (http://www.who.int/patientsafety/research/methodological_guide/en/index.html).

Global patient safety research priorities

Patient safety is a global issue affecting countries at all levels of development. Understanding the magnitude of the problem and the main contributing factors is essential in order to devise appropriate solutions. The WHO Patient Safety project convened an international multistakeholder working group to identify a set of global priorities for patient safety research using a modified Delphi technique to build consensus. Priorities were based on the severity and frequency of the patient safety issue, magnitude of harm and its distribution, and the impact the issue has on the efficiency of the health system as a whole. The priorities are broad areas that have substantial knowledge gaps for which it is believed that further knowledge will significantly contribute to improving patient safety and reducing harm. Fifty topics have been identified and prioritized according to developing, transitional, and developed countries. Among the top priorities are development and testing of locally effective and affordable solutions, cost-effectiveness of risk-reducing strategies, lack of communication and coordination, and latent organizational failures (www.who.int/patientsafety/research/priority_setting/en/index/html).

It is important to foster research in developing countries where needs may be greater but also to help understand the patient safety issues through multicountry studies. WHO has established the Patient Safety Small Research Grants program to stimulate research on patient safety priority areas by providing seed funding for small research projects.

Sharing results for quality management in disease-specific areas is another way to expand global capacity. For example, Groene and Suñol (2010) assessed quality and safety requirements for cross-border cardiovascular patients, to compare with hospital characteristics and quality improvement systems in 315 hospitals in the Czech Republic, France, Poland, and Spain. The study assessed an area of quality and safety concern in the increasing globalization of health care, managing differing views and languages for informed consent, maintaining contact with the patient's local health care providers, and coordinating case management.

The way forward: leveraging collaborations to improve quality and safety

The World Health Professions Alliance issued four areas with recommendations for action that include involving patients and the community, training health professionals, organizational system standards, and governmental oversight for reporting systems, standards, and data sharing (www.whpa.org). What are ways to begin to explore these and other questions to share what we know about quality and safety globally? The questions in Textbox 17.2 can be the start of discussions.

The recommendation from the IOM 2003 report on health professions education for the future provides a first consideration for global implications of

> **Textbox 17.2   The way forward: questions for global discussion**
>
> ● How do we design systems to insure quality and safety standards?
> ● How do we prepare students and educators to be prepared for leading and working in systems focused on quality and safety?
> ● What are teaching and learning pedagogies that create lasting changes in behavior and attitudes related to quality and safety?
> ● What are common themes in hospital redesign and regulatory standards across countries?
> ● What are cultural considerations that impact quality and safety, particularly the competencies patient-centered care, teamwork and collaboration, and evidence-based standards?
> ● How do we develop learning collaboratives that can share local strategies for global sharing and applications?
> ● What are key research dissemination strategies that can speed translation of results to improve practice?

quality and safety. Educator development is a key to preparing clinicians, administrators, leaders, and current students across the health professions in the core quality and safety competencies. Most current educators completed their formal training prior to the emphasis on quality and safety improvements and thus lack the vocabulary, conceptual understanding, and knowledge of the regulations required in clinical settings as well as application to their own educational programs, where evidence-based approaches are equally important. Educators across academic and health care delivery settings can use innovative partnerships to integrate didactic learning with clinical learning opportunities (Sherwood, 2012).

In the United States, the Consortium of Universities for Global Health was formed by 50 universities to define the field of global health, standardize curricula, expand research, and coordinate projects in low-resource countries (Consortium of Universities for Global Health, 2009). How can international perspectives on quality and safety be included in global health curricula to increase collaboration in this significant but complex topic (www.icn.ch)? How can we leverage private and nongovernmental organizations to participate in educational approaches as well as project implementation to improve quality and safety across borders?

Quality collaboratives have been proposed as a strategy to speed cross-country sharing for health care improvement (Øvretveit et al., 2002). Wilson, Berwick, and Cleary (2003) interviewed 15 leaders of health care in seven countries to develop a framework for a multiorganizational quality improvement collaborative and reported seven essentials of effective collaboration: sponsorship, topic, ideas for improvements, participants, senior leadership support, preliminary work and learning, and strategies for learning about and making improvements. Collaboratives can be a way to speed development of new approaches and share results, such as that used by the U.S.-based Quality and Safety Education for Nurses Learning Collaborative for demonstration projects to speed integration of quality and safety competencies in nursing education (Cronenwett, Sherwood, & Gelmon, 2009). Reid and Catchpole (2011) summarized the relationship and interdependence of four key areas of the health care system that could offer topics for collaboration in advancing the quality and safety agenda:

- Policy, practice, systems of work, and process
- Workspace design, and equipment design, procurement, maintenance, and training
- The professions, culture, and human factors
- Leadership, management, and the role of oversight boards

Nursing has the unique opportunity to realize new roles and leadership for nurses and midwives around the world to help shape the future of health care by leading the way in quality and safety improvements (Sherwood, 2010). It demands radical redesign of nursing education to match the rapid changes in health care delivery, to move out of traditional modes of education to interactive, transformational pedagogies (Benner, Sutphen, Leonard, & Day, 2010). We have the opportunity to examine and document how nurses and midwives around the world provide evidence-based care and education by engaging in scholarly investigation to determine effective pedagogies, outcomes of care interventions, strategies for reporting and investigating errors, solutions to system malfunctions that lead to work-arounds, and communication that promotes interprofessional teamwork (Sherwood, 2012). It is an opportunity of global proportions, and we need to be proactive in bringing together nurses and other health professionals to explore ways to share what we know, share our scarce resources for research, and provide a stronger voice within our countries and across borders to provide best practice care.

Summary

The magnitude of the issues in health care quality and safety in all areas of the globe mandate collaboration, partnerships, and sharing to be able to speed progress toward better health for all. The World Health Organization, the World Alliance for Patient Safety, and the International Council of Nurses are examples of the global agencies promoting quality and safety improvements through programs, core curricula, collaboration, research training, and assessments that are bringing together clinicians, consumers, educators, regulatory agencies, and governmental agencies to focus attention on improvements in developing and transitional countries as well as in developed countries. This chapter has presented only a slice of the work ongoing all over the world to honor the commitment of health professionals to first, do no harm. Working together, we can seek improvement solutions by transforming health professions education, train educators, and promote scholarly development to determine evidence-based strategies. Quality and safety are issues of global proportion and require global solutions.

References

Andermann, A., Ginsburg, L., Norton, P., Arora, N., Bates, D., Wu, A., Larizgoitia, I., & Patient Safety Research Training and Education Expert Working Group of WHO Patient Safety. (2011). Core competencies for patient safety research: A cornerstone for global capacity strengthening. *BMJ Quality and Safety, 20*(1), 96–101.

Barnsteiner, J. (2012). Safety. In G. Sherwood & J. Barnsteiner (Eds.), *Quality and safety in nursing: A competency approach to improving outcomes.* Hoboken, NJ: Wiley-Blackwell.

Benner, P., Sutphen, M., Leonard, V., & Day, L. (2010). Educating nurses: A call for radical transformation. San Francisco: Jossey-Bass.

Butterworth, T., Jones, K., & Jordan, S. (2011) Building capacity and capability in patient safety, innovation and service imporvement: An English case study. *Journal of Research in Nursing, 16*(3), 243–251.

Cheng, L., Sun, N., Li, Y., Zhang, Z., Wang, L., Zhou, J., et al. (2011, February 18). International comparative analyses of incidents reporting systems for healthcare risk management. *Journal of Evidence-Based Medicine.* doi: 10.1111/j.1756–5391.2011.01119.x. [Epub ahead of print]

Consortium of Universities for Global Health. (2009). *Saving lives: Universities transforming global health.* Retrieved July 25, 2011, from http://cugh.org/about/landing

Cronenwett, L. (2012). A National Initiative: Quality and Safety Education for Nurses (QSEN). In G. Sherwood & J. Barnsteiner (Eds.), *Quality and safety in nursing: A competency approach to improving outcomes.* Hoboken, NJ: Wiley-Blackwell.

Cronenwett, L., Sherwood, G., Barnsteiner, J., Disch, J., Johnson, J., Mitchell, P., et al. (2007). Quality and safety education for nurses. *Nursing Outlook, 55*(3), 122–131.

Cronenwett, L., Sherwood, G., & Gelmon, S. (2009). Improving quality and safety education: The QSEN Learning Collaborative. *Nursing Outlook, 57*(6), 304–312.

Cronenwett, L., Sherwood, G., Pohl, J., Barnsteiner, J., Moore, S., Taylor Sullivan, D. T., et al. (2009). Quality and safety education for advanced practice nursing practice. *Nursing Outlook, 57*(6), 338–348.

Davis, K., Schoen, C., Schoenbaum, S. C., Doty, M. M., Holmgren, A. L., Kriss, J. L., & Shea, K. K. (2007, May). Mirror, mirror on the wall: An international update on the comparative performance of American health care. *The Commonwealth Fund.* Retrieved July 25, 2011, from http://www.commonwealthfund.org/Content/Publications/Fund-Reports/2007/

Emanuel, L., Walton, M., Hatlie, M., Lau, D., Shaw, T., Shalowitz, J., & Combes, J. (2008). The patient safety education project: An international collaboration. In K. Henriksen, J. B. Battles, M. A. Keyes, & M. L. Grady (Eds.). *Advances in patient safety: New directions and alternative approaches: Vol. 2. Culture and redesign.* Rockville, MD: Agency for Healthcare Research and Quality.

Groene, O., Klazinga, N., Wagner, C., Arah, O. A., Thompson, A., Bruneau, C., Suñol, R. (2010). Deepening our understanding of quality improvement in Europe research project investigating organizational quality improvement systems, patient empowerment, organizational culture, professional involvement and the quality of care in European hospitals: the "Deepening our Understanding of Quality Improvement in Europe (DUQuE)" project. *BMC Health Services Research*, *24*(10), 281.

Groene, O., Lombarts, M. J., Klazinga, N., Alonso, J., Thompson, A., & Suñol, R. (2009). Is patient-centredness in European hospitals related to existing quality improvement strategies? Analysis of a cross-sectional survey (MARQuIS study). *Quality and Safety in Health Care*, *18*(Suppl. 1), i44–i50.

Groene, O., & Suñol, R. (2010). Factors associated with the implementation of quality and safety requirements for cross-border care in acute myocardial infarction: Results from 315 hospitals in four countries. *Health Policy*, *98*(2/3), 107–113.

Hellings, J., Schrooten, W., Klazinga, N. S., & Vleugels, A. (2010). Improving patient safety culture. *International Journal of Health Care Quality Assurance*, *23*(5), 489–506.

Institute of Medicine. (2000). *To err is human: Building a safer health system*. Committee on Quality of Health Care in America, Institute of Medicine. Washington, DC: National Academies Press.

Institute of Medicine. (2001). *Crossing the quality chasm: A new health system for the 21st century*. Committee on Quality of Health Care in America, Institute of Medicine. Washington, DC: National Academies Press.

Institute of Medicine. (2003). *Health professions education: A bridge to quality*. Committee on Quality of Health Care in America, Institute of Medicine. Washington, DC: National Academies Press.

Institute of Medicine. (2008). *The U.S. commitment to global health: Recommendations for the new administration*. Board on Global Health. Washington, DC: Author. Retrieved July 25, 2011, from http://www.iom.edu/ Reports/2008/The-US-Commitment-to-Global-Health-Recommendations-for-the-New-Administration.aspx

Institute of Medicine. (2009). *The U.S. commitment to global health: Recommendations for the public and private sectors*. Board on Global Health. Washington, DC: Author. Retrieved July 25, 2011, from http://www.iom.edu/ Reports/2009/The-US-Commitment-to-Global-Health-Recommendations-for-the-Public-and-Private-Sectors.aspx

International Council of Nurses. (2008). *Positive practice environments for health care professionals: Quality workplaces for quality care*. Retrieved from http:// www.ppecampaign.org/content/campaign-toolkit

Johnson, J. (2012). Quality improvement. In G. Sherwood & J. Barnsteiner (Eds.), *Quality and safety in nursing: A competency approach to improving outcomes*. Hoboken, NJ: Wiley-Blackwell.

Lombarts, M. J., Rupp, I., Vallejo, P., Klazinga, N. S., & Suñol, R. (2009). Differentiating between hospitals according to the "maturity" of quality improvement systems: A new classification scheme in a sample of European hospitals. *Quality and Safety in Health Care*, *18*(Suppl 1), i38–i43.

Lombarts, M. J., Rupp, I., Vallejo, P., Suñol, R., & Klazinga, N. S. (2009). Application of quality improvement strategies in 389 European hospitals: Results of the MARQuIS project. *Quality and Safety in Health Care*, *18*(Suppl 1), i28–i37.

ØVretveit, J., Bate, P., Cleary, P., Cretin, S., Gustafson, D., McInnes, K, et al. (2002). Quality collaboratives: Lessons from research. *Quality and Safety in Health Care*, *11*(4), 345–351.

Reid, J., & Catchpole, L. (2011). Patient safety: A core value of nursing—So why is achieving it so difficult? *Journal of Research in Nursing*, *16*(3), 209–223.

Sherwood, G. (2010). New views of quality and safety offer new roles for nurses and midwives. *Nursing and Health Sciences, 12*(3), 281–283.

Sherwood, G. (2012). The imperative to transform education to transform practice. In G. Sherwood & J. Barnsteiner (Eds.), *Quality and safety in nursing: A competency approach to improving outcomes*. Hoboken, NJ: Wiley-Blackwell.

Sun, N., Wang, L., Zhou, J., Yuan, Q., Zhang, Z., Li, Y., Liang, M., Cheng, L., Gao, G., & Cui, X. International comparative analyses of healthcare risk management. J Evid Based Med. 2011 Feb 15. doi: 10.1111/j.1756–5391.2011.01118.x. [Epub ahead of print]

Suñol, R., Vallejo, P., Groene, O., Escaramis, G., Thompson, A., Kutryba, B., & Garel, P. (2009). Implementation of patient safety strategies in European hospitals. *Quality and Safety in Health Care, 18* (Suppl 1), i57–i61.

Wilson, T., Berwick, D. M., & Cleary, P. D. (2003). What do collaborative improvement projects do? Experience from seven countries. *Joint Commission Journal on Quality and Safety, 29*(2), 85–93.

World Health Organization (n.d.-a). *10 Facts on patient safety*. Retrieved July 25, 2011, from http://www.who.int/features/factfiles/patient_safety/en/

World Health Organization (n.d.-b). *Patient safety solutions*. Retrieved July 25, 2011, from http://www.who.int/patientsafety/implementation/solutions/patient safety/en/

World Health Organization. (2004). *World Alliance for Patient Safety*. Retrieved from http://www.who.int/patientsafety/worldalliance/en/

World Health Organization. (2009). *Global standards for the initial education of nurses and midwives*. Geneva, Switzerland: World Health Organization. Available at http://www.who.int/patientsafety/en/

World Health Organization. (2011). *Core competencies to carry out patient safety research*.Retrievedfrom http://www.who.int/patientsafety/research/strengthening_capacity/training_leaders/en/

World Health Professions Alliance. (2002). *Fact sheet: Patient safety*. Retrieved from http://www.whpa.org/factptsafety.htm

Appendix A
Prelicensure Competencies

Table A.1 Patient-centered care
Definition: Recognize the patient or designee as the source of control and full partner in providing compassionate and coordinated care based on respect for patient's preferences, values, and needs.

Knowledge	Skills	Attitudes
Integrate understanding of multiple dimensions of patient centered care: • patient/family/community preferences, values • coordination and integration of care • information, communication, and education • physical comfort and emotional support • involvement of family and friends • transition and continuity	Elicit patient values, preferences, and expressed needs as part of clinical interview, implementation of care plan, and evaluation of care Communicate patient values, preferences, and expressed needs to other members of health care team Provide patient-centered care with sensitivity and respect for the diversity of human experience	Value seeing health care situations "through patients' eyes" Respect and encourage individual expression of patient values, preferences, and expressed needs Value the patient's expertise with own health and symptoms Seek learning opportunities with patients who represent all aspects of human diversity Recognize personally held attitudes about working with patients from different ethnic, cultural, and social backgrounds Willingly support patient-centered care for individuals and groups whose values differ from own

(*Continued*)

Quality and Safety in Nursing: A Competency Approach to Improving Outcomes, First Edition. Edited by Gwen Sherwood and Jane Barnsteiner.
© 2012 John Wiley & Sons, Inc. Published 2012 by John Wiley & Sons, Inc.

Table A.1 (*Continued*)

Knowledge	Skills	Attitudes
Describe how diverse cultural, ethnic, and social backgrounds function as sources of patient, family, and community values		
Demonstrate comprehensive understanding of the concepts of pain and suffering, including physiologic models of pain and comfort	Assess presence and extent of pain and suffering Assess levels of physical and emotional comfort Elicit expectations of patient and family for relief of pain, discomfort, or suffering Initiate effective treatments to relieve pain and suffering in light of patient values, preferences, and expressed needs	Recognize personally held values and beliefs about the management of pain or suffering Appreciate the role of the nurse in relief of all types and sources of pain or suffering Recognize that patient expectations influence outcomes in management of pain or suffering
Examine how the safety, quality, and cost effectiveness of health care can be improved through the active involvement of patients and families Examine common barriers to active involvement of patients in their own health care processes Describe strategies to empower patients or families in all aspects of the health care process	Remove barriers to presence of families and other designated surrogates based on patient preferences Assess level of patient's decisional conflict and provide access to resources Engage patients or designated surrogates in active partnerships that promote health, safety and well-being, and self-care management	Value active partnership with patients or designated surrogates in planning, implementation, and evaluation of care Respect patient preferences for degree of active engagement in care process Respect patient's right to access to personal health records

Table A.1 (*Continued*)

Knowledge	Skills	Attitudes
Explore ethical and legal implications of patient-centered care Describe the limits and boundaries of therapeutic patient-centered care	Recognize the boundaries of therapeutic relationships Facilitate informed patient consent for care	Acknowledge the tension that may exist between patient rights and the organizational responsibility for professional, ethical care Appreciate shared decision making with empowered patients and families, even when conflicts occur
Discuss principles of effective communication Describe basic principles of consensus building and conflict resolution Examine nursing roles in assuring coordination, integration, and continuity of care	Assess own level of communication skill in encounters with patients and families Participate in building consensus or resolving conflict in the context of patient care Communicate care provided and needed at each transition in care	Value continuous improvement of own communication and conflict resolution skills

Table A.2 Teamwork and collaboration

Definition: Function effectively within nursing and interprofessional teams, fostering open communication, mutual respect, and shared decision making to achieve quality patient care.

Knowledge	Skills	Attitudes
Describe own strengths, limitations, and values in functioning as a member of a team	Demonstrate awareness of own strengths and limitations as a team member	Acknowledge own potential to contribute to effective team functioning
	Initiate plan for self-development as a team member	Appreciate importance of intra- and interprofessional collaboration
	Act with integrity, consistency, and respect for differing views	
Describe scopes of practice and roles of health care team members	Function competently within own scope of practice as a member of the health care team	Value the perspectives and expertise of all health team members
Describe strategies for identifying and managing overlaps in team member roles and accountabilities	Assume role of team member or leader based on the situation	Respect the centrality of the patient/family as core members of any health care team
Recognize contributions of other individuals and groups in helping patient/family achieve health goals	Initiate requests for help when appropriate to situation	Respect the unique attributes that members bring to a team, including variations in professional orientations and accountabilities
	Clarify roles and accountabilities under conditions of potential overlap in team member functioning	
	Integrate the contributions of others who play a role in helping patient/family achieve health goals	

Table A.2 (*Continued*)

Knowledge	Skills	Attitudes
Analyze differences in communication style preferences among patients and families, nurses, and other members of the health team Describe impact of own communication style on others Discuss effective strategies for communicating and resolving conflict	Communicate with team members, adapting own style of communicating to needs of the team and situation Demonstrate commitment to team goals Solicit input from other team members to improve individual, as well as team, performance Initiate actions to resolve conflict	Value teamwork and the relationships upon which it is based Value different styles of communication used by patients, families, and health care providers Contribute to resolution of conflict and disagreement
Describe examples of the impact of team functioning on safety and quality of care	Follow communication practices that minimize risks associated with handoffs among providers and across transitions in care	Appreciate the risks associated with handoffs among providers and across transitions in care
Explain how authority gradients influence teamwork and patient safety	Assert own position/perspective in discussions about patient care Choose communication styles that diminish the risks associated with authority gradients among team members	
Identify system barriers and facilitators of effective team functioning Examine strategies for improving systems to support team functioning	Participate in designing systems that support effective teamwork	Value the influence of system solutions in achieving effective team functioning

Table A.3 Evidence-based practice (EBP)
Definition: Integrates best current evidence with clinical expertise and patient/family preferences and values for delivery of optimal health care.

Knowledge	Skills	Attitudes
Demonstrate knowledge of basic scientific methods and processes	Participate effectively in appropriate data collection and other research activities	Appreciate strengths and weaknesses of scientific bases for practice
Describe EBP to include the components of research evidence, clinical expertise and patient/family values	Adhere to Institutional Review Board (IRB) guidelines Base individualized care plan on patient values, clinical expertise and evidence	Value the need for ethical conduct of research and quality improvement Value the concept of EBP as integral to determining best clinical practice
Differentiate clinical opinion from research and evidence summaries	Read original research and evidence reports related to area of practice	Appreciate the importance of regularly reading relevant professional journals
Describe reliable sources for locating evidence reports and clinical practice guidelines	Locate evidence reports related to clinical practice topics and guidelines	
Explain the role of evidence in determining best clinical practice Describe how the strength and relevance of available evidence influences the choice of interventions in provision of patient-centered care	Participate in structuring the work environment to facilitate integration of new evidence into standards of practice Question rationale for routine approaches to care that result in less than desired outcomes or adverse events	Value the need for continuous improvement in clinical practice based on new knowledge
Discriminate between valid and invalid reasons for modifying evidence-based clinical practice based on clinical expertise or patient/family preferences	Consult with clinical experts before deciding to deviate from evidence-based protocols	Acknowledge own limitations in knowledge and clinical expertise before determining when to deviate from evidence-based best practices

Table A.4 Quality improvement

Definition: Use data to monitor the outcomes of care processes and use improvement methods to design and test changes to continuously improve the quality and safety of health care systems.

Knowledge	Skills	Attitudes
Describe strategies for learning about the outcomes of care in the setting in which one is engaged in clinical practice	Seek information about outcomes of care for populations served in care setting Seek information about quality improvement projects in the care setting	Appreciate that continuous quality improvement is an essential part of the daily work of all health professionals
Recognize that nursing and other health professions students are parts of systems of care and care processes that affect outcomes for patients and families Give examples of the tension between professional autonomy and system functioning	Use tools (such as flow charts, cause-effect diagrams) to make processes of care explicit Participate in a root cause analysis of a sentinel event	Value own and others' contributions to outcomes of care in local care settings
Explain the importance of variation and measurement in assessing quality of care	Use quality measures to understand performance	Appreciate how unwanted variation affects care
	Use tools (such as control charts and run charts) that are helpful for understanding variation Identify gaps between local and best practice	Value measurement and its role in good patient care
Describe approaches for changing processes of care	Design a small test of change in daily work (using an experiential learning method such as Plan-Do-Study-Act)	Value local change (in individual practice or team practice on a unit) and its role in creating joy in work
	Practice aligning the aims, measures, and changes involved in improving care	Appreciate the value of what individuals and teams can to do to improve care
	Use measures to evaluate the effect of change	

Table A.5 Safety
Definition: Minimizes risk of harm to patients and providers through both system effectiveness and individual performance.

Knowledge	Skills	Attitudes
Examine human factors and other basic safety design principles as well as commonly used unsafe practices (such as work-arounds and dangerous abbreviations) Describe the benefits and limitations of selected safety-enhancing technologies (such as, barcodes, computer provider order entry, medication pumps, and automatic alerts/alarms) Discuss effective strategies to reduce reliance on memory	Demonstrate effective use of technology and standardized practices that support safety and quality Demonstrate effective use of strategies to reduce risk of harm to self or others Use appropriate strategies to reduce reliance on memory (such as forcing functions, checklists)	Value the contributions of standardization/reliability to safety Appreciate the cognitive and physical limits of human performance
Delineate general categories of errors and hazards in care Describe factors that create a culture of safety (such as open communication strategies and organizational error reporting systems)	Communicate observations or concerns related to hazards and errors to patients, families, and the health care team Use organizational error reporting systems for near miss and error reporting	Value own role in preventing errors
Describe processes used in understanding causes of error and allocation of responsibility and accountability (such as root cause analysis and failure mode effects analysis)	Participate appropriately in analyzing errors and designing system improvements Engage in root cause analysis rather than blaming when errors or near misses occur	Value vigilance and monitoring (even of own performance of care activities) by patients, families, and other members of the health care team
Discuss potential and actual impact of national patient safety resources, initiatives, and regulations	Use national patient safety resources for own professional development and to focus attention on safety in care settings	Value relationship between national safety campaigns and implementation in local practices and practice settings

Table A.6 Informatics
Definition: Use information and technology to communicate, manage knowledge, mitigate error, and support decision making.

Knowledge	Skills	Attitudes
Explain why information and technology skills are essential for safe patient care	Seek education about how information is managed in care settings before providing care Apply technology and information management tools to support safe processes of care	Appreciate the necessity for all health professionals to seek lifelong, continuous learning of information technology skills
Identify essential information that must be available in a common database to support patient care Contrast benefits and limitations of different communication technologies and their impact on safety and quality	Navigate the electronic health record Document and plan patient care in an electronic health record Employ communication technologies to coordinate care for patients	Value technologies that support clinical decision making, error prevention, and care coordination Protect confidentiality of protected health information in electronic health records
Describe examples of how technology and information management are related to the quality and safety of patient care Recognize the time, effort, and skill required for computers, databases, and other technologies to become reliable and effective tools for patient care	Respond appropriately to clinical decision-making supports and alerts Use information management tools to monitor outcomes of care processes Use high-quality electronic sources of health care information	Value nurses' involvement in design, selection, implementation, and evaluation of information technologies to support patient care

From "Quality and Safety Education for Nurses," by L. Cronenwett, G. Sherwood, J. Barnsteiner, J. Disch, J. Johnson, P. Mitchell, D. T. Sullivan, and J. Warren, 2007, *Nursing Outlook*, 55(3), pp. 122–131. Reprinted with permission from Elsevier Ltd.

Appendix B

QSEN Graduate/Advanced Practice Nursing Competencies (bolded and italicized words are different knowledge, skills, and attitudes from the prelicensure competencies)

Table B.1   Patient-centered care

Definition: Recognize the patient or designee as the source of control and full partner in providing compassionate and coordinated care based on respect for patient's preferences, values, and needs.

Knowledge	Skills	Attitudes
Analyze multiple dimensions of patient-centered care: • Patient/family/community preferences, values • Coordination and integration of care • Information, communication, and education • Physical comfort and emotional support • Involvement of family and friends	Elicit patient values, preferences, and expressed needs as part of clinical interview, *diagnosis,* implementation of care plan, and evaluation of care Communicate patient values, preferences, and expressed needs to other members of health care team Provide patient-centered care with	Value seeing health care situations "through patients' eyes" Respect and encourage individual expression of patient values, preferences, and expressed needs Value the patient's expertise with own health and symptoms *Honor* learning opportunities with

(Continued)

Quality and Safety in Nursing: A Competency Approach to Improving Outcomes,
First Edition. Edited by Gwen Sherwood and Jane Barnsteiner.
© 2012 John Wiley & Sons, Inc. Published 2012 by John Wiley & Sons, Inc.

Table B.1 *(Continued)*

Knowledge	Skills	Attitudes
• transition and continuity *Analyze* how diverse cultural, ethnic, spiritual, and social backgrounds function as sources of patient, family, and community values *Analyze social, political, economic, and historical dimensions of patient care processes and the implications for patient-centered care* *Integrate knowledge of psychological, spiritual, social, developmental and physiological models* of pain and suffering *Analyze* ethical and legal implications of patient-centered care Describe the limits and boundaries of therapeutic patient-centered care	sensitivity, empathy, and respect for the diversity of human experience *Ensure that the systems within which one practices support patient-centered care for individuals and groups whose values differ from the majority or one's own* *Assess and treat pain and suffering in light of patient values, preferences, and expressed needs* *Respect* the boundaries of therapeutic relationships *Acknowledge the tension that may exist between patient preferences and organizational and professional responsibilities for ethical care* Facilitate informed patient consent for care	patients who represent all aspects of human diversity *Seek to understand* one's personally held attitudes about working with patients from different ethnic, cultural, and social backgrounds Willingly support patient-centered care for individuals and groups whose values differ from own *Value cultural humility* *Seek to understand one's personally held values and beliefs about the management of pain or suffering* *Value* shared decision making with empowered patients and families, even when conflicts occur
Analyze strategies that empower patients or families in all aspects of the health care process *Analyze features of physical facilities that support or pose barriers to patient-centered care*	Engage patients or designated surrogates in active partnerships *along the health illness continuum* *Create or change organizational cultures so that patient and family preferences are assessed and supported*	Respect patient preferences for degree of active engagement in care process *Honor* active partnerships with patients or designated surrogates in planning, implementation, and evaluation of care

Table B.1 (*Continued*)

Knowledge	Skills	Attitudes
Analyze reasons for common barriers to active involvement of patients and families in their own health care processes	Assess level of patient's decisional conflict and provide access to resources ***Eliminate*** barriers to presence of families and other designated surrogates based on patient preferences	Respect patient's right to access to personal health records ***Value system changes that support patient-centered care***
Integrate principles of effective communication ***with knowledge of quality and safety competencies*** ***Analyze*** principles of consensus building and conflict resolution ***Analyze advanced practice nursing roles in assuring coordination, integration, and continuity of care*** ***Describe process of reflective practice***	***Continuously analyze and improve*** own level of communication skill in encounters with patients, families, and teams ***Provide leadership in*** building consensus or resolving conflict in the context of patient care Communicate care provided and needed at each transition in care ***Incorporate reflective practices into own repertoire***	Value continuous improvement of own communication and conflict resolution skills ***Value consensus*** ***Value the process of reflective practice***

Table B.2 Teamwork and collaboration

Definition: Function effectively within nursing and interprofessional teams, fostering open communication, mutual respect, and shared decision making to achieve quality patient care.

Knowledge	Skills	Attitudes
Analyze own strengths, limitations, and values as a member of a team *Analyze impact of own advanced practice role and its contributions to team functioning*	Demonstrate awareness of own strengths and limitations as a team member *Continuously plan for improvement in use of self in effective team development and functioning*	Acknowledge own contributions to effective *or ineffective* team functioning
	Act with integrity, consistency, and respect for differing views	
Describe scopes of practice and roles of all health care team members *Analyze* strategies for identifying and managing overlaps in team member roles and accountabilities	Function competently within own scope of practice as a member of the health care team Assume role of team member or leader based on the situation *Guide the team in managing areas* of overlap in team member functioning	Respect the unique attributes that members bring to a team, including variation in professional orientations, competencies and accountabilities
	Solicit input from other team members to improve individual, as well as team, performance *Empower* contributions of others who play a role in helping patients/families achieve health goals	Respect the centrality of the patient/family as core members of any health care team
Analyze strategies that influence the ability to initiate and sustain effective partnerships with members of nursing and inter-professional teams *Analyze impact of cultural diversity on team functioning*	*Initiate and sustain effective health care teams* Communicate with team members, adapting own style of communicating to needs of the team and situation	Appreciate importance of interprofessional collaboration *Value collaboration with nurses and other members of the nursing team*

Table B.2 (*Continued*)

Knowledge	Skills	Attitudes
Analyze differences in communication style preferences among patients and families, *advanced practice* nurses, and other members of the health team *Describe impact of own communication style on others*	*Communicate respect for team member competence in communication* Initiate actions to resolve conflict	Value different styles of communication
Describe examples of the impact of team functioning on safety and quality of care	Follow communication practices that minimize risks associated with handoffs among providers and across transitions in care	Appreciate the risks associated with handoffs among providers and across transitions in care
Analyze authority gradients and their influence on teamwork and patient safety	Choose communication styles that diminish the risks associated with authority gradients among team members Assert own position/perspective *and supporting evidence* in discussions about patient care	*Value the solutions obtained through systematic, interprofessional collaborative efforts*
Identify system barriers and facilitators of effective team functioning	*Lead or* participate in the design *and implementation* of systems that support effective teamwork	Value the influence of system solutions in achieving team functioning
Examine strategies for improving systems to support team functioning	*Engage in state and national policy initiatives aimed at improving teamwork and collaboration*	

Table B.3 Evidence-based practice
Definition: Integrate best current evidence with clinical expertise and patient/family preferences and values for delivery of optimal health care

Knowledge	Skills	Attitudes
Demonstrate knowledge of *health research* methods and processes	*Use health research methods and processes, alone or in partnership with scientists, to generate new knowledge for practice*	Appreciate strengths and weaknesses of scientific bases for practice Value the need for ethical conduct of research and quality improvement
Describe evidence-based practice to include the components of research evidence, clinical expertise, and patient/family values	Adhere to Institutional Review Board guidelines *Role model clinical decision making* based on evidence, clinical expertise, and patient/family preferences and values	Value *all components of evidence-based practice*
Identify efficient and effective search strategies to locate reliable sources of evidence	*Employ efficient and effective search strategies to answer focused clinical questions*	*Value development of search skills for locating evidence for best practice*
Identify principles that comprise the critical appraisal of research evidence	*Critically appraise* original research and evidence summaries related to area of practice	*Value knowing the evidence base for practice specialty* *Value public policies that support evidence-based practice*
Summarize current evidence regarding major diagnostic and treatment actions within the practice specialty	*Exhibit contemporary knowledge of best evidence related to practice specialty*	
Determine evidence gaps within the practice specialty	*Promote research agenda for evidence that is needed in practice specialty* *Initiate changes in approaches to care when new evidence warrants evaluation of other options for improving outcomes or decreasing adverse events*	

Table B.3 *(Continued)*

Knowledge	Skills	Attitudes
Analyze how the strength of available evidence influences the provision of care (assessment, diagnosis, treatment, and evaluation)	*Develop guidelines for clinical decision making* regarding departure from established protocols/standards of care	Acknowledge own limitations in knowledge and clinical expertise before determining when to deviate from evidence-based best practices
Evaluate organizational cultures and structures that promote evidence-based practice	*Participate in designing systems that support evidence-based practice*	Value the need for continuous improvement in clinical practice based on new knowledge

Table B.4 Quality improvement
Definition: Use data to monitor the outcomes of care processes and use improvement methods to design and test changes to continuously improve the quality and safety of health care systems.

Knowledge	Skills	Attitudes
Describe strategies *for improving* outcomes of care in the setting in which one is engaged in clinical practice	*Use a variety of sources of information to review outcomes of care and identify potential areas for improvement*	Appreciate that continuous quality improvement is an essential part of the daily work of all health professionals
Analyze the impact of context (such as access, cost, or team functioning) on improvement efforts	*Propose appropriate aims for quality improvement efforts* *Assert leadership in shaping the dialogue about and providing leadership for the introduction of best practices*	
Analyze ethical issues associated with quality improvement	*Assure ethical oversight of quality improvement projects*	Value the need for ethical conduct of quality improvement
Describe features of quality improvement projects that overlap sufficiently with research, thereby requiring institutional review board oversight	*Maintain confidentiality of any patient information used to determine outcomes of quality improvement efforts*	

(Continued)

Table B.4 *(Continued)*

Knowledge	Skills	Attitudes
Describe the benefits and limitations of quality improvement data sources, and measurement and data analysis strategies	*Design and use databases as sources of information for improving patient care* *Select and use relevant benchmarks*	*Appreciate the importance of data that allows one to estimate the quality of local care*
Explain common causes of variation in outcomes of care in the practice specialty	*Select and* use tools (such as control charts and run charts) that are helpful for understanding variation Identify gaps between local and best practice	Appreciate how unwanted variation affects outcomes of care processes
Describe common quality measures in the practice specialty	*Use findings from* root cause analyses to design and implement system improvements *Select and use quality measures to understand performance*	Value measurement and its role in good patient care
Analyze the differences between micro-system and macro-system change *Understand principles of change management*	*Use principles of change management to implement and evaluate care processes at the micro-system level*	Appreciate the value of what individuals and teams can to do to improve care *Value local systems improvement (in individual practice, team practice on a unit, or in*
Analyze the strengths and limitations of common quality improvement methods	Design, *implement, and evaluate* tests of change in daily work (using an experiential learning method such as Plan-Do-Study-Act) *Align the aims, measures, and changes involved in improving care* Use measures to evaluate the effect of change	*the macro-system) and its role in professional job satisfaction* *Appreciate that all improvement is change but not all change is improvement*

Table B.5 Safety

Definition: Minimize risk of harm to patients and providers through both system effectiveness and individual performance.

Knowledge	Skills	Attitudes
Describe human factors and other basic safety design principles as well as commonly used unsafe practices (such as workarounds and dangerous abbreviations)	*Participate as a team member to design, promote, and model effective use* of technology and standardized practices that support safety and quality	Value the contributions of standardization and reliability to safety *Appreciate the importance of being a safety mentor and role model*
Describe the benefits and limitations of selected safety-enhancing technologies (such as barcodes, computer provider order entry, and electronic prescribing)	*Participate as a team member to design, promote, and model* effective use of strategies to reduce risk of harm to self and others	Appreciate the cognitive and physical limits of human performance
Evaluate effective strategies to reduce reliance on memory	*Promote a practice culture conducive to highly reliable processes built on human factors research*	
	Use appropriate strategies to reduce reliance on memory (such as forcing functions, checklists)	
Delineate general categories of errors and hazards in care	Communicate observations or concerns related to hazards and errors to patients, families, and the health care team	Value own role in reporting and preventing errors
Identify best practices for organizational responses to error	*Identify and correct system failures and hazards in care*	*Value systems approaches to improving patient safety in lieu of blaming individuals*
Describe factors that create *a just culture* and culture of safety	*Design and implement micro-system changes in response to identified hazards and errors*	*Value the use of organizational error reporting systems*
Describe best practices that promote patient and provider safety in the practice specialty	*Engage in a systems focus* rather than blaming individuals when errors or near misses occur	

(Continued)

Table B.5 *(Continued)*

Knowledge	Skills	Attitudes
	Report errors and support members of the health care team in being forthcoming about errors and near misses	
Describe processes used to analyze causes of error and allocation of responsibility and accountability (such as root cause analysis and failure mode effects analysis)	Participate appropriately in analyzing errors and designing, *implementing, and evaluating* system improvements	Value vigilance and monitoring of care, including one's own performance, by patients, families, and other members of the health care team
Describe methods of identifying and preventing verbal, physical, and psychological harm to patients and staff	*Prevent escalation of conflict* *Respond appropriately to aggressive behavior*	*Value prevention of assaults and loss of dignity for patients, staff, and aggressors*
Analyze potential and actual impact of national patient safety resources, initiatives, and regulations	Use national patient safety resources: • for own professional development • to focus attention on safety in care settings • *to design and implement improvements in practice*	Value relationship between national patient safety campaigns and implementation in local practices and practice settings

Table B.6 Informatics
Definition: Use information and technology to communicate, manage knowledge, mitigate error, and support decision making.

Knowledge	Skills	Attitudes
Contrast benefits and limitations of common information technology strategies used in the delivery of patient care	*Participate in the selection, design, implementation, and evaluation of information systems*	*Value the use of information and communication technologies in patient care*
Evaluate the strengths and weaknesses of information systems used in patient care	*Communicate the integral role of information technology in nurses' work*	
	Model behaviors that support implementation and appropriate use of electronic health records	
	Assist team members in adopting information technology by piloting and evaluating proposed technologies	
Formulate essential information that must be available in a common database to support patient care in the practice specialty	*Promote access to patient care information for all professionals who provide care to patients*	*Appreciate the need for consensus and collaboration in developing systems to manage information for patient care*
Evaluate benefits and limitations of different communication technologies and their impact on safety and quality	*Serve as a resource for how to document nursing care at basic and advanced levels*	*Value the confidentiality and security of all patient records*
	Develop safeguards for protected health information	
	Champion communication technologies that support clinical decision making, error prevention, care coordination, and protection of patient privacy	

(Continued)

Table B.6 *(Continued)*

Knowledge	Skills	Attitudes
Describe and critique taxonomic and terminology systems used in national efforts to enhance interoperability of information systems and knowledge management systems	*Access and evaluate high-quality electronic sources of health care information* *Participate in the design of clinical decision-making supports and alerts* *Search, retrieve, and manage data to make decisions using information and knowledge management systems* *Anticipate unintended consequences of new technology*	*Value the importance of standardized terminologies in conducting searches for patient information* *Appreciate the contribution of technological alert systems* *Appreciate* the time, effort, and skill required for computers, databases, and other technologies to become reliable and effective tools for patient care

From "Quality and Safety Education for Advanced Nursing Practice," by L. Cronenwett, G. Sherwood, J. Pohl, J. Barnsteiner, S. Moore, D. T. Sullivan, D. Ward, and J. Warren, 2009, *Nursing Outlook*, 57(6), pp. 122–131. Reprinted with permission from Elsevier Ltd.

Quality and Safety Education for Nurses: Results of a National Delphi Study to Developmentally Level KSAs

Table C.1 Patient-centered care

Competency	Curricular Introduction			Curricular Emphasis		
Knowledge	Beg	Inter	Adv	Beg	Inter	Adv
Integrate understanding of multiple dimensions of patient-centered care: *Patient/family/community preferences, values	X				X	
*Coordination and integration of care	X					X
*Information, communication, and education	X				X	
*Physical comfort and emotional support	X			X		
*Involvement of family and friends	X				X	
*Transition and continuity		X				X
Describe how diverse cultural, ethnic, and social backgrounds function as sources of patient, family, and community values	X				X	

(Continued)

Quality and Safety in Nursing: A Competency Approach to Improving Outcomes, First Edition. Edited by Gwen Sherwood and Jane Barnsteiner.
© 2012 John Wiley & Sons, Inc. Published 2012 by John Wiley & Sons, Inc.

Table C.1 (*Continued*)

Competency	Curricular Introduction			Curricular Emphasis		
Knowledge	Beg	Inter	Adv	Beg	Inter	Adv
Demonstrate comprehensive understanding of the concepts of pain and suffering, including physiologic models of pain and comfort	X				X	
Examine how the safety, quality, and cost-effectiveness of health care can be improved through the active involvement of patients and families		X				X
Examine common barriers to active involvement of patients in their own health care processes		X			X	
Describe strategies to empower patients or families in all aspects of the health care process		X			X	
Explore ethical and legal implications of patient-centered care	X				X	
Describe the limits and boundaries of therapeutic patient-centered care	X					X
Discuss the principles of effective communication	X			X		
Describe basic principles of consensus building and conflict resolution	X					X
Examine nursing roles in assuring coordination, integration, and continuity of care	X					X
Skills						
Elicit patient values, preferences, and expressed needs as part of clinical interview, implementation of care plan, and evaluation of care	X				X	
Communicate patient values, preferences, and expressed needs to other members of health care team	X				X	
Provide patient-centered care with sensitivity and respect for the diversity of human experience	X				X	
Assess presence and extent of pain and suffering	X				X	
Assess levels of physical and emotional comfort	X			X		
Elicit expectations of patient and family for relief of pain, discomfort, or suffering	X				X	

Table C.1 (*Continued*)

Competency	Curricular Introduction			Curricular Emphasis		
Knowledge	Beg	Inter	Adv	Beg	Inter	Adv
Initiate effective treatments to relieve pain and suffering in light of patient values, preferences, and expressed needs	X				X	
Remove barriers to presence of families and other designated surrogates based on patient preferences		X				X
Assess level of patient's decisional conflict and provide access to resources		X				X
Engage patients or designated surrogates in active partnerships that promote health, safety and well-being, and self-care management		X				X
Recognize the boundaries of therapeutic relationships	X				X	
Facilitate informed patient consent for care	X				X	
Assess own level of communication skill in encounters with patients and families	X				X	
Participate in building consensus or resolving conflict in the context of patient care		X				X
Communicate care provided and needed at each transition in care		X			X	
Attitudes						
Value seeing health care situations "through patients' eyes"	X			X		
Respect and encourage individual expression of patient values, preferences, and expressed needs	X				X	
Value the patient's expertise with own health and symptoms	X				X	
Seek learning opportunities with patients who represent all aspects of human diversity	X				X	
Recognize personally held attitudes about working with patients from different ethnic, cultural, and social backgrounds	X			X		

(*Continued*)

Table C.1 *(Continued)*

Competency	Curricular Introduction			Curricular Emphasis		
Knowledge	Beg	Inter	Adv	Beg	Inter	Adv
Willingly support patient-centered care for individuals and groups whose values differ from own	X				X	
Recognize personally held values and beliefs about the management of pain or suffering	X				X	
Appreciate the role of the nurse in relief of all types and sources of pain or suffering	X				X	
Recognize that patient expectations influence outcomes in management of pain or suffering	X				X	
Value active partnership with patients or designated surrogates in planning, implementation, and evaluation of care		X			X	
Respect patient preferences for degree of active engagement in care process	X				X	
Respect patient's right to access to personal health records	X				X	
Acknowledge the tension that may exist between patient rights and the organizational responsibility for professional, ethical care		X				X
Appreciate shared decision making with empowered patients and families, even when conflicts occur		X				X
Value continuous improvement of own communication and conflict resolution skills	X					X

Table C.2 Teamwork and collaboration

Competency	Curricular Introduction			Curricular Emphasis		
Knowledge	Beg	Inter	Adv	Beg	Inter	Adv
Describe own strengths, limitations, and values in functioning as a member of a team		X				X
Describe scopes of practice and roles of health care team members	X				X	
Describe strategies for identifying and managing overlaps in team member roles and accountabilities		X				X
Recognize contributions of other individuals and groups in helping patient/family achieve health goals		X			X	
Analyze differences in communication style preferences among patients and families, nurses, and other members of the health team		X				X
Describe impact of own communication style on others	X				X	
Discuss effective strategies for communicating and resolving conflict		X				X
Describe examples of the impact of team functioning on safety and quality of care		X				X
Explain how authority gradients influence teamwork and patient safety		X				X
Identify system barriers and facilitators of effective team functioning		X				X
Examine strategies for improving systems to support team functioning			X			X
Skills						
Demonstrate awareness of own strengths and limitations as a team member	X					X
Initiate plan for self-development as a team member		X			X	
Act with integrity, consistency, and respect for differing views	X				X	
Function competently within own scope of practice as a member of the health care team	X					X

(Continued)

Table C.2 *(Continued)*

Competency Knowledge	Curricular Introduction			Curricular Emphasis		
	Beg	Inter	Adv	Beg	Inter	Adv
Assume role of team member or leader based on the situation		X				X
Initiate requests for help when appropriate to situation	X				X	
Clarify roles and accountabilities under conditions of potential overlap in team-member functioning		X				X
Integrate the contributions of others who play a role in helping patient/family achieve health goals		X				X
Communicate with team members, adapting own style of communicating to needs of the team and situation	X					X
Demonstrate commitment to team goals	X				X	
Solicit input from other team members to improve individual, as well as team, performance		X				X
Initiate actions to resolve conflict		X				X
Follow communication practices that minimize risks associated with handoffs among providers and across transitions in care	X				X	
Assert own position/perspective in discussions about patient care		X				X
Choose communication styles that diminish the risks associated with authority gradients among team members		X				X
Participate in designing systems that support effective teamwork			X			X
Attitudes						
Acknowledge own potential to contribute to effective team functioning	X				X	
Appreciate importance of intra- and interprofessional collaboration	X				X	
Value the perspectives and expertise of all health team members	X				X	
Respect the centrality of the patient/family as core members of any health care team	X				X	

Table C.2 (*Continued*)

Competency	Curricular Introduction			Curricular Emphasis		
Knowledge	Beg	Inter	Adv	Beg	Inter	Adv
Respect the unique attributes that members bring to a team, including variations in professional orientations and accountabilities		X			X	
Value teamwork and the relationships upon which it is based	X				X	
Value different styles of communication used by patients, families, and health care providers	X				X	
Contribute to resolution of conflict and disagreement		X				X
Appreciate the risks associated with handoffs among providers and across transitions in care	X				X	
Value the influence of system solutions in achieving effective team functioning		X				X

Table C.3 Evidence-based practice (EBP)

Competency	Curricular Introduction			Curricular Emphasis		
Knowledge	Beg	Inter	Adv	Beg	Inter	Adv
Demonstrate knowledge of basic scientific methods and processes	X				X	
Describe EBP to include the components of research evidence, clinical expertise, and patient/ family values	X				X	
Differentiate clinical opinion from research and evidence summaries		X				X
Describe reliable sources for locating evidence reports and clinical practice guidelines	X				X	
Explain role of evidence in determining best clinical practice	X				X	
Describe how the strength and relevance of available evidence influences the choice of interventions in provision of patient-centered care		X				X

(Continued)

Table C.3 (Continued)

Competency	Curricular Introduction			Curricular Emphasis		
Knowledge	Beg	Inter	Adv	Beg	Inter	Adv
Discriminate between valid and invalid reasons for modifying evidence-based clinical practice based on clinical expertise or patient/family preferences			X			X
Skills						
Participate effectively in appropriate data collection and other research activities		X				X
Adhere to institutional review board guidelines		X				X
Base individualized care plan on patient values, clinical expertise, and evidence	X				X	
Read original research and evidence reports related to area of practice		X			X	
Locate evidence reports related to clinical practice topics and guidelines		X			X	
Participate in structuring the work environment to facilitate integration of new evidence into standards of practice			X			X
Question rationale for routine approaches to care that result in less than desired outcomes or adverse events		X				X
Consult with clinical experts before deciding to deviate from evidence-based protocols		X				X
Attitudes						
Appreciate strengths and weaknesses of scientific bases for practice		X			X	
Value the need for ethical conduct of research and quality improvement	X				X	
Value the concept of EBP as integral to determining best clinical practice	X				X	
Appreciate the importance of regularly reading relevant professional journals	X					X

Table C.3 *(Continued)*

Competency	Curricular Introduction			Curricular Emphasis		
Knowledge	Beg	Inter	Adv	Beg	Inter	Adv
Value the need for continuous improvement in clinical practice based on new knowledge	X					X
Acknowledge own limitations in knowledge and clinical expertise before determining when to deviate from evidence-based best practices	X					X

Table C.4 Quality Improvement

Competency	Curricular Introduction			Curricular Emphasis		
Knowledge	Beg	Inter	Adv	Beg	Inter	Adv
Describe strategies for learning about the outcomes of care in the setting in which one is engaged in clinical practice		X				X
Recognize that nursing and other health professions students are parts of systems of care and care processes that affect outcomes for patients and families	X				X	
Give examples of the tension between professional autonomy and system functioning			X			X
Explain the importance of variation and measurement in assessing quality of care			X			X
Describe approaches for changing processes of care			X			X
Skills						
Seek information about outcomes of care for populations served in care setting		X				X
Seek information about quality improvement projects in the care setting		X				X
Use tools (such as flow charts, cause-effect diagrams) to make processes of care explicit		X				X

(Continued)

Table C.4 *(Continued)*

Competency	Curricular Introduction			Curricular Emphasis		
Knowledge	Beg	Inter	Adv	Beg	Inter	Adv
Participate in root cause analysis of sentinel event			X			X
Use quality measures to understand performance		X				X
Use tools (such as control charts and run charts) that are helpful for understanding variation		X				X
Identify gaps between local and best practice		X				X
Design a small test of change in daily work (using an experiential learning method such as Plan-Do-Study-Act)		X				X
Practice aligning the aims, measures, and changes involved in improving care			X			X
Use measures to evaluate the effect of change			X			X
Attitudes						
Appreciate that continuous quality improvement is an essential part of the daily work of all health professionals	X				X	
Value own and others' contributions to outcomes of care in local care settings	X				X	
Appreciate how unwanted variation affects care		X				X
Value measurement and its role in good patient care		X			X	
Value local change (in individual practice or team practice on a unit) and its role in creating joy in work		X				X
Appreciate the value of what individuals and teams can do to improve care	X					X

Table C.5 Safety

Competency	Curricular Introduction			Curricular Emphasis		
Knowledge	Beg	Inter	Adv	Beg	Inter	Adv
Examine human factors and other basic safety design principles as well as commonly used unsafe practices (such as work-arounds and dangerous abbreviations)	X					X
Describe the benefits and limitations of selected safety-enhancing technologies (such as barcodes, computer provider order entry, medication pumps, and automatic alerts/alarms)	X				X	
Discuss effective strategies to reduce reliance on memory	X			X		
Delineate general categories of errors and hazards in care		X			X	
Describe factors that create a culture of safety (such as open communication strategies and organizational error reporting systems)	X				X	
Describe processes used in understanding causes of error and allocation of responsibility and accountability (such as root cause analysis and failure mode effects analysis)		X				X
Discuss potential and actual impact of national patient safety resources, initiatives, and regulations		X				X
Skills						
Demonstrate effective use of technology and standardized practices that support safety and quality	X				X	
Demonstrate effective use of strategies to reduce risk of harm to self or others	X				X	
Use appropriate strategies to reduce reliance on memory (such as forcing functions, checklists)	X				X	
Communicate observations or concerns related to hazards and errors to patients, families, and the health care team	X				X	

(Continued)

Table C.5 *(Continued)*

Competency	Curricular Introduction			Curricular Emphasis		
Knowledge	Beg	Inter	Adv	Beg	Inter	Adv
Use organizational error reporting systems for near-miss and error reporting	X				X	
Participate appropriately in analyzing errors and designing system improvements		X				X
Engage in root-cause analysis rather than blaming when errors or near-misses occur			X			X
Use national patient safety resources for own professional development and to focus attention on safety in care settings		X				
Attitudes						
Value the contributions of standardization/reliability to safety	X				X	
Appreciate the cognitive and physical limits of human performance	X			X		
Value own role in preventing errors	X			X		
Value vigilance and monitoring (even of own performance of care activities) by patients, families, and other members of the health care team	X				X	
Value relationship between national safety campaigns and implementation in local practices and practice settings		X				X

Table C.6   Informatics

Competency	Curricular Introduction			Curricular Emphasis		
Knowledge	Beg	Inter	Adv	Beg	Inter	Adv
Explain why information and technology skills are essential for safe patient care	X			X		
Identify essential information that must be available in a common database to support patient care	X				X	
Contrast benefits and limitations of different communication technologies and their impact on safety and quality		X				X
Describe examples of how technology and information management are related to the quality and safety of patient care		X				X
Recognize the time, effort, and skill required for computers, databases, and other technologies to become reliable and effective tools for patient care		X				X
Skills						
Seek education about how information is managed in care settings before providing care		X				X
Apply technology and information management tools to support safe processes of care	X				X	
Navigate the electronic health record	X				X	
Document and plan patient care in an electronic health record	X				X	
Employ communication technologies to coordinate care for patients		X			X	
Respond appropriately to clinical decision-making supports and alerts		X			X	
Use information management tools to monitor outcomes of care processes		X				X
Use high-quality electronic sources of health care information	X				X	

(Continued)

Table C.6 *(Continued)*

Competency	Curricular Introduction			Curricular Emphasis		
Knowledge	Beg	Inter	Adv	Beg	Inter	Adv
Attitudes						
Appreciate the necessity for all health professionals to seek lifelong, continuous learning of information technology skills	X					X
Value technologies that support clinical decision making, error prevention, and care coordination	X				X	
Protect confidentiality of protected health information in electronic health records	X			X		
Value nurses' involvement in design, selection, implementation, and evaluation of information technologies to support patient care		X				X

From *Quality and Safety Education for Nurses: Results of a National Delphi Study of Developmentally Level KSAs*, by A. Barton, G. Armstrong, and G. Preheim, 2009. Denver: University of Colorado. Reprinted with permission from the authors.

Glossary

Achieving Competence Today (ACT)–an interdisciplinary teaching program that focuses on quality, safety, and health systems improvement.

Adverse event–unintentional harm caused by health care management rather than the underlying condition of the patient.

Adverse reaction–unexpected harm resulting from a justified action where the correct process was followed for the context in which the event occurred.

Agency for Healthcare Research and Quality (AHRQ)–the nation's lead federal agency for research on health care quality, costs, outcomes, and patient safety. AHRQ is the health services research arm of the U.S. Department of Health and Human Services, complementing the biomedical research mission of its sister agency, the National Institutes of Health. The agency is home to research centers that specialize in major areas of healthcare research, including clinical practice and technology assessment, health care organization and delivery systems, and primary care. AHRQ is a major source of funding and technical assistance for health services research and research training at leading U.S. universities and other institutions. As a science partner, the agency works with the public and private sectors to build the knowledge base for what works–and does not work–in health and health care and to translate this knowledge into everyday practice and policy making.

American Health Information Community (AHIC)–a federally chartered advisory committee that makes recommendations to the secretary of the U.S. Department of Health and Human Services on how to make health records digital and interoperable, encourage market-led adoption, and ensure that the privacy and security of those records are protected at all times. In 2009 AHIC became the National eHealth Collaborative, a new public-private partnership to continue the work of the AHIC (www.nationalehealth.org).

Applicability of study findings–whether the effects of the study are appropriate for a particular patient situation.

Quality and Safety in Nursing: A Competency Approach to Improving Outcomes,
First Edition. Edited by Gwen Sherwood and Jane Barnsteiner.
© 2012 John Wiley & Sons, Inc. Published 2012 by John Wiley & Sons, Inc.

Background questions–questions that need to be answered as a foundation for asking the searchable, answerable foreground question. They are questions that ask for general information about a clinical issue and they have two components: the starting place of the question (e.g., what, where, when, why, and how), and the outcome of interest (e.g., the clinical diagnosis).

Benchmark (benchmarking)–Benchmarking is a way for hospitals and doctors to analyze quality data, both internally and against data from other hospitals and doctors, to identify best practices of care and improve quality.

Benefits versus risks–one way to interpret guideline recommendations. For decisions in which it is clear that benefits far outweigh downsides or downsides far outweigh benefits, the risk/benefit discussion allows the provider to offer a strong recommendation.

Best practices–Best practices are the most up-to-date patient care interventions, which result in the best patient outcomes and minimize patient risk of death or complications.

Bracketing–identifying and suspending previously acquired knowledge, beliefs, and opinions about a phenomenon.

Call-out–technique for communicating important or critical information by intentionally verbalizing a step in a process.

Care delivery outcomes–the outcomes that are influenced by the delivery of clinical care.

Care coordination–an interdisciplinary approach to the care of a patient.

Caregiver–a person who helps in identifying, preventing, or treating illness or disability.

Carrier–an entity which may underwrite or administer a range of health benefit programs; may refer to an insurer or a managed health plan.

Case-control study–a type of research that retrospectively compares characteristics of an individual who has a certain condition (e.g., hypertension) with one who does not (e.g., a matched control or similar person without hypertension); often conducted for the purpose of identifying variables that might predict the condition (e.g., stressful lifestyle, sodium intake).

Case series–a report on a series of patients with an outcome of interest. No control group is involved.

Centers for Medicare and Medicaid Services (CMS; formerly Health Care Financing Administration [HCFA])–federal agency that seeks to ensure effective, up-to-date health care coverage and to promote quality care for beneficiaries. Ultimately, CMS is working to transform and modernize the health care system.

Check-back—a process that uses closed-loop communication to ensure that information conveyed by the sender is understood by the receiver as intended.

Clinical practice guidelines—a set of systematically developed statements, usually based on scientific evidence, that help physicians and their patients make decisions about appropriate health care for specific medical conditions. Clinical practice guidelines briefly identify and evaluate the most current information about prevention, diagnosis, prognosis, therapy, risk/benefit, and cost effectiveness.

Cochrane Collaboration—a worldwide association of groups that create and maintain systematic reviews of the literature for specific topic areas.

Cohort study—involves the identification of two groups (cohorts) of patients, one that did receive the exposure of interest and one that did not, and following these cohorts forward for the outcome of interest.

Collaboration—process of joint decision making among independent parties involving joint ownership of decisions and collective responsibility for outcomes. The essence of collaboration involves working across professional boundaries.

Commission on Systemic Operability—Authorized by the Medicare Modernization Act of 2003, the commission was charged with developing strategies to make health care information instantly accessible at all times, by consumers and their health care providers. The group's 12 recommendations and a discussion of the benefits of an interoperable network and the barriers to creating such a network were published in 2005 in a report titled "Ending the Document Game: Connecting and Transforming Your Healthcare Through Information Technology" (http://endingthedocumentgame.gov).

Committee—a relatively stable, formally composed group that has an identified purpose as part of an organizational structure.

Communication—a process by which information is exchanged between individuals through a common system of symbols, signs, or behavior.

Computerized physician order entry (CPOE)—CPOE is a computerized system that allows a physician's orders for services such as medications, laboratory tests and other tests to be entered electronically instead of being recorded on order sheets or prescription pads. This allows for the order to be compared against standards for dosing and to be checked for any patient allergies or interactions with other medications, or other potential problems if the order is filled. However, some people prefer to call this **computerized provider order entry system**, thereby recognizing that more than physicians enter orders.

Confidence interval (CI)—the range around a study's result within which we would expect the true value to lie. CIs account for the sampling error between the study population and the wider population the study is supposed to represent.

Confounding variable—a variable that is not the one in which you are interested but that may affect the results of trial.

Connectivity—the physical network and operating rules allowing computerized health information to be stored at one point and retrieved at another by an authorized user. For some people in the health information technology field, connectivity implies having uniform privacy laws protecting individually identifiable medical information from being accessed by unauthorized persons.

Consumer—A consumer is an individual who uses, is affected by, or is entitled or compelled to use a health-related service.

Consumer Assessment of Healthcare Providers and Systems (CAHPS)—develops and supports the use of a comprehensive and evolving family of standardized surveys that ask consumers and patients to report on and evaluate their experiences with health care. These surveys cover topics that are important to consumers, such as the communication skills of providers and the accessibility of services. CAHPS originally stood for the Consumer Assessment of Health Plans Study, but as the products have evolved beyond health plans, the name has evolved as well to capture the full range of survey products and tools.

Consumer engagement—the situation in which consumers take an active role in their own health care, from understanding their own conditions and available treatments, to seeking out and making decisions based on information about the performance of health care providers.

Consumer-driven (or directed) care—a form of health insurance that combines a high-deductible health plan with a tax-favored Health Savings Account, Flexible Spending Account, or Health Reimbursement Account to cover out-of-pocket expenses. These accounts are "consumer driven" in that they give participants greater control over their own health care, allowing individuals to determine on a personal basis how they choose to spend their health care account funds.

Coordination of care—comprises mechanisms that ensure patients and clinicians have access to, and take into consideration, all required information on a patient's conditions and treatments to ensure that the patient receives appropriate health care services.

Core measures–specific clinical measures that, when viewed together, permit a robust assessment of the quality of care provided in a given focus area, such as acute myocardial infarction.

Critically appraised topic (CAT)–a short summary of an article from the literature, created to answer a specific clinical question.

Crew Resource Management (CRM)–a training program to improve team functioning in high-stakes industries such as aviation, nuclear power, and health care.

Cultural competence–the knowledge, skills, and attitudes necessary for providing quality care to diverse populations.

Culture–shared knowledge and behavior of people who interact within distinct social settings and subsystems.

Culture of safety–minimizes risk of harm to patients and providers through both system effectiveness and individual performance and recognizes the influence of systems and human factors.

Database of Abstracts of Reviews of Effects (DARE)–database that includes abstracts of systematic reviews that have been critically appraised by reviewers at the NHS Centre for Reviews and Dissemination at the University of York, England.

Data collection–the acquisition of health care information or facts based on patient and consumer race, ethnicity, and language. Data collection provides health care providers with the ability to perform benchmarking measures on health care systems to determine areas where improvement is needed in providing care.

Decision analysis–the application of explicit, quantitative methods to analyze decisions under conditions of uncertainty.

Delegation–process of transferring authority to a competent individual for completing selected nursing tasks/activities/functions. To assign is to direct an individual to do activities within an authorized scope of practice. Assignment (noun) describes the distribution of work that each staff member is to accomplish in a given work period.

Department of Health and Human Services (HHS)–principal federal agency for protecting the health of all Americans and providing essential human services, especially for those who are least able to help themselves.

Design—the overall plan for a study that includes strategies for controlling confounding variables, strategies for when the intervention will be delivered (in experimental studies), and how often and when the data will be collected.

Disease management—an approach designed to improve the health and quality of life for people with chronic illnesses by working to keep the conditions under control and prevent them from getting worse.

Disease registry—a large collection or registry belonging to a health care system that contains information on different chronic health problems affecting patients within the system. A disease registry helps to manage and log data on chronic illnesses and diseases. All data contained within the disease registry are logged by health care providers and are available to providers to perform benchmarking measures on health care systems.

Disparities (in care)—differences in the delivery of health care, access to health care services, and medical outcomes based on ethnicity, geography, gender, and other factors that do not include socioeconomic status or insurance coverage. Understanding and eliminating the causes of health care disparities is an ongoing effort of many groups and organizations.

Disruptive behavior—behavior that interferes with the ability of everyone on the team to provide safe and effective care, undermines the confidence of any member of the health care team in effectively caring for patients, undermines patients' confidence in the health care team or organization, causes concern for anyone's physical safety, and undermines effective teamwork.

Diversity—racial, cultural, or ethnic variation in the demographics of a place, organization, or profession.

Effectiveness—a measure of the benefit resulting from an intervention for a given health problem under usual conditions of clinical care for a particular group.

Effective care—includes health care services that are of proven value and have no significant trade-offs. The benefits of the services so far outweigh the risks that all patients with specific medical needs should receive them. These services, such as beta-blockers for heart attack patients, are backed by well-articulated medical theory and strong evidence of efficacy, determined by clinical trials or valid cohort studies.

Efficacy—a measure of the benefit resulting from an intervention for a given health problem under the ideal conditions of an investigation.

Electronic Health (Medical) Record (EHR or EMR)—a computerized medical file that contains the history of a patient's medical care, commonly abbreviated as EHR, in contrast to PHR, which stands for personal health record. An EHR or EMR enables patients to transport their health care information with them at all times.

Emergency department–the department within a health care facility that is intended to provide rapid treatment to victims of sudden injury or illness. Emergency departments across the nation struggle with overcrowding, long patient wait periods, and shortages of health care professionals.

Error–the failure of a planned action to be completed as intended or the use of an incorrect plan to achieve an aim.

Evidence-based clinical practice guidelines–specific practice recommendations that are based on a methodologically rigorous review of the best evidence on a specific topic.

Evidence-based decision making–the integration of best research evidence in making decisions about patient care, which should also include the clinician's expertise as well as patient preferences and values.

Evidence-based medicine–the use of the current, best available scientific research and practices with demonstrated effectiveness in daily medical decision making, including individual clinical practice decisions, by well-trained, experienced clinicians. Evidence is central to developing performance measures for the most common and costly health conditions. The measures allow consumers to compare medical providers and learn which ones routinely offer the highest quality, safest, and most effective care.

Event–something that happens to or involves a patient.

Event rate–the proportion of patients in a group in whom an event is observed.

Exclusion criteria–characteristics possessed by individuals that would exclude them from participating in a study.

Failure Mode Effect Analysis (FMEA)–a procedure of analysis of potential failure modes within a system, and classification by severity or determination of the consequences of failures on the system.

Family-centered rounds–nursing rounds that include the patient's family with the patient's consent.

Foreground questions–those questions that can be answered from scientific evidence regarding diagnosing, treating, or assisting patients with understanding their prognosis, focusing on specific knowledge.

Fully operational electronic health record system–system that collects patient information, displays test results, allows providers to enter medical orders and prescriptions, and helps doctors make treatment decisions.

Generalizability–the extent to which the findings from a study can be generalized or applied to the larger population (i.e., external validity).

Grading the strength of recommendations:

Level I evidence–evidence that is generated from systematic reviews or meta-analyses of all relevant randomized controlled trials or evidence-based clinical practice guidelines based on systematic reviews of randomized controlled trials; the strongest level of evidence to guide clinical practice.

Level II evidence–evidence generated from a least one well-designed randomized clinical trial (i.e., a true experiment).

Level III evidence–evidence obtained from well-designed controlled trials without randomization.

Level IV evidence–evidence from well-designed case-control and cohort studies.

Level V evidence–evidence from systematic reviews of descriptive and qualitative studies.

Level VI evidence–evidence from a single descriptive or qualitative study.

Level VII evidence–evidence from the opinion of authorities and/or reports of expert committees.

Group–any collection of interconnected individuals working together for some purpose.

Handoff–a time when information is transferred, along with authority and responsibility, during transitions in care across the continuum; provides an opportunity to ask questions, clarify, and confirm responses.

Health care associated harm–harm arising from or associated with plans or actions taken during the provision of health care rather than an underlying disease or injury.

Health information exchange (HIE)–the mobilization of health care information digitally across organizations within a region or community. HIE provides the capability to move clinical information between separate health care information systems while maintaining the meaning of the information being exchanged.

Health information technology (HIT)–a global term (which encompasses electronic health records and personal health records) to indicate the use of computers, software programs, electronic devices and the internet to store, retrieve, update, and transmit information about patients' health.

Health IT Policy Committee–This federal advisory committee makes recommendations to the Office of the National Coordinator for Health Information Technology (ONC) on a policy framework for the development and adoption of a nationwide health information infrastructure, including standards for the exchange of patient medical information (http://healthit.hhs.gov/portal/server.pt/community/healthit_hhs_gov__health_it_policy_committee/1269).

Health IT Standards Committee–This federal advisory committee makes recommendations to ONC on standards, implementation specifications, and certification criteria for the electronic exchange and use of health information (http://healthit.hhs.gov/portal/server.pt/community/healthit_hhs_gov__health_it_standards_committee/1271).

Health literacy–the degree to which individuals have the capacity to obtain, process, and understand basic information and services needed to make appropriate decisions regarding their health.

Health Plan Employer Data and Information Set (HEDIS) Measures–a set of health care quality measures designed to help purchasers and consumers determine how well health plans follow accepted care standards for prevention and treatment. Formerly known as the Health Plan Employer Data Information Set, health plans can receive accreditation on HEDIS measures from certain organizations, such as the National Committee on Quality Assurance.

Heterogeneity–in systematic reviews, the amount of incompatibility between trials included in the review, whether clinical (i.e., the studies are clinically different) or statistical (i.e., the results are different from one another).

High-reliability organization (HRO)–organization that maintains culture of safety, fosters a learning environment and evidence-based care, promotes positive working environments, and is committed to improving quality and safety. It incorporates the following: direct involvement of top and middle leadership, safety and quality efforts that are aligned with the organization strategic plan, an established infrastructure for safety and continuous improvement, and active engagement of staff across the organization.

Hierarchy of evidence–a mechanism for determining which study designs have the most power to predict cause and effect. The highest level of evidence is systematic reviews of randomized clinical trials, and the lowest level of evidence is expert opinion and consensus statements.

Hospital Consumer Assessment of Healthcare Providers and Systems (H-CAHPS or CAHPS Hospital Survey)—a standardized survey instrument and data collection methodology for measuring patients' perspectives of hospital care. While many hospitals collect information on patient satisfaction, there is no national standard for collecting or publicly reporting this information that would enable valid comparisons to be made across all hospitals. H-CAHPS is a core set of questions that can be combined with customized, hospital-specific items to produce information that complements the data hospitals currently collect to support improvements in internal customer service and quality-related activities.

Improving Performance in Practice (IPIP)—This initiative is a project within the North Carolina Academy of Family Physicians. The program seeks to establish a designated quality improvement consultant (QIC) to work onsite with the practice leadership team to develop a practice-specific redesign plan utilizing the resources of collaborating experts.

Incident characteristics—selected attributes of an incident.

Incident type—descriptive term for a category made up of incidents of a common nature grouped because of shared, agreed features.

Inclusion criteria—essential characteristics of potential participants established by the investigator that must be possessed in order to be considered for a study.

Informed decision-making (IDM)—IDM is a term used to describe a process designed to help patients understand the nature of the disease or condition being addressed; understand the clinical service being provided including benefits, risks, limitations, alternatives, and uncertainties; consider their own preferences and values; participate in decision making at the level they desire; and make decisions consistent with their own preferences and values, or choose to defer a decision until a later time.

Institute for Healthcare Improvement (IHI)—independent nonprofit organization helping to lead the improvement of health care throughout the world. Founded in 1991 and based in Cambridge, Massachussetts, IHI works to accelerate improvement by building the will for change, cultivating promising concepts for improving patient care, and helping health care systems put those ideas into action.

Institute of Medicine (IOM)—nonprofit organization and honorific membership organization that works outside the framework of government to ensure scientifically informed analysis and independent guidance on matters of bio-medical science, medicine, and health. The institute provides unbiased, evidence-based, and authoritative information and advice concerning health and science policy to policy makers, professionals, leaders in every sector of society, and the public at large. IOM's book on quality and safety, *Crossing the Quality Chasm: A New Health System for the 21st Century*, partially funded by the Robert Wood Johnson Foundation, reported that a huge divide exists between the care we should receive and the care that we get. *Crossing the Quality Chasm* introduces the notion that health care needs to take a page from industry and use its engineering improvement methods to aim for top quality, efficiency, and safety. The report lays out six goals that would become akin to a mantra for the quality improvement movement: care should be "safe, effective, patient-centered, timely, efficient, and equitable." IOM's 2003 landmark report, *Unequal Treatment: Confronting Racial and Ethnic Disparities in Health Care*, demonstrates the reality and effect of health disparities and quality-of-care differences for persons of racial and ethnic minorities.

Integrative reviews—systematic summaries of the accumulated state of knowledge about a concept, including highlights of important issues left unresolved.

Interdisciplinary teams—individuals from at least two different disciplines who coordinate their expertise to deliver care to patients. More recently, the term used is *interprofessional team*.

Interoperability—the ability of different information technology systems and software applications to communicate; to exchange data accurately, effectively, and consistently; and to use the information that has been exchanged.

Interprofessional team—a team made up of individuals from at least two distinct professions or disciplines.

Knowledge translation—exchange, synthesis, and application of knowledge within a complex system of interactions among researchers and users to improve health, provide more effective health services and products, and strengthen the health care system.

Medical error—a mistake that harms a patient. Adverse drug events, hospital-acquired infections, and wrong-site surgeries are examples of preventable medical errors.

Medical Subject Headings (MeSH)—a thesaurus of medical terms used by many databases and libraries to index and classify medical information.

Meta-analysis—a process of using quantitative methods to summarize the results from the multiple studies, obtained and critically reviewed using a rigorous process (to minimize bias) for identifying, appraising, and synthesizing studies to answer a specific clinical question and draw conclusions about the data gathered, to gain a summary statistic (i.e., a measure of a single effect) that represents the effect of the intervention across the multiple studies.

Microsystem—small, functional, frontline units that provide most health care to most people. They are the essential building blocks of larger organizations and of the health system. They are the place where patients and providers meet. The quality and value of care produced by a large health system can be no better than the services generated by the small systems of which it is composed.

Misuse—occurs when an appropriate process of care has been selected, but a preventable complication arises and the patient does not receive the full potential benefit of the service. Avoidable complications of surgery or medication use are misuse problems. A patient who suffers a rash after receiving penicillin for strep throat, despite having a known allergy to that antibiotic, is an example of misuse. A patient who develops a pneumothorax after an inexperienced operator attempted to insert a subclavian line would represent another example of misuse.

Mitigating factor—an action or circumstance that prevents or moderates the progression of an incident toward harming a patient.

Model of care—a conceptual object or diagram that provides an outline of how to plan all current and future facility and clinical service. It is important that the model of care be designed and evaluated for its ability to be replicated within the health care system. Models of care can help guide and direct a patient's experience within a health care system.

Multidisciplinary (or interprofessional) teams—health care teams made up of health care professionals as well as health educators and/or community leaders.

National Committee on Vital and Health Statistics—a federal committee that makes recommendations to the Secretary of Health and Human Services on health data, statistics, privacy, national health information policy, and the department's strategy to best address those issues (www.ncvhs.hhs.gov).

National Guidelines Clearinghouse—a comprehensive database of up-to-date, English-language, evidence-based clinical practice guidelines, developed in partnership with the American Medical Association, the American Association of Health Plans, and the Association for Healthcare Research and Quality.

Nationwide Health Information Network (NHIN)—the technologies, standards, laws, policies, programs, and practices that enable health information to be shared among health decision makers, including consumers and patients, to promote improvements in health and health care. The vision for NHIN is said to have begun in 1991 with the publication of an Institute of Medicine report, "The Computer-Based Patient Record." The path to a national network of health care information is through the successful establishment of regional health information organizations. This has been a core component of the work of ONC (Office of the National Coordinator for Health Information Technology) to insure patient information is available at the point of care, regardless of the location of the patient and his or her data.

Near miss—an incident that did not cause harm; events, situations, or incidents that could have caused adverse consequences and harmed a patient but did not. Sometimes referred to as a "good catch."

Never event/serious reportable event—medical errors with serious consequences for which we have the knowledge to prevent, identified by the National Quality Forum.

Office of the National Coordinator for Health Information Technology (ONC)—principal federal entity charged with coordination of nationwide efforts to implement and use the most advanced health information technology and the electronic exchange of health information. The position of National Coordinator was created in 2004, through an executive order, and legislatively mandated in the Health Information Technology for Economic and Clinical Health Act (HITECH Act) of 2009 (healthit.hhs.gov).

Opinion leaders—individuals typically highly knowledgeable and well respected in a system; as such, they are often able to influence change.

Outcome—the result of a process, including outputs, effects, and impacts.

Outcomes management—the use of process and outcomes data to coordinate and influence actions and processes of care that contribute to patient achievement of targeted behaviors or desired effects.

Outcomes measurement—a generic term used to describe the collection and reporting of information about an observed effect in relation to some care delivery process or health promotion action.

Outcomes research—the use of rigorous scientific methods to measure the effect of some intervention on some outcome(s).

Overuse—describes a process of care in circumstances where the potential for harm exceeds the potential for benefit. Prescribing an antibiotic for a viral infection like a cold, for which antibiotics are ineffective, constitutes overuse. The potential for harm includes adverse reactions to the antibiotics and increases in antibiotic resistance among bacteria in the community. Overuse can also apply to diagnostic tests and surgical procedures.

Partnership–an explicit relationship with clear roles and responsibilities between two people who share a common goal or vision.

Patient activation–the situation in which patients believe they have important roles to play in self-managing care, collaborating with providers, and maintaining their health; they know how to manage their condition and maintain functioning and prevent health declines; and they have the skills and behavioral repertoire to manage their condition, collaborate with their health providers, maintain their health functioning, and access appropriate and high-quality care.

Patient-centered care–considers patients' cultural traditions, personal preferences and values, family situations, and lifestyles. Responsibility for important aspects of self-care and monitoring is put in patients' hands–along with the tools and support they need. Patient-centered care also ensures that transitions between different health care providers and care settings are coordinated and efficient. When care is patient-centered, unneeded and unwanted services can be reduced.

Patient-centered environment of care–a care setting that is safe and clean, and that guards patient privacy. It also engages all the human senses with color, texture, artwork, music, aromatherapy, views of nature, and comfortable lighting, and considers the experience of the body, mind, and spirit of all who use the facility. Space is provided for loved ones to congregate, as well as for peaceful contemplation, meditation, or prayer; and patients, families, and staff have access to a variety of arts and entertainment that serve as positive diversions. At the heart of the environment of care, however, are the human interactions that occur within the physical structure to calm, comfort, and support those who inhabit it. Together the design, aesthetics, and these interactions can transform an institutional, impersonal, and alien setting into one that is truly healing (Picker Institute).

Patient-centered rounds–regular patient visits in which health care professionals are careful to provide medical information to the patient, answer questions, and involve the patient in decisions (IOM).

Patient registry–a patient database maintained by a hospital, doctors' practice, or health plan that allows providers to identify their patients according to disease, demographic characteristics, and other factors. Patient registries can help providers better coordinate care for their patients, monitor treatment and progress, and improve overall quality of care.

Patient safety–freedom, for a patient, from unnecessary harm or potential harm associated with health care.

Patient safety incident—an event or circumstance that could have resulted, or did result, in unnecessary harm to a patient.

Patient satisfaction—a measurement designed to obtain reports or ratings from patients about services received from an organization, hospital, physician, or health care provider.

Patient values and preferences—values the patient holds; concerns the patient has regarding the clinical decision/treatment/situation, choices the patient has/prefers regarding the clinical decision/treatment/situation.

Pay-for-performance (P4P)—a method for paying hospitals and physicians based on their demonstrated achievements in meeting specific health care quality objectives. The idea is to reward providers for the quality—not the quantity—of care they deliver.

Payer—the entity that assumes the risk of paying for medical treatments. Examples of payers include uninsured patients, self-insured employers, health plans, or HMOs.

Performance measures—sets of established standards against which health care performance is measured. Performance measures are now widely accepted as a method for guiding informed decision making as a strong impetus for improvement.

Personal health record (PHR)—a health record that is "owned" and maintained by an individual patient, rather than by payers or providers. Though the term has been around for several decades, it has recently received renewed attention with the adoption of electronic health records. Many health care organizations are offereing PHRs to their patients to support their healthy life style and disease management activities.

PICO format—a process in which clinical questions are phrased in a manner that yields the most relevant information; P = patient population; I = intervention of interest; C = Comparison intervention or status; O = outcome.

Physician Quality Reporting Initiative (PQRI)—a measure authorized through the Medicare, Medicaid, and SCHIP Extension Act of 2007. It is a financial incentive for health care professionals to improve the quality of care that they provide.

Prevalence—the baseline risk of a disorder in the population of interest.

Preventable adverse event—an event whose outcome, under the circumstances, was avoidable.

Process Improvement–techniques and strategies used to make the processes implemented to solve health care problems better. Process improvement can occur in emergency room or hospital settings as well as in other health-system environments.

Productive pairs–individuals who come together and develop a partnership to accomplish a shared goal.

Provider incentives–inducements that motivate the regulation of health care. Examples of incentives include monetary rewards for providers who meet specific benchmark standards for their patient care.

p **value**–the probability that a particular result would have happened by chance.

Publication or reporting bias–a bias in a systematic review caused by incompleteness of the search, such as omitting non-English language sources or unpublished trials (inconclusive trials are less likely to be published than conclusive ones but are not necessarily less valid)

Public reporting–information about physician and physician group performance available for consumers to use to compare the performance of local physicians/physician groups. The expectation is that a comparative public report of local physicians' performance in treating people with chronic illnesses will motivate and improve performance.

Purchasers–the entity that not only pays the premium for health care costs but also controls the premium dollar before paying it to the provider. Included in the category of purchasers or payers are patients, businesses, and managed care organizations. While patients and businesses function as ultimate purchasers, managed care organizations and insurance companies serve a processing or payer function.

Quality and Safety Education for Nurses (QSEN)–project that defined quality and safety competencies (derived from the IOM), including patient-centered care, teamwork and collaboration, evidence-based practice, quality improvement, safety, and informatics (www.QSEN.org).

Quality of care–a measure of the ability of a doctor, hospital, or health plan to provide services for individuals and populations that increase the likelihood of desired health outcomes and are consistent with current professional knowledge. Good quality health care means doing the right thing at the right time, in the right way, for the right person, and getting the best possible results. According to the mantra for the quality improvement movement, care should be "safe, effective, patient-centered, timely, efficient, and equitable."

Quality of life–the amount of happiness and balance in an individual's life. Attention to good health will create a better quality of life.

Quality improvement (QI)—term first coined in the private sector, when corporations began looking at ways to streamline and improve processes and systems. The most well-known example of quality improvement methodology is the "Six Sigma" method of change, developed by engineers at Motorola. In the health care context, the goal of quality improvement strategies is for patients to receive the appropriate care at the appropriate time and place with the appropriate mix of information and supporting resources. In many cases, health care systems are designed in such a way as to be overly cumbersome, fragmented, and indifferent to patients' needs. Quality improvement tools range from those that simply make recommendations but leave decision making largely in the hands of individual physicians (e.g., practice guidelines) to those that prescribe patterns of care (e.g., critical pathways). Typically, quality improvement efforts are strongly rooted in evidence-based procedures and rely extensively on data collected about processes and outcomes.

Quality indicator—agreed-upon process or outcome measure that is used to determine the level of quality achieved. It is a measurable variable (or characteristic) that can be used to determine the degree of adherence to a standard or achievement of quality goals.

Quality measures—mechanisms used to assign a quantity to quality of care by comparison to a criterion.

Randomized controlled clinical trial—A group of patients is randomized into an experimental group and a control group. These groups are followed up for the variables/outcomes of interest.

Rapid-cycle change—A quality improvement method that identifies, implements, and measures changes made to improve a process or a system. At the onset, the team sets an outcome measure based on the system's goals. Improvement occurs through small, rapid PDSA (Plan-Do-Study-Act) cycles to advance practice change. This model requires targeting a specific area to change; planning changes on the basis of sound science, theory, and evidence; piloting several changes with small patient groups; measuring the effects of changes; and acting according to the data. The fundamental concept of rapid-cycle improvement is that health care processes—once defined, in place, and in effect—should be continually improved by instituting a constant cycle of innovations or improvements.

Red rules—standards for a particular process without exception.

Regional health information organization (RHIO)—a multistakeholder organization, operating in a specific geographical area, that enables the exchange and use of health information, in a secure manner, for the purpose of promoting the improvement of health quality, safety, and efficiency. Officials from the U.S. Department of Health and Human Services see RHIOs as the building blocks for the National Health Information Network (NHIN). When complete, the NHIN will provide universal access to electronic health records. As a result of the Health Information Technology for Economic and Clinical Health Act (HITECH Act) of 2009, RHIOs have been replaced with State health information exchange initiatives (http://healthit.hhs.gov/portal/server.pt/community/healthit_hhs_gov_state_health_information_exchange_program/1488).

Report card–an assessment of the quality of care delivered by health plans. Report cards provide information on how well a health plan treats its members, keeps them healthy, and provides access to needed care. Report cards can be published by states, private health organizations, consumer groups, or health plans.

Research utilization–process by which empirical findings from one or more studies are transformed into nursing interventions and/or tools that support clinical decision making such as guidelines, protocols, or algorithms.

Return on investment (ROI)–the amount of improvement in care brought about by a certain investment. ROI can also refer to the theory that if you invest in health care quality now, then the quality of care for patients will improve in the future.

Right care–made up of the treatments that, according to evidence-based guidelines, are effective and appropriate for a given condition. Indicators used to define right care are often grouped into two categories: prevention and chronic care.

Root cause analysis (RCA)–set of problem solving methods used to identify the series of actions and circumstances that led to an outcome, usually used to dissect a problem occurrence, although it could also trace the path of success.

Safety–safe, effective care requires understanding the complexity of care delivery, the limits of human factors, safety design principles, characteristics of high-reliability organizations, and patient safety resources.

Safety science–applies an organizational framework to minimize risk of harm to patients and providers through both system effectiveness and individual performance by applying human factors.

Safe zones–designated areas where critical functions requiring concentration, such as medication preparation, are being performed and the clinician is not to be interrupted.

SBAR (situation, background, assessment, recommendation)–a structured communication framework that helps health care providers clearly, consistently, and succinctly communicate pertinent information about patient care situations.

Sentinel event—any unexpected event in a health care setting that causes death or serious injury to a patient and is not related to the natural course of the patient's illness.

Standard of care—the expected level and type of care provided by the average caregiver under a certain given set of circumstances. These circumstances are supported through findings from expert consensus and based on specific research and/or documentation in scientific literature.

STEEEP—Institute of Medicine acronym for six measures of health care quality based on whether care is safe, timely, effective, efficient, equitable, and patient centered.

Systematic review—an article in which the authors have systematically searched for, appraised, and summarized all of the medical literature for a specific topic.

Systems—a set of interdependent components that interact to achieve a common goal.

Task force—a group convened to accomplish a specific objective within a designated period of time.

Team—a small number of consistent people committed to a relevant shared purpose.

TeamSTEPPS (Team Strategies and Tools to Enhance Performance and Patient Safety)—a training program developed by the Department of Defense and AHRQ that consists of content and exercises on leadership, situation monitoring, mutual support, and communication. It has been widely used outside of health care and, increasingly, within health care settings.

Teamwork—a joint action by two or more people, in which each person contributes with different skills and expresses his or her individual interests and opinions to the unity and efficiency of the group in order to achieve common goals.

Throughput—the ability of a medical facility, such as an emergency department, to complete a patient input and output cycle (i.e., to provide patients with the full cycle of care)

Translational research—activities designed to transform ideas, insights, and discoveries generated through basic science inquiry and from clinical or population studies into effective and widely available clinical applications.

396 ■ Glossary

Transparency–the process of collecting and reporting health care cost, performance, and quality data in a format that can be accessed by the public and is intended to improve the delivery of services and ultimately improve the health care system as a whole.

Triad for Optimal Patient Safety (TOPS)–a multidisciplinary training program.

Underuse–the failure to provide a health care service when it would have produced a favorable outcome for a patient. Standard examples include failure to provide appropriate preventive services to eligible patients (e.g., Pap smears, flu shots for elderly patients, screening for hypertension) and proven medications for chronic illnesses (steroid inhalers for asthmatics; aspirin, beta-blockers and lipid-lowering agents for patients who have suffered a recent myocardial infarction).

Validity–the extent to which a variable or intervention measures what it is supposed to measure or accomplishes what it is supposed to accomplish. The *internal validity* of a study refers to the integrity of the experimental design. The *external validity* of a study refers to the appropriateness by which its results can be applied to nonstudy patients or populations.

Value purchasing–a broad strategy used by some large employers to get more value for their health care dollars by demanding that health care providers meet certain quality objectives or supply data documenting their use of best practices and quality treatment outcomes.

Violation–deliberate deviation from an operating procedure, standard, or rules.

Work flow–a repeatable pattern of activity enabled by the organization of resources, defined roles, and information into a process that can be documented and learned. Improvements in work flow for health care providers will lessen the burden of providing health care and will lead to greater quality health care overall.

Index

Page references followed by *b, f, or t denote* boxes, figures, and tables respectively.

Quality and Safety in Nursing: A Competency Approach to Improving Outcomes,
First Edition. Edited by Gwen Sherwood and Jane Barnsteiner.
© 2012 John Wiley & Sons, Inc. Published 2012 by John Wiley & Sons, Inc.